RHEUMATOLOGIC
REHABILITAT[...]S

VOLUME 2
ADULT RHEUMATIC DISEASES

EDITORS
Jeanne L. Melvin
MS, OTR, FAOTA
Kathleen M. Ferrell
MLA, PT

AOTA® **The American Occupational Therapy Association, Inc.**

MT

Joseph C. Isaacs, CAE, Executive Director
Chris Bluhm, CPA, CMA, Associate Executive Director, Business Operations Division
Jennifer J. Jones, Director of Publications

Krishni Patrick, MA, Editor, Books
Joyce Raynor, Production Editor
Robert A. Sacheli, Manager, Creative Services
Sarah E. Ely, Book Production Coordinator

The American Occupational Therapy Association, Inc.
4720 Montgomery Lane
PO Box 31220
Bethesda, Maryland 20824-1220
To order call: 1-877-404-AOTA
www.aota.org

Disclaimers
This publication is designed to provide accurate and authoritative information in regard to the subject matter covered. It is sold or distributed with the understanding that the publisher is not engaged in rendering legal, accounting, or other professional service. If legal advice or other expert assistance is required, the services of a competent professional person should be sought.
—*From the Declaration of Principles jointly adopted by the American Bar Association and a
Committee of Publishers and Associations*

It is the objective of The American Occupational Therapy Association to be a forum for free expression and interchange of ideas. The opinions expressed by the contributors to this work are their own and not necessarily those of either the editors or The American Occupational Therapy Association.

ISBN 1-56900-139-1

Cover Illustration © David Rini

Composition by World Comp Inc., Sterling, Virginia

Printed by Boyd Printing Company, Albany, New York

10/8/03

Dedication

John H. Bland, MD

Professor Emeritus at the University of Vermont College of Medicine, Dr. Bland is a dedicated and superb physician, researcher, and educator. He has few equals in terms of conquering and then communicating the fascinating complexities of a topic. His skill in communication has helped heal his patients, inspire his students and colleagues, and empower the readers of his publications, which include a dozen books on a broad range of topics: renal function, cartilage, osteoarthritis, healthy aging, fitness training, self-management of arthritis, and mosses and lichen. His 30 years of research on the cervical spine culminated in the textbook, *Disorders of the Cervical Spine.* Dr. Bland is additionally a world-class skier, marathon runner, and equestrian.

Table of Contents

Preface to the *Rheumatologic Rehabilitation Series*

The specialty practice area of rheumatologic rehabilitation has been created in large part by the Association of Rheumatology Health Professionals (ARHP), which was founded to support interdisciplinary communication and education. The effect of the ARHP and its philosophy is manifest in the concept of this series and in the spirit of cooperation shown by the contributing authors, many of whom joined this project specifically because it is an interdisciplinary educational endeavor.

This series is the direct result of the first ARHP Fellowship (1973–1974) from the ARHP and the Arthritis Foundation, which made it possible for me to research and write *Rheumatic Disease in the Adult and Child: Occupational Therapy and Rehabilitation* (Melvin, 1977), which was published in 1977 and then continued into three editions. Although the present series was initially intended to be a revision and expansion of that textbook to include physical therapy, there is now little left of the previous text except organizational design, some illustrations, and a few paragraphs in volumes 2 and 3.

This series focuses on educating physical and occupational therapy practitioners because these two professions share knowledge bases in the areas of anatomy, physiology, rheumatology, and rehabilitation to be competent in the physical rehabilitation of persons with rheumatic diseases. Additionally, these practitioners often work together to achieve the desired outcomes for this patient population. But, of course, we hope that all professionals interested in the rehabilitation of persons with rheumatic diseases will find this series useful.

We tackle the task of educating practitioners about rheumatologic rehabilitation in an unprecedented format. First, the content is divided into five volumes so that practitioners in adult, pediatric, hand, and orthopedic practice areas can select the volumes most relevant to their interests. The theoretical and research basis for evaluation and treatment is presented in volume 1 to facilitate the use of this material in occupational therapy and physical therapy curricula. Second, all of the disease chapters in volumes 2 and 3 demonstrate the team approach because they are written collaboratively by a rheumatologist, a physical therapist, and an occupational therapist. In volume 5, *Surgical Rehabilitation*, most chapters are authored by an orthopedic surgeon, an occupational therapist, a physical therapist, and an orthopedic nurse. Third, each chapter in all of the volumes have been reviewed from both physical therapy and occupational therapy perspectives by the coeditors.

Eighty-six authors from all health professions involved in caring for persons with rheumatic diseases have contributed to this series, which testifies to the editors' commitment to training practitioners in the multidisciplinary approach to treatment. The size of this series and the number of contributing authors reflect the growth of rheumatologic rehabilitation in all of the treating disciplines (e.g., rheumatology, orthopedic surgery, nursing, patient education, psychology, social work, and pedorthics). In each of these fields, research is being conducted that directly affects the practice of occupational and physical therapy. It is no longer sufficient or even possible to learn about rheumatologic rehabilitation as a specialty area in physical therapy or occupational therapy from within a single practice area. For physical therapy and occupational therapy, the new frontiers in rheumatologic rehabilitation during the next 20 years will not necessarily be in advanced interventions unique to each field but rather will be in integrating into practice the research from the areas of patient education, wellness studies, pain management, adherence research, fatigue management, and outcome and functional evaluation. In volume 1, we have invited leading researchers and clinicians from all these fields to share the latest research and methodologies that are specifically relevant to physical and occupational therapy intervention. Within the fields of physical therapy and occupational therapy, we have invited both specialists in rheumatologic rehabilitation and in evaluation or treatment outside of arthritis treatment who could broaden the approach to treatment in rheumatology.

Jeanne L. Melvin, MS, OTR, FAOTA
Program Manager, Chronic Pain and Fibromyalgia Programs
Cedars-Sinai Medical Center
Beverly Hills, California

Preface to Volume 2: *Adult Rheumatic Diseases*

It is essential to the successful treatment of people with rheumatic diseases that therapists work closely with the referring physician and integrate therapy with medical management. This requires an understanding of medical management. Volume II is designed specifically to help therapists and other health professionals develop this understanding.

The book starts with the foundations of practice. We invited Betts Carpenter, MD, PhD, an instructor of immunology, to explain the process of joint inflammation and to put immunology into a functional context that is accessible for therapists—what happens when a joint is inflamed. She has created an original chapter that wonderfully accomplishes this task. John Bland, MD, a renown clinician and researcher in osteoarthritis and cartilage physiology, took on the task of explaining the pathophysiology of cartilage and joint structures in a manner that is easy to understand an eminently usable for therapists. This is in stark contrast to most existing chapters on the subject. Eric Gall, MD, who has been a major supporter of rehabilitation for arthritis, explains in lucid language the pro's and con's of the current medications being used to manage arthritis and how drugs can enhance therapy outcomes. The chapter on radiographic imaging is written by Tom Learch, MD, who started his career as an OTR working in rheumatology. He is now a radiologist specializing in musculoskeletal disease and brings a unique focus to the subject of radiographic imaging and what is most important for therapists to know about it.

This volume contains a chapter on each of the eight major rheumatic diseases: osteoarthritis, fibromyalgia, rheumatoid arthritis, systemic lupus erythematosus, systemic sclerosis, psoriatic arthritis, ankylosing spondylitis, polymyositis; and it contains one chapter on nineteen of the "less common" diseases. Every chapter is authored by a team consisting of a leading rheumatologist in that disease, a physical therapist and an occupational therapist. We believe this team approach breaks new ground in rehabilitation literature. It has taken more work to integrate the material of three authors, but now the roles of these three clinicians whose task it is to improve physical function in the patient can all be seen in the same chapter. This should make clear the significance of integrating and coordinating the care given by each member of the clinical team and can provide an opportunity for each to learn about the others' roles and contributions to the rehabilitation process. This is even more important in the era of managed care. When a patient with severe polyarticular RA has only 12 physical therapy and 12 occupational therapy visits per year, therapists and physicians must really work together to accomplish all the therapy that is needed. If patients are not on an optimal drug regimen, they may not be able to fully participate in therapy, thus wasting precious visits; or if therapists are not aware of the course or prognosis of specific symptoms, therapy can be in vain.

We hope these chapters will be shared among team members and used in the training of rheumatology and internal medicine fellows.

Jeanne L. Melvin, MS, OTR, FAOTA
Program Manager, Chronic Pain and Fibromyalgia Programs
Cedars-Sinai Medical Center
Beverly Hills, California

Reference

Melvin, J. L. (Ed.). (1977). *Rheumatic disease in the adult and child* (1st ed.). Philadelphia: F. A. Davis.

About the Authors

Frank C. Arnett, MD, is Professor at the Division of Rheumatology/Department of Medicine, University of Texas, Houston, Texas.

Thomas D. Beardmore, MD, is Chief, Rheumatology at Rancho Los Amigos National Rehabilitation Center, Downy, California.

John H. Bland, MD, is Professor Emeritus at the Department of Medicine/Rheumatology, College of Medicine, University of Vermont, Burlington, Vermont.

A. Betts Carpenter, MD, PhD, is Professor and Vice Chairman of the Department of Pathology, Marshall University School of Medicine, Huntington, West Virginia.

Cathy S. Elrod, MS, PT, is Assistant Professor, Physical Therapy Program, Marymount University, Arlington, Virginia.

Kathleen M. Ferrell, MLA, PT, is Associate Director, Regional Arthritis Center, Washington University, St. Louis, Missouri.

Mary Lou Galantino, PhD, PT, is Associate Professor, Physical Therapy Program, PROS Division, The Richard Stockton College of New Jersey, Pomona, New Jersey.

Eric P. Gall, MD, is Professor and Chairman of the Department of Medicine, FUHS/The Chicago Medical School, North Chicago, Illinois.

Victoria Gall, MEd, PT, formerly with Orthopedic and Rheumatology Services, Brigham and Women's Hospital, Boston, Massachusetts, is currently in the Peace Corps in Turkmenistan.

Dafna D. Gladman, MD, FRCPC, is Professor of Medicine and Deputy Director, Centre for Prognosis Studies in the Rheumatic Diseases, Toronto Western Hospital, University Health Network, Toronto, Ontario, Canada.

Scott Hasson, EdD, PT, FACSM, is Chairperson, Department of Physical Therapy, University of Connecticut, Storrs, Connecticut.

Thomas J. Learch, MD, OTR, is Assistant Professor, Department of Radiology, University of Southern California University Hospital, Los Angeles, California.

E. Carwile LeRoy, MD, is Professor of Medicine and Chairman of Microbiology and Immunology Department, Medical University of South Carolina, Charleston, South Carolina.

James S. Louie, MD, is Chief of Rheumatology, Harbor-UCLA Medical Center in Torrance, California.

Jeanne L. Melvin, MS, OTR, FAOTA, is Program Manager, Chronic Pain and Fibromyalgia Programs, Cedars-Sinai Medical Center, Los Angeles, California.

Leslie Miller-Porter, PT, is a Senior Clinician at Rancho Los Amigos National Rehabilitation Center, Downy, California.

Proton Rahman, MD, FRCPC, MSC, is Assistant Professor of Medicine at Memorial University of Newfoundland, St. John's, Newfoundland, Canada.

I. Jon Russell, MD, PhD, is Associate Professor of Medicine, Division of Clinical Immunology, University of Texas Health Science Center, San Antonio, Texas.

Marilyn Sanford, PhD, PT, is Clinical Associate Professor and Chairman of the Department of Physical Therapy, University of Missouri, Columbia, Missouri.

Mima Siegel, PT, is Senior Physical Therapist, Cedars-Sinai Medical Center, Los Angeles, California.

Stuart L. Silverman, MD, FACP, FACR, is a Clinical Professor of Medicine, UCLA School of Medicine, Los Angeles, California.

Dena Slonaker, MSEd, OTR, CHT, is Rheumatology and Hand Rehabilitation Specialist at Health South, Encino, California.

Ranjana Sood, MD, is a rheumatologist and works in San Jose, California.

Judy R. Sotosky, MEd, PT, is a consultant in private practice in Virginia Beach, Virginia.

Sara E. Walker, MD, MACP, is Professor of Internal Medicine at Harry S Truman Memorial Veterans Hospital and at University of Missouri, Columbia, Missouri.

Terri Wolfe, OTR/L, CHT, is Owner and Director of the Hand and Arthritis Rehab Center, Erie, Pennsylvania.

Y. Lynn Yasuda, MSEd, OTR, FAOTA, is Interim Director, Education and Staff Development Department at Rancho Los Amigos National Rehabilitation Center, Downy, California.

1

THE IMMUNE SYSTEM AND INFLAMMATORY JOINT DISEASE

A. Betts Carpenter, MD, PhD

W̲hen initially examining a patient with a new onset of rheumatoid arthritis (RA) who has multiple red swollen joints, do you ever wonder about what has been happening inside the joint to cause this? What initiated this disease? Is the disease the result of a defective immune system? What is the role of stress and genetics in the disease process? This chapter will examine some of these questions, provide a blueprint for the immune system, and examine how the immune system is responsible for many of the problems that we see daily in our patients. A glossary of terms used throughout the chapter is found in Appendix A at the end of this chapter.

Inflammation

Inflammation is the basis of many of the clinical symptoms that characterize patients with rheumatic diseases. By definition, inflammation is the response of the body to injured tissues (Abbas, Lichtman, & Pober, 1994; Cotran, Kumar, & Robbins, 1994; Roitt, Brostoff, & Male, 1996; Stites, Terr, & Parslow, 1994; Talaro & Talaro, 1996). It is a complex process that can be initiated in many different ways from various foreign insults (e.g., microbes, altered cells, and foreign particles). Myriad cells and soluble inflammatory mediators can be involved. Signs of inflammation are redness, heat, swelling, and pain. Because the bloodstream contains the major components that combat inflammation (white blood cells and antibodies), changes in blood vessel flow and in the vasculature itself understandably play a major role in the inflammatory process (Cotran et al., 1994). In response to tissue injury, the capillary and postcapillary venules containing the inflammatory cells respond to the injury through several events. The endolethial cells lining the vessel walls are disrupted, allowing fluid and cells to flow into the extravascular spaces and to the site of injury. The increased flow of blood and the presence of fluid in the tissues are responsible for the heat and swelling characteristic of the inflammatory process. The cells recruited into the area (neutrophils, platelets, mast cells, eosinophils, basophils, and lymphocytes) add to the inflammatory response because of the release of various mediators (Abbas et al., 1994; Arai et al., 1990; Cotran et al., 1994; Roitt et al., 1996; Stites et al., 1994; Talaro & Talaro, 1996). Some of the mediators are preformed and are in cytoplasmic granules or are formed from the metabolism of lipids that comprise the cell membrane. The mediators have many effects, including increased vascular permeability, increased pain, recruitment of additional cells, and contraction of smooth muscle, and they induce the release of additional mediators. One group of important mediators includes the vaso-active amines (histamine, serotonin, adenosine) and nitric oxide, which have variable effects on the vasculature such as vasodilatation and increased vascular permeability. Other important systems in the inflammatory process include the complement pathway, the kinin or contact system, and the clotting cascade. These systems interact with one another to promote the inflammatory process. The arachidonic acid pathway is activated when the lipids in cell membrane are acted on, which results in a complex series of chemical reactions that cause the release of several important compounds (e.g., prostaglandins and leukotrienes). These compounds have various effects, most importantly the promotion of inflammation. Much of the drug therapy used for rheumatic diseases focuses on inhibiting the release of the metabolites of arachidonic acid. For example, both corticosteroids and non-steroidal anti-inflammatory drugs (NSAIDs) act to inhibit the production of these compounds.

The inflammatory process can be acute or chronic (Abbas et al., 1994; Cotran et al., 1994; Stites et al., 1994; Talaro & Talaro, 1996). Acute inflammation often occurs as the initial response to highly virulent organisms and is characterized by a cellular infiltrate of primarily neutrophils. Most often, the acute inflammatory reaction resolves the noxious assault and restores the tissues to normal physiological integrity and functioning. However, in numerous pathological situations, the inflammatory response does not resolve but rather becomes chronic. This chronic response occurs after the initial response and is characterized by an infiltrate composed primarily of lymphocytes, plasma cells, and macrophages. There are many factors that determine whether an acute inflammatory reaction will become chronic. Chronicity may be due to the characteristics of the inciting agent (e.g., persistent, intracellular), to factors in the host (e.g., genetic background such as human lymphocyte antigen [HLA] type and or dysregulation in the immune system), or both.

Pathogenesis of RA

Inflammation is a process that can be induced by various initiating factors, and the precise biochemical process varies depending on the etiology. In this discussion, the pathogenesis of RA (Brostoff, Scadding, Male, & Roitt, 1991; Harris, 1989; Roitt et al., 1996; Sell, 1996; Winchester, 1995) will be used as a model for understanding the most common form of inflammation seen in rheumatic disease. So how do we explain the hot inflamed joint in RA (Figure 1)? The process begins before any clinical manifestations when a foreign substance (an antigen) enters the joint cavity. No one antigen has been identified as the only causative factor in RA. There are many candidates, including substances such as viruses, bacteria, other microorganisms, and components of the body termed altered self-antigens. Altered self-antigens are substances that have been changed in some way such that the immune system does not view them as part of the

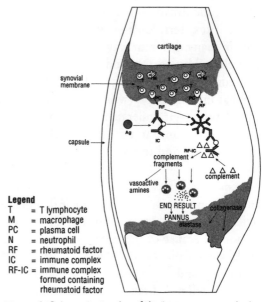

Legend
T   = T lymphocyte
M   = macrophage
PC = plasma cell
N   = neutrophil
RF = rheumatoid factor
IC = immune complex
RF-IC = immune complex formed containing rheumatoid factor

Figure 1. Schematic drawing of the immune process in the joint of a patient with RA.

body but rather views them as foreign substances. Our immune system is programmed to respond to foreign invaders and to eliminate or mitigate their effects on the host. One way that the immune system responds is through the recruitment of one of its major players, the B lymphocyte. The task of the B lymphocyte is to secrete protein substances called *immunoglobulins*, which are termed *antibodies* when they are directed toward a specific antigen. Immunoglobulins are grouped into five classes: IgG, IgM, IgA, IgE, and IgD. Once antibodies are secreted in response to a particular antigen, they can bind to this foreign antigen and facilitate its destruction. When antigen binds to the antibodies, it forms a structure called an *immune complex* (antigen–antibody complex).

Once these complexes are formed, they attract a protein substance called *complement*, which is composed of multiple proteins that facilitate the work of antibodies. This is a cascade system of approximately 25 serum proteins that normally are inactive, but, on activation, they act sequentially to mediate numerous biological effects (Abbas et al., 1994; Ruddy, 1989; Stites et al., 1994; Talaro & Talaro, 1996). One action of the complement system is to lyse (break up) foreign invaders that are coated with antibodies. In addition, complement is important in the inflammatory process because it attracts other inflammatory cells to the site and can enhance the ability of *macrophages* (scavenger cells) to engulf and destroy foreign invaders.

In addition to attracting complement to the area, immune complexes can induce the formation of additional antibodies. The rheumatoid factor (RF) is an example of this. When the initial antigen–antibody complex forms, previously unexposed parts of the antibody become exposed and can act as antigens, and this stimulates a second antibody response to the new antigenic site (Sell, 1996). This antibody, termed *rheumatoid factor*, is classically in the IgM class and is directed against antigenic sites on the initial antibody, which is in the IgG class. Although RF is used as a marker of RA, it does not appear to be the "pathogenic substance" but rather is one player in a complex scenario (Harris, 1989; Winchester, 1995). RF is present in approximately 75% of patients with RA, but its presence does not establish or rule out the diagnosis of RA. In fact, in nearly 25% of patients who fulfill the criteria for RA, RF is not detected, although it can be present in persons with no joint disease. Although RF can be detected in the synovial fluid of RA joints, and cells producing RF can be found in synovial tissue, the exact role of RF in the pathogenesis of RA has not been clearly established (Harris, 1989; Roitt et al., 1996; Sell, 1996; Winchester, 1995). Most cells in the synovial tissue are not plasma cells producing RF but rather are helper T-cells (Harris, 1989; Roitt et al., 1996; Winchester, 1995). Future studies will better define the role of RF in the pathogenesis of RA.

As a result of immune complex formation and the activation of complement, many events occur that are part of the process of inflammation (Abbas et al., 1994; Cotran et al., 1994; Roitt et al., 1996; Stites et al., 1994; Talaro & Talaro, 1996). Various inflammatory cells such as neutrophils, platelets, eosinophils, macrophages, and lymphocytes are recruited. One of the effects of this is the production of soluble mediators termed *cytokines* that are released from the infiltrating inflammatory cells (Abbas et al., 1994; Arai et al., 1990). Cytokines have various actions that include recruiting additional inflammatory cells and inducing an increase in vascular permeability. With increasing vascular permeability, there is increased blood flow into the joint space. This increased amount of blood brings additional fluid and inflammatory cells into the area. This increased fluid, coupled with a disruption of the endolethial cell layer lining the vessels walls, contributes to the development of swelling in the area. The inflammatory cells, especially neutrophils, release their contents (e.g., lysosomal enzymes) and further potentiate the inflammatory process. In addition, the B lymphocytes in the area differentiate to plasma cells that act as antibody factories to make additional RF that can increase the inflammatory process through further immune complex formation and activation of complement. The end result of all these cells and their products acting together is a hot, red, and swollen joint. Over time, these events result in the transformation of the joint cavity from an area with a thin layer of bland stromal cells embedded in a connective tissue matrix into a thick, boggy, irregular tissue referred to as pannus. Pannus looks quite similar to a lymph node, the home of many cells of the immune system.

The above sequence of events constitutes the initial acute phase of RA, which is primarily a humoral or antibody-mediated process (Abbas et al., 1994; Cotran et al., 1994; Roitt et al., 1996; Stites et al., 1994; Talaro & Talaro, 1996). Most patients are not seen by rheumatologists or occupational therapists and physical therapists during this initial acute phase. When this initial episode does not resolve spontaneously, the disease often evolves into a protracted or chronic phase. The exact reasons for this transformation are not known, and reasons likely differ among patients. Some proposed factors that could be responsible include genetics, characteristics of the inciting antigen, and alterations in the regulatory processes of the immune system. The chronic phase is mediated by the other major division of the immune system, the cellular immune system, in which the major players are T lymphocytes and macrophages (Abbas et al., 1994; Cotran et al., 1994; Roitt et al., 1996; Stites et al., 1994; Talaro & Talaro, 1996). Cytokines are released from T lymphocytes and have many far-reaching effects. Especially relevant to the joint cavity, cytokines can activate and cause proliferation of synovial fibroblasts and endolethial cells present in the joint. To further potentiate the process, these fibroblasts and endolethial cells can themselves produce additional mediators such as arachidonic aid and vasoactive amines (histamine, serotonin). Cytokines can further activate synovial cells, chrondrocytes, and osteocytes, which have a major role in cartilage destruction and bone remodeling. In addition, substances on the surface of synovial cells called cellular adhesion molecules increase and act as a cellular "adhesive tape" to adhere inflammatory cells in the joint cavity. Macrophages present in the joint space lead to further damage by releasing osteoclast activating factor, which then leads to further bone destruction. The inflammatory cells and their products continue to proliferate, and eventually the synovial lining becomes the thickened and irregular tissue pannus. Pannus erodes and covers the articular cartilage and can itself produce collagenase and elastase and lead to further bone destruction.

The above model provides a framework for the immunological processes working together to produce disease. However, all of the immunological players participating in this scenario normally play a crucial role in the body's ability to survive in a hostile environment. As seen in children born with a severely compromised immune system or in patients with AIDS who acquire a severely impaired immune system, without some intervention, humans can only survive a limited time without a functioning immune system. So what goes wrong in a patient with RA? What occurs to make this normally protective system malfunction and cause disease?

Innate Immunity

To understand RA fully, additional understanding of the normal functioning of the immune system is necessary. In a healthy person, all members of the immunological army protect the body from the many foreign invaders with which we are constantly confronted. Our first line of defense is our innate immune system (Abbas et al., 1994; Stites et al., 1994; Talaro & Talaro, 1996). This is innate in a species and does not require previous exposure to an antigen, which makes the system quick to act and effective. The innate immune system consists of natural physical barriers, a special group of lymphocytes termed natural killer (NK) cells, and phagocytic cells, which directly attack and "eat" foreign invaders (phagocytosis). The major phagocytes in the body are white blood cells and include monocytes, macrophages, and neutrophils (polymorphonuclear leukocytes). Monocytes circulate in the peripheral blood and, once they go into the tissues, are termed macrophages or histiocytes. Monocytes and macrophages comprise one of the major cell populations involved in protecting the body from intracellular organisms such as mycobacteria, various viruses, fungi, and some parasites (Abbas et al., 1994; Johnson, 1988; Stites et al., 1994; Talaro & Talaro, 1996). Various microbes such as encapsulated bacteria do not readily bind to the surface of phagocytes for engulfment. However, on being coated with substances such as products of the complement system and antibodies, the particles are recognized as foreign and can bind to the macrophage cell surface. This process is called *opsonization* and facilitates the process of phagocytosis. In addition to their role in innate immunity, macrophages have a major role in how cells communicate with one another. Macrophages can produce cytokines that affect cell interactions and recruit inflammatory cells to sites of injury.

Neutrophils are the other major phagocytic cells (Johnson, 1988; Roitt et al., 1996; Stites et al., 1994; Talaro & Talaro, 1996). They comprise the major population of white blood cells in the peripheral blood (up to 80%). They are short-lived cells and survive only 1–2 days in the bloodstream. Neutrophils have a multilobed nucleus and various storage cytoplasmic granules containing digestive enzymes and proteins used to break down particles that have been phagocytized. Neutrophils provide one of the first lines of defense against foreign invaders and are one of the first cell populations present in tissues with an acute infection. Neutrophils mediate their effects via phagocytosis or release of granules either intracellularly or extracellularly.

NK cells are a distinctive population of cells that are separate from T or B lymphocytes (Abbas et al., 1994; Herberman, Reynolds, & Ortaldo, 1986; Roitt et al., 1996; Stites et al., 1994; Talaro & Talaro, 1996; Trinchieri, 1989). They have large cytoplasmic granules and are thus called large granular lymphocytes. One of their major roles includes killing tumor cells and virally infected cells. One difference between NK cells and T lymphocytes that can kill tumor cells is that NK cells can kill when they first see the tumor, whereas T lymphocytes must have previously been exposed to the tumor cells before they will kill them.

Acquired Immunity

The other major division of the immune system is the acquired or specific immune system, which is generally the system we are referring to when we speak of the immune system (Abbas et al., 1994; Stites et al., 1994; Talaro & Talaro, 1996). Acquired immunity has a great degree of specificity and requires previous exposure to foreign pathogens. Therefore, it is referred to as specific immunity. The cells mediating this part of the immune system are white blood cells termed lymphocytes. The acquired immune system is further divided into two compartments, humoral and cellular, which relate to the response of distinctive types of lymphocytes. Humoral responses are those mediated by B lymphocytes that produce specific antibodies whose function is to neutralize foreign substances termed *antigens*. Humoral immunity is predominantly concerned with protection against bacterial pathogens. Cellular responses are those mediated by T lymphocytes that instead of antibodies produce soluble factors for the immune response. Cellular responses are mainly involved in immunity against fungi, parasites, and intracellular parasites. The major T-lymphocyte subpopulations are T-helper cells and cytotoxic or suppressor cells. T-helper cells, as the name implies, mediate the work of T lymphocytes. They are crucial in our defense against infectious agents. T-helper cells are killed specifically by infection with HIV; thus, the depletion of the action of these cells is largely responsible for the susceptibility to infections in patients with AIDS. The other major subpopulation, suppressor cytotoxic cells, has dual functions. They can kill tumor cells and virally infected cells, and they have suppressor activity and thus can dampen the activity of an overactive immune system. It must be added that, although traditionally these cells are termed cytotoxic or suppressor cells, many immunologists object to the use of these terms because suppressor cells are not universally accepted as a distinct cellular entity. Through the use of antibodies specific to the T lymphocyte subpopulations, we can enumerate the numbers of these different populations in the peripheral blood of patients. This is especially useful in patients with AIDS and with certain types of cancer, but generally is not done with rheumatology patients except for research purposes.

Cytokines are soluble mediators produced by T lymphocytes in addition to various other cell types (Abbas et al., 1994; Arai et al., 1990; Stites et al., 1994; Talaro & Talaro, 1996). Most of these substances are produced in small amounts and act either on adjacent cells or on the cell that produces them. In addition, some act on distant cells and tissues. As is seen in the initial discussion of the pathogenesis of RA, cytokines have a wide variety of effects on many cellular functions and cell populations. Their major roles include mediating effects induced by infectious agents, regulation of lymphocyte growth, and mediating inflammatory reactions. The major groups of cytokines consist of the interleukins (IL) and are numbered IL-1 to IL-12. Some additional cytokines include tumor necrosis factor (TNF), T lymphocyte transforming factor, and interferons. Only a few of the cytokines will be discussed here.

IL-1 and TNF are two cytokines structured quite differently; however, they have similar physiological effects (Abbas et al., 1994; Lehner, Ganz, Selsted, Babior, & Curnotte, 1988; Stites et al., 1994; Talaro & Talaro, 1996). IL-1 is produced most predominately by macrophages and activated T lymphocytes. IL-1 and TNF are important mediators of inflammatory responses and cause fever; thus, they are termed endogenous pyrogens. Both of these cytokines act on hepatocytes to induce the synthesis of plasma proteins termed acute phase reactants, which are increased in many inflammatory diseases, infection, cancer, and trauma. IL-1 and TNF have several effects on cells important in rheumatic disease such as synovial cells, chondrocytes, and osteoclasts (osteophages). These two cytokines can induce bone resorption by osteoclasts, increase cartilage turnover by chondrocytes, and cause proliferation of fibroblasts and synovial cells. Studies have shown increased levels of IL-1 and TNF in joint fluid from patients with RA (Harris, 1989; Stites et al., 1994; Winchester, 1995). There has been interest in treating patients with RA with inhibitors of these cytokines. A new drug, etanercept (ENBREL™) is a soluble recombinant TNF receptor that acts as an inhibitor of TNF. Etanercept is approved for use in patients with moderate to severe active RA who have had an inadequate response to other disease-modifying drugs and has shown major positive effects. (Moreland et al., 1999). (See chapter 3 in this volume for more information on these new drugs.)

IL-2 is a crucial cytokine that is a growth factor for T lymphocytes. Activated T lymphocytes produce IL-2, which then acts on the same cell that produced it to stimulate further growth. In addition, IL-2 stimulates the growth of nearby cells. IL-2 has been used to treat some patients with cancer.

IL-6 is the final cytokine to be discussed. Various cells, including macrophages, produce IL-6. It stimulates hepatocytes to increase the production of fibrinogen, which causes erythrocytes to stack. An increase in this protein is measured by the erythrocyte sedimentation rate (ESR), which frequently is used in rheumatology patients to evaluate inflammation and follow their disease course. As expected, increased IL-6 levels are found in rheumatic diseases such as RA. In addition to its immunological effects, IL-6 has many endocrine and metabolic actions. It is a stimulator of the hypothalamic-pituitary-adrenal axis, and its levels are decreased by the administration of glucocorticoids (Papanicolaou et al., 1998).

Autoimmunity

A review of the inflammatory process helps us to understand what happens in an inflamed joint, but it does not clarify what originally initiated this process. To understand this in the context of the inflammatory rheumatic diseases, we must examine the role of autoimmunity. Autoimmunity is defined as pathological changes that occur due to the immune system reacting against itself (Abbas et al., 1994; Brostoff et al., 1991; Roitt et al., 1996; Stites et al., 1994; Talaro & Talaro, 1996). Before discussing autoimmunity further, one must understand the way in which the cells of the immune system communicate with one another and how the immune system can differentiate what is self and what is foreign. Both of these tasks are accomplished through markers or receptors on the cell surface that allow cells to recognize one another and communicate. A single cell can have multiple receptors on its surface. These receptors play pivotal roles in both cell-to-cell communication and in the recognition of self and foreign substances. This is similar to the many ways in which we identify people: by the color of their hair, eyes, the way they speak, and any unique identifying physical characteristics. Autoimmunity represents the loss of the ability of the immune system to differentiate foreign invaders from its own body. The ability to recognize our body as self, and thus not cause potential danger, is termed self-tolerance (Cotran et al., 1994; Harris, 1989; Roitt et al., 1996; Sell, 1996; Winchester, 1995). Immunologists agree that autoimmunity is the loss of self-tolerance. Most of our self-tolerance occurs during the fetal period in our bone marrow and thymus. In these organs, lymphocytes that recognize the self as foreign are killed or inactivated. However, there are some self-reactive lymphocytes that escape being killed. Thus, there is a continuing effort throughout life to keep these cells under control and prevent the emergence of autoimmune diseases.

So if self-tolerance is present, then how does autoimmunity occur? There are many theories to explain autoimmune disease (Abbas et al., 1994; Brostoff et al., 1991; Roitt et al., 1996; Stites et al., 1994; Talaro & Talaro, 1996). One explanation relates to differences in the depletion of self-reactive T and B lymphocytes in fetal life. It appears that there is more complete purging of autoreactive T lymphocytes than B lymphocytes during the neonatal period. Consequently, we all have some "escapee" self-reactive B lymphocytes present that failed to be depleted. Normally, these self-reactive B lymphocytes do no harm because all of the autoreactive T lymphocytes potentially available to provide help to these B lymphocytes have been previously depleted. However, because we know that autoimmune disease occurs, the remaining T lymphocytes must be "tricked" into providing help to the self-responsive B lymphocytes. One way in which this can occur is when we are infected with microbial antigens that are similar to self-antigens. Due to the similarity between the microbial and self-antigens, the T lymphocytes think they are assisting B lymphocytes in responding to microbes when actually they are providing help to self-reactive B lymphocytes, and autoimmunity ensues. This is one explanation for the association of autoimmune disease after bacterial and viral infections. Another mechanism of autoimmunity is widespread activation of previously unresponsive self-reactive lymphocytes by substances that stimulate many clones of lymphocytes, so-called "polyclonal activators." Infectious agents such as gram-negative bacteria containing lipopolysaccharide can act as polyclonal activators. In addition, tissue injury and inflammation can lead to autoimmunity by causing the release of self-antigens that normally are sequestered. Because these antigens have been hidden from the immune system, they have never been identified as self. Thus, on release, they are viewed as foreign and can induce an autoimmune response. There can be alterations of self-antigens by either a microbial agent or by injury or inflammation so that they are now recognized as foreign. In addition, there are various genetic factors that have a role in the autoimmune system. In summary, there is not one theory that explains all autoimmune diseases. In most situations, disease results from a complex interplay between environmental factors including exposure to microbial antigens in a genetically susceptible host.

Many rheumatic diseases are characterized by detectable circulating levels of antibodies that can react with our body's own tissues and thus are called autoantibodies. These are quite useful in diagnosis, in following disease activity, and in prognosis (Brostoff et al., 1991; Naparstek & Poltz, 1993; Stites et al., 1994). For example, in systemic lupus erythematosus (SLE), the presence of antibody against double-stranded DNA (anti-DNA) is used clinically both for initial diagnosis and to follow a patient's disease activity. Anti-DNA immune complexes have been found deposited in the kidneys and in the skin and generally are believed to be an important factor in the pathology of SLE (Kotzin & O'Dell, 1995). In addition, RF is used clinically to evaluate patients with RA.

Several caveats must be kept in mind when evaluating the role of autoantibodies in disease states (Naparstek & Poltz, 1993; Roitt et al., 1996; Sell, 1996; Winchester, 1995). The presence of autoantibodies does not mean that autoimmune disease is present. Low levels of autoantibodies are found in many healthy persons. Even when high levels of autoantibodies are found associated with disease, they may not necessarily have a pathogenic role in the disease. Many studies demonstrate that the number of autoantibodies increases as we age, and, more commonly, autoantibodies can be seen in healthy women. In addition, genetic background has an important effect on autoantibody production. For example, clinically normal (without SLE) relatives of patients with SLE have a greater number of positive autoantibodies than the general population. Therefore, one must evaluate the role of autoantibodies in the light of age, gender, and genetic background. This should not dampen one's enthusiasm for evaluating autoantibodies, but autoantibodies should be evaluated in the proper context because they are important in many diseases.

Role of Genetics

The Human Genome Project had vastly increased our knowledge of the human genome, and consequently patients increasingly may query caregivers regarding the role of genetics in their disease process. Understandably, patients are concerned about the risk of their offspring developing a rheumatic disease. The following section will aid in addressing some of these concerns.

Just as our physical characteristics are determined by areas of DNA called genes, cells are identified by their physical characteristics, in this case, their surface receptors, which are determined by the genes present in DNA. One set of genes that encodes a set of receptors that are important in cell recognition and communication is located on human chromosome 6, which is termed the HLA complex or, in the mouse, the major histocompatibility complex (Campbell & Trowsdale, 1993; Salazar & Yunis, 1995). The term *HLA* is derived from the fact that these receptors were first identified on the surface of white blood cells. The HLA is divided into three divisions or classes (classes I, II, and III). Class I is important in organ transplantation, and the products of these genes, class I antigens, are present as surface receptors on all nucleated cells of the body. Class II is most important in immune system cell communication and plays an important role in organ translation. Class II surface receptors are present only on the surface of immune system cells. Class III controls proteins of the complement system that defend against foreign invaders. These genes code for surface receptors that have a vital role in recognition of self and thus are important in rejecting any foreign tissues. For this reason, the testing and measurement of HLA is important in organ transplantation because if differences between an organ and its recipient are too great, the transplanted organ will be rejected.

In addition to their role in organ transplantation, HLAs play an important role in susceptibility to various diseases (Campbell & Trowsdale, 1993; Salazar & Yunis, 1995). Certain human diseases occur more frequently in persons carrying particular HLA markers. Many of these diseases have immunological components and include several rheumatic diseases: RA, SLE, ankylosing spondylitis (AS), Reiter's syndrome, psoriatic arthritis, and Sjögren's syndrome. Some of the non-rheumatic diseases associated with the HLA include some inherited errors of metabolism such as 21-hydroxylase deficiency, insulin-dependent diabetes, and other autoimmune diseases such as autoimmune endocrinopathies. Possession of a particular HLA confers increased susceptibility to develop a particular disease. However, this is only an increased susceptibility and not a predictable transmission rate as in an autosomal dominant or recessive disorders such as Huntington's chorea or cystic fibrosis. The association of a particular HLA with disease is most often expressed as a relative risk, which is the increased risk resulting from having a particular genetic marker versus not having it. For example, if you have HLA DR-4, which is associated with a relative risk of 5 for RA, this means you have a five times greater risk of developing RA than if you lacked DR-4. Table 1 lists rheumatic diseases associated with HLAs and their relative risks.

The strongest association between an HLA and disease is between HLA B-27 and AS (Lipsky, 1995). If a person has HLA B-27, the relative risk of developing AS is 90. However, this figure is somewhat misleading. Although approximately 90% of persons with AS possess B-27 in a population study of B-27–positive subjects, only 1% to 2% of these will develop AS. Therefore, possessing the B-27 antigen only confers an increased risk for AS; this does not mean the person will develop the disease because there are many factors other than genetic ones that are involved in the development of AS. HLA B-27 is increased in patients with Reiter's syndrome, which includes arthritis, urethritis, and conjunctivitis.

Table 1. Association of HLA With Rheumatic Diseases

Disease	HLA	Relative Risk*
Ankylosing spondylitis	B-27	69–90
Reiter's syndrome	B-27	37
Rheumatoid arthritis	DR-4	2.7–6
Sjögren's syndrome	DR-2	5.2–9.7
	DR-3	3.6
Systemic lupus erythematosus	DR-2	2.3
	DR-3	2.5–5.8

*Relative risk refers to increased risk conferred from possessing a particular HLA versus lacking this antigen.

There has been much interest in the role of heredity in the development of RA (Stites et al., 1994). If one family member has the disease, then there is a two times greater risk that a second affected family member will be found. Many studies have examined the relationship between HLAs and RA, and an association exists between HLA DR-4 and RA with a relative risk of 5. In addition to studying the role of HLA, there has been interest in twin studies because these studies allow one to examine the effect of genes and environment on disease susceptibility (Jarvinen & Aho, 1994; Silman et al., 1993). By examining the concordance in monozygotic (genetically identical) twins versus that of dizygotic (nonidentical) twins, a disease determined entirely by genetics would be expected to show almost complete concordance in identical twins. Therefore, by comparing the frequency of disease in these two groups, one can roughly approximate the relative importance of genetic and environmental factors in the susceptibility to disease. By using molecular-based techniques, the association between the HLA system and RA has been better defined, and genotypes strongly associated with RA have been discovered. Patients with a particular amino acid sequence on the HLA DR-B1 chain have a strong association with severe, erosive, and seropositive RA. It now appears that HLA is more strongly associated with the progression of disease and its severity than with the onset of disease symptoms. To read further about this topic, the reader is referred to several references (Jawaheer et al., 1994; Ollier & MacGregor, 1995; Symmons, Ollier, Brennan, & Silman, 1996). Due to the multifactorial nature of causation in RA, genetic testing is generally not recommended routinely for patients or their offspring. However, this is a controversial topic with some researchers in disagreement. For a full discussion of this topic, refer to a recent article by Symmons et al. (1996). Although physicians may order genetic testing for some persons, HLA typing is used most often for large epidemiological studies of the disease. Clearly more work is needed to elucidate the complex interaction between HLA and many other factors that interact to result in disease.

In SLE, the development of disease is partially hereditary (Kotzin & O'Dell, 1995). As in RA, there are most likely multiple genes involved that interact with as-yet-unknown environmental factors. Twin studies in SLE have shown concordance rates from 25% to 60% for monozygotic twins versus 2% to 5% for dizygotic twins. Regarding HLA, there has been an association between HLA DR-2 and DR-3. In addition, there is an association between complement deficiencies and SLE. Patients with deficiencies of C4 and C2 have an increased risk of developing SLE, and patients with SLE have an increased frequency of C2 and C4 deficiency. Genetic studies with molecular techniques are further defining the role of genetics in SLE.

Role of Stress and Immunity in Rheumatic Disease

Nearly all health professionals working with rheumatology patients have at one time or another been questioned about the role of stressful or traumatic events in either causing or exacerbating rheumatic disease. There are several reports in the literature that examine these questions; however, there is no absolute consensus about the data. This is a complex topic affected by many variables that are difficult to control. For example, numerous studies examining these questions use nondirective interviews to collect psychosocial data. This method of data collection is difficult to control and may be subject to bias. In addition, many studies are retrospective and are influenced by a patient's recollection of feelings or events that occurred that may not be reproducible data. Because the intent of this section is to examine the interaction between stress and the immune system and its interplay with rheumatic disease, only a brief summary will be given concerning the role of psychosocial factors in rheumatology. Because most studies have been done with RA and SLE, studies in these diseases will be emphasized.

Numerous studies have examined whether emotionally stressful events can precipitate or exacerbate rheumatic disease. Reports of the percentage of patients with RA with precipitating psychosocial factors at the onset of their disease vary widely from 22% to 100% (Rimon & Laakso, 1985; Solomon, 1981). In 1969, Rimon published a study of stress and RA exacerbations with 100 patients with RA (Rimon, 1969). More than half of these subjects (55%) associated a major life event with the first symptoms of RA, whereas 45% of patients had no association. Rimon published a 15-year follow-up of these patients, and he proposed two categories of patients with RA: a disease group in which psychological factors are strongly associated and genetic influences are minor, and a second group in which there is a strong association with hereditary factors and less influence by psychological events (Rimon & Laakso, 1985). A more recent study examining life events and RA found no evidence of an excess of events in the 12 months preceding the onset of disease (Conway, Creed, & Symmons, 1995). This was confirmed by Haller, Holzner, Mur, and Gunther (1997), who examined the effect of life events in 48 patients with RA and found that the course of RA was not affected by the number of life events nor by the degree of stress caused by these events. In contrast, Potter and Zautra (1997) reported a case study in which major life events were associated with decreased symptoms, and smaller life events related to symptom increases. Furthermore, these same authors examined the role of changes in interpersonal stress on disease activity in 41 women with RA. They found that increases in interpersonal stress were associated with increases in disease activity (Zautra et al., 1997). A recent longitudinal study of 216 patients with RA found that pain and disability were most strongly related to mental distress (Smedstad, Valgum, Moum, & Kvien, 1997). Another study of 91 patients with RA found that a decrease in psychological stress 1 year after diagnosis was related to male gender, less severe disease at onset, and strong social support (Evers, Kraaimaat, Geenen, & Bijlsma, 1997).

Many older studies have examined personality variables to determine whether certain variables predispose to RA (Geist, 1966; Polley, Swenson, & Steinhilber, 1970). Many of these studies were uncontrolled and not scientifically valid. Although some early studies suggested that there were some personality characteristics that predisposed to RA, most investigators now agree that personality characteristics of patients with RA before the onset of their disease do not differ from that of control subjects (Anderson, Bradley, Young, McDaniel, & Wise, 1985; Wallace, 1987).

Patients had more stress at the onset of disease compared with subjects with osteoarthritis (Latman & Walls, 1996).

The role of depression in RA has been extensively studied, and there is not agreement in the literature regarding the magnitude of the problem (Hawley & Wolfe, 1993; Katz & Yelin, 1994; Parker & Wright, 1995; Smedstad, Valgum, Kvien, & Moum, 1995; Smith, Christensen, Peck, & Ward, 1994; Wolfe & Hawley, 1993). Although the prevalence of depression in RA is not precisely known, it has been estimated to range from 15% to 34% (Creed, Murphy, & Jayson, 1990; Katz & Yelin, 1993). However, in one large 10-year longitudinal study of more than 6,000 patients, the depression scores in patients with RA did not differ from that of clinic patients (Hawley & Wolfe, 1993). Several studies that reported higher rates of depression in patients with RA found this to be related to factors such as pain (Smedstad et al., 1995), inability to perform valued activities (Katz & Yelin, 1995), and disability (Wolfe & Hawley, 1993). A recent study examining the relationships among age, depression, and RA found that younger subjects (less than 45 years of age) are at higher risk for depressive symptoms (Wright et al., 1998).

In examining the role of stress in RA, one must consider the contribution of the disease itself to the feelings of stress in a patient's life (Anderson et al., 1985; Wallace, 1987). With a chronic disease such as RA, there are many effects on life resulting from pain, sexual dysfunction, altered mobility, economic and occupational disability, and social stressors. Although these factors can clearly affect a person's psychological well-being, studies vary in the degree of psychological dysfunction reported for patients with RA. The disparity between the results of multiple studies examining these questions suggests that there is not a universal effect of stress on all persons with RA; rather, there is great variability between patients. Due to the complexities of the disease, it is difficult to conclusively demonstrate a cause-and-effect relationship among rheumatic disease, stress, and psychological factors. In summary, although a great deal of work has been done in this area, additional large prospective controlled studies must be conducted before we can conclusively determine the effects of these factors.

In the last two decades, there has been increased interest in the relationship between stress and the immune systems. In our fast-paced society, we constantly refer to stress in our lives. In a biomedical sense, stress is defined as any aversive stimuli (emotional, physical, and mental) that disturb our usual equilibrium (Chrousos, 1995; Moos & Solomon, 1964; Rabin, Cohen, Ganguli, Lysle, & Cunnick, 1989; Wilder, 1995). Our body's ability to respond to stress is crucial to our survival as a species. Our stress system consists of parts of the brain, especially the pituitary, the hypothalamus, peripheral tissues, and nerves (Chrousos, 1995; Rabin et al., 1989). The diverse components of the stress system communicate mainly by hormones, which are soluble substances that stimulate a cascade of biochemical activity. Essentially these chemical messengers tell an organ whether it should increase or decrease production of additional hormones. Stress hormones released from the brain interact primarily with the adrenal glands located above the kidneys. On stimulation, the adrenal gland releases multiple hormones including epinephrine (adrenaline), norepinephrine (nonadrenaline), and cortisol. Epinephrine and norepinephrine are the major hormones that control the visceral functions of the body. Epinephrine is the "fight or flight" stress hormone, and we all experience the effects of this hormone whenever we are physically or psychologically threatened in some way. The pounding of the heart and sweating that many people feel when speaking in front of a large group is one common example of how epinephrine affects our body. On the other hand, cortisol is an equally important hormone, but we are not conscious of its many actions. The most relevant action of cortisol in rheumatic disease is its action as an anti-inflammatory compound. Cortisol inhibits many functions of the immune system, primarily influencing the cellular immune system. It dampens the inflammatory response by inhibiting the expression of cellular adhesion molecules, decreasing the production of many cytokines, and suppressing the release of prostaglandins.

Our stress system constantly monitors our bodily functions and our response to the environment (Chrousos, 1995). When our body is at rest, signals are sent to our stress system from many parts of the body. One important interaction is with the immune system. Lymph nodes have been shown to be directly innervated by peripheral nerves. One possible route of interaction between the central nervous system (CNS) and the immune system may be nerves terminating in lymphoid organs that affect immune function. Another important interaction occurs via cytokines that can activate the stress system, and, alternatively, the stress system can affect cytokine release. This is a bidirectional interaction with the stress system affecting the immune system and vice versa.

Many studies have examined the role of stress and autoimmunity (Chrousos, 1995; Rabin et al., 1989; Wilder, 1995), and several authors have hypothesized that stress leads to immunosuppression that could then lead to autoimmune disease. In the case of RA, contrasting hypotheses are suggested. McFarlane and Brooks (1990) proposed that, because RA disease activity is characterized by excessive immunoreactivity, stress could have a beneficial effect on disease activity by suppressing an overactive immune system. Alternatively, O'Leary (1990) suggested that stress could selectively impair the ability of the immune system to suppress itself; thus, increased stress could lead to more active disease. Harrington and associates (1993) published a study that supports McFarlane and Brooks' hypothesis. In a study of 14 patients with RA, they examined the changes in a global parameter of cellular immunity and soluble IL-2 receptor (sIL-2R), along with indicators of daily stress, joint inflammation, and pain (Harrington et al., 1993). The measurement of sIL-2R has been shown in several studies to correlate with increased activation of T lymphocytes. Both serum and synovial fluid levels of sIL-2R in patients with RA have been shown to correlate with disease activity. This study confirmed the association between joint inflammation and serum levels of sIL-2R. Stress as measured by increases in mood disturbances was linked with a decrease in sIL-2R levels, which suggests that stress had an immunosuppressive effect. Reports of increased pain were unrelated to changes in sIL-2R levels and joint swelling. The authors extended this study in 1997 and proposed a dual pathway model of stressor effects on RA disease activity (Affleck et al., 1997). They suggested that psychological stressors could have a dual and even opposing effect on RA disease activity. Their recent study in 50 patients with RA examined the validity of a dual pathway model of stress by examining the linkage of daily event stressors to RA disease activity. Although their across-person analyses failed to support linkages, they did find that the model was supported in within-person analyses. Increases in daily event stressors were associated with increased joint pain. However, increased stressors resulted in decreased joint inflammation as measured by decreased sIL-2R levels. These results are intriguing; however, additional studies are needed to shed light on this topic.

In a recent review of stress and the immune system, Chrousos (1995) proposed that defects in the stress system could have two effects. If the stress system becomes excessively activated in response to inflammation, the result is immunosuppression. As a result, this can lead to increased susceptibility to infection but decreased susceptibility to autoimmune disease. Alternatively, less stimulation of the stress system can lead to excessive activity of the immune system, which results in a decreased susceptibility to infection but an increased activity of or susceptibility to autoimmune disease. This proposal is supported by studies reporting a subgroup of patients with RA who have a decreased ability to respond to stimulation; thus, they represent a population susceptible to autoimmune disease (Katz & Yelin, 1994). Although the immune system of these patients was stimulated, as evidenced by high levels of cytokines, their stress system did not respond normally to the inflammation because they had low levels of stress hormones in their bloodstream. In addition, these same patients showed hyporesponsiveness of their stress system to major stressors, such as major surgery (Katz & Yelin, 1994). Although detailed genetic studies have not been performed on these types of patients, it appears that the hyporesponsiveness of the stress system is genetically determined. Additional studies are needed to evaluate this association. Further support for a decreased cortisol responsiveness is obtained from studies showing that the white blood cells of patients with RA have up to a 50% decrease in the number of cortisol receptors on their surface (Chrousos, 1995). Thus, this would lead to a hyporesponsiveness of white blood cells to the immunoresponsive effects of cortisol. Additional studies have examined this topic by examining the hypothalamic-pituitary-adrenal axis in patients with RA (Crofford et al., 1997; Jorgenson, Bressot, Bologna, & Sany, 1995).

Conclusion

It is clear from this brief summary of stress, the immune system, and rheumatic disease that there is far from consensus in the literature on this topic. In fact, it is difficult to predict the effects of stress on disease. Is stress a positive or negative force in terms of its effects on the immune system? The answer to this question is not clear from the available data. The complexity of the disease process in many of the rheumatic diseases confounds our interpretation. Stress may affect autoimmune disease differently depending on the stage of disease (Rubin & Hawker, 1993). For example, at the onset of autoimmune disease, immunosuppression induced by stress may lead to heightened disease activity and may even account for the initiation of the disease. This may occur via increased susceptibility to a microbe responsible for initiating an immune response that ultimately leads to the autoimmune disease. Alternatively, later in the disease course, stress-included immunosuppression could have beneficial effects by allowing a dampening of an overactive immune system. In addition, changes induced by the disease process itself could alter a person's response to a small amount of stress, which may be immunosuppressive at one point and immunostimulatory at another time. In support of these concepts, McFarland and Brooks (1990) proposed that different phases of RA should be considered separately when evaluating the effects of stress. They considered these phases to be the loss of immunological tolerance, the initiation of inflammation in the joint, and the chronic phase of the disease. The interaction of stress and immunity in rheumatology will not be understood until many well-controlled prospective studies are completed.

Although much work is clearly needed in the area of stress and the immune system, major strides have been made in our understanding of the pathogenesis of rheumatic disease. Major advances occur daily in understanding the human genome, and we certainly expect to increase our knowledge greatly in these areas in the next few years. Hopefully, this brief outline of the immune system will provide caregivers with an increased understanding of many of the new and exciting discoveries to come in the next few years that they can share with their patients.

References

Abbas, A. K., Lichtman, A. H., & Pober, J. S. (1994). *Cellular and molecular immunology.* Philadelphia: Saunders.

Affleck, G., Urrows, S., Tennen, H., Higgins, P., Pav, D., & Aloisi, R. (1997). A dual pathway model of daily stressor effects on rheumatoid arthritis. *Annals of Behavioral Medicine, 19*(2), 161–170.

Anderson, K. O., Bradley, L. A., Young, L. D., McDaniel, L. K., & Wise, C. M. (1985). Rheumatoid arthritis: Review of psychological factors related to etiology, effects, and treatment. *Psychological Bulletin, 98,* 358–387.

Arai, K., Lee, F., Miyajima, A., Miyatake, S., Arai, N., & Yokota, T. (1990). Cytokines: Coordinators of immune and inflammatory responses. *Annual Reviews of Biochemistry, 59,* 783-836.

Brostoff, J., Scadding, G. K., Male, D., & Roitt, I. M. (1991). *Clinical immunology.* London: Gower Medical.

Campbell, R. D., & Trowsdale, J. (1993). Map of the human MHC. *Immunology Today, 14,* 349–352.

Chrousos, G. P. (1995). The hypothalamic-pituitary-adrenal axis and immune-mediated inflammation. *New England Journal of Medicine, 20,* 1351–1362.

Conway, S. C., Creed, F. H., & Symmons, D. P. (1995). Life events and the onset of rheumatoid arthritis. *Journal of Psychosomatic Research, 39,* 507–508.

Cotran, R. S., Kumar, V., & Robbins, S. L. (1994). Inflammation and repair. In R. S. Cotran, V. Kumar, & S. L. Robbins (Eds.), *Pathologic basis of disease* (5th ed., pp. 51–92). Philadelphia: Saunders.

Creed, F., Murphy, S., & Jayson, M. V. (1990). Measurement of psychiatric disorder in rheumatoid arthritis. *Journal of Psychosomatic Research, 34,* 79–87.

Crofford, L. J., Kalogeras, K. T., Mastorakos, G., Magiakou, M. A., Wells, J., Kanik, K. S., Gold, P. W., Chrousos, G. P., & Wilder, R. L. (1997). Circadian relationships between interleukin (IL)-6 and hypo-thalamic-pituitary-adrenal axis hormones: Failure of IL-6 to cause sustained hypercortisolism in patients with early untreated rheumatoid arthritis. *Journal of Clinical Endocrinology and Metabolism, 82*(4), 1279–1283.

Evers, A. W., Kraaimaat, F. W., Geenen, R., & Bijlsma, J. W. (1997). Determinants of psychological distress and its course in the first year after diagnosis in rheumatoid arthritis patients. *Journal of Behavioral Medicine, 20*(5), 489–504.

Geist, H. (1966). *The psychological aspects of rheumatoid arthritis.* Springfield, IL: Thomas.

Haler, C., Holzner, B., Mur, E., & Gunther, V. (1997). The impact of life events on patients with rheuma-toid arthritis: A psychological myth? *Clinical Experiments in Rheumatology, 15*(2), 175–179.

Harrington, L., Affleck, G., Urrows, S., Tennan, H., Higgins, P., Zautra, A., & Hoffman, S. (1993). Tempo-ral covariation of soluble interleukin-2 receptor levels, daily stress, and disease activity in rheumatoid arthritis. *Arthritis and Rheumatism, 36,* 199–203.

Harris, E. D., Jr. (1989). Pathogenesis of rheumatoid arthritis. In W. N. Kelley, E. D. Harris, Jr., S. Ruddy, & C. B. Sledge (Eds.), *Textbook of rheumatology* (pp. 905–942). Philadelphia: Saunders.

Hawley, D. J., & Wolfe, F. (1993). Depression is not more common in rheumatoid arthritis: A 10 year longitudinal study of 6,153 patients with rheumatic disease. *Journal of Rheumatology, 20*, 2025–2031.

Herberman, R. B., Reynolds, C. W., & Ortaldo, J. (1986). Mechanisms of cytoxicity by natural killer (NK) cells. *Annual Reviews of Immunology, 4*, 651–680.

Jarvinen, P., & Aho, K. (1994). Twin studies in rheumatic diseases. *Seminars in Arthritis and Rheumatism, 24*(1), 19–28.

Jawaheer, D., Thomson, W., MacGregor, A. J., Carthy, D., Davidson, J., Dyer, P. A., Silman, A. J., & Ollier, W. E. (1994). "Homozygosity" for the HLA-DR shared epitope contributes to the highest risk for rheumatoid arthritis concordance in identical twins. *Arthritis and Rheumatism, 37*(5), 681–686.

Johnson, R. B. (1988). Monocytes and macrophages. *New England Journal of Medicine, 318*, 747–752.

Jorgensen, C., Bressot, N., Bologna, C., & Sany, J. (1995). Dysregulation of the hypothalamo-pituitary axis in rheumatoid arthritis. *Journal of Rheumatology, 22*, 1829–1833.

Katz, P. P., & Yelin, E. H. (1993). Prevalence and correlates of depressive symptoms among persons with rheumatoid arthritis. *Journal of Rheumatology, 20*, 790–796.

Katz, P. P., & Yelin, E. H. (1994). Life activities with rheumatoid arthritis with and without depressive symptoms. *Arthritis Care and Research, 7*, 67–77.

Katz, P. P., & Yelin, E. H. (1995). The development of depressive symptoms among women with rheumatoid arthritis. *Arthritis and Rheumatism, 38*, 49–56.

Kotzin, B. L., & O'Dell, J. R. (1995). Systemic lupus erythematosus. In M. M. Frank, K. F. Austen, H. N. Claman, & E. R. Unanue (Eds.), *Samter's immunologic diseases* (pp. 667–757). New York: Little, Brown.

Latman, N. S., & Walls, R. (1996). Personality and stress: An exploratory comparison of rheumatoid arthritis and osteoarthritis. *Archives of Physical Medicine and Rehabilitation, 77*(8), 796–800.

Lehner, R. I., Ganz, T., Selsted, M. E., Babior, B. M., & Curnotte, J. T. (1988). Neutrophils and host defense. *Annals of Internal Medicine, 109*, 127–142.

Lipsky, P. E. (1995). The spondyloarthropathies. In M. M. Frank, K. F. Austen, H. N. Claman, & E. R. Unanue (Eds.), *Samter's immunologic diseases* (pp. 769–790). New York: Little, Brown.

McFarlane, A. C., & Brooks, P. M. (1990). Psychoimmunology and rheumatoid arthritis: Concepts and methodologies. *International Journal of Psychiatry and Medicine, 20*, 306–322.

Moos, R. H., & Solomon, G. F. (1964). Personality correlates of the rapidity of progression of rheumatoid arthritis. *Annals of Rheumatic Diseases, 23*, 145–151.

Moreland, L. W., Schiff, M. H., Baumgartner, S. W., Tindall, E. A., Fleischmann, R. M., Bulpitt, K. J., Weaver, A. L., Keystone, E. C., Furst, D. E., Mease, P. J., Ruderman, E. M., Horwitz, D. A., Arkfeld, D. G., Garrison, L., Burge, D. J., Blosch, C. M., Lange, M. L., McDonnell, N. D., & Weinblatt, M. E. (1999). Etanercept therapy in rheumatoid arthritis: A randomized, controlled trial. *Annals of Internal Medicine, 130*, 478–486.

Naparstek, Y., & Poltz, P. H. (1993). The role of autoantibodies in autoimmune diseases. *Annual Reviews of Immunology, 11*, 79–104.

O'Leary, A. (1990). Stress, emotion, and human immune function. *Psychological Bulletin, 108*, 363–382.

Ollier, W. E., & MacGregor, A. (1995). Genetic epidemiology of rheumatoid disease. *British Medical Bulletin, 51*(2), 267–285.

Papanicolaou, D. A., Wilder, R. L., Manolagas, S. C., & Chrousos, G. P. (1998). The pathophysiologic roles of interleukin-6 in human disease. *Annals of Internal Medicine, 128*(2), 127–137.

Parker, J. C., & Wright, G. E. (1995). The implications of depression for pain and disability in rheumatoid arthritis. *Arthritis Care and Research, 8,* 279–283.

Polley, H. F., Swenson, W., & Steinhilber, R. M. (1970). Personality characteristics of patients with rheumatoid arthritis. *Psychosomatics, 11,* 45–49.

Potter, P. T., & Zautra, A. J. (1997). Stressful life events' effects on rheumatoid arthritis disease activity. *Journal of Consultation and Clinical Psychology, 65*(2), 319–323.

Rabin, B. S., Cohen, S., Ganguli, R., Lysle, D. T., & Cunnick, J. E. (1989). Bidirectional interaction between the central nervous system and the immune system. *Critical Reviews in Immunology, 9,* 279–312.

Rimon, R. (1969). A psychosomatic approach to rheumatoid arthritis: A clinical study of 100 female patients. *Acta Rheumatica Scandinavia, 13,* 1–154.

Rimon, R., & Laakso, R. L. (1985). Life stress and rheumatoid arthritis. *Psychotherapy and Psychosomatics, 43,* 38–43.

Roitt, I., Brostoff, J., & Male, D. (1996). *Immunology.* St. Louis, MO: Mosby.

Rubin, L. A., & Hawker, G. A. (1993). Stress and the immune system: Preliminary observations in rheumatoid arthritis using an in vivo marker of immune activity. *Arthritis and Rheumatism, 39,* 204–207.

Ruddy, S. (1989). Complement. In W. N. Kelley, E. D. Harris, Jr., S. Ruddy, & C. B. Sledge (Eds.), *Textbook of rheumatology* (pp. 241–252). Philadelphia: Saunders.

Salazar, M., & Yunis, E. J. (1995). MHC: Gene structure and function. In M. M. Frank, K. F. Austen, H. N. Claman, & E. R. Unanue (Eds.), *Samter's immunologic diseases* (pp. 101–116). New York: Little, Brown.

Sell, S. (1996). *Immunology, immunopathology and immunity.* Stamford, CT: Appleton & Lange.

Silman, A. J., MacGregor, A. J., Thomson, W., Holligan, S., Carthy, D., Farhan, A., & Ollier, W. E. (1993). Twin concordance rates for rheumatoid arthritis: Results from a nationwide study. *British Journal of Rheumatology, 32*(10), 903–907.

Smedstad, L. M., Vaglum, P., Kvien, T. K., & Moum, T. (1995). The relationship between self-reported pain and sociodemographic variables, anxiety, and depressive symptoms in rheumatoid arthritis. *Journal of Rheumatology, 22,* 514–520.

Smedstad, L. M., Valgum, P., Moum, T., & Kvien, T. K. (1997). The relationship between psychological distress an traditional clinical variables: A 2-year prospective study of 216 patients with early rheumatoid arthritis. *British Journal of Rheumatology, 36*(12), 1304–1311.

Smith, T. W., Christensen, A. J., Peck, J. R., & Ward, J. R. (1994). Cognitive distortion, helplessness, and depressed mood in rheumatoid arthritis: A four year longitudinal analysis. *Health Psychology, 13,* 213–217.

Solomon, G. F. (1981). Emotional and personality factors in the onset and course of autoimmune disease, particularly rheumatoid arthritis. In R. Ader (Ed.), *Psychoneuroimmunology* (pp. 159–180). New York: Academic Press.

Stites, D. P., Terr, A. I., & Parslow, T. G. (1994). *Basic and clinical immunology.* Norwalk, CT: Appleton & Lange.

Symmons, D. P., Ollier, W.E., Brennan, P., & Silman, A. J. (1996). Should patients with recent onset rheumatoid arthritis be offered genetic screening? *Annals of Rheumatic Diseases, 55*(7), 407–410.

Talaro, K., & Talaro, A. (1996). *Foundations in microbiology* (pp. 423–542). Dubuque, IA: Wm. C. Brown.

Trinchieri, G. (1989). Biology of natural killer cells. *Advances in Immunology, 47,* 187–376.

Wallace, D. J. (1987). The role of stress and trauma in rheumatoid arthritis and systemic lupus erythematosus. *Seminars in Arthritis and Rheumatism, 26,* 153–156.

Wilder, R. L. (1995). Neuroendocrine-immune system interactions and autoimmunity. *Annual Reviews of Immunology, 13*, 307–318.

Winchester, R. (1995). Rheumatoid arthritis. In M. M. Frank, K. F. Austen, H. N. Claman, & E. R. Unanue (Eds.), *Samter's immunologic diseases* (pp. 699–757). New York: Little, Brown.

Wolfe, F., & Hawley, D. J. (1993). The relationship between clinical activity and depression in rheumatoid arthritis. *Journal of Rheumatology, 20*, 2032–2037.

Wright, G. E., Parker, J. C., Smarr, K. L., Johnson, J. C., Hewett, J. E., & Walker, S. E. (1998). Age, depressive symptoms, and rheumatoid arthritis. *Arthritis and Rheumatism, 41*(2), 298–305.

Zautra, A. J., Hoffman, J., Potter, P., Matt, K. S., Yocum, D., & Castro, L. (1997). Examination of changes in interpersonal stress as a factor in disease exacerbations among women with rheumatoid arthritis. *Annals of Behavioral Medicine, 19*(3), 279–286.

Appendix A
Glossary

Antibodies: The name given to immunoglobulins when they are produced in response to a particular invader.

Antigen: A foreign substance that induces the formation of an antibody that can then bind to it and facilitate its destruction.

Antigenic sites: The parts of a foreign substance that the immune system recognizes as foreign and that induce the formation of an antibody.

B lymphocyte: One of the major types of lymphocytes originating in the bone marrow. In its terminally differentiated form (plasma cell), it secretes antibodies that provide protection from foreign invaders, primarily bacteria.

Cellular immune system: The division of the immune system composed of T lymphocytes and macrophages. This system provides the major defense against viruses, parasites, intracellular bacteria, fungi, and cancer cells. The major mediators are cytokines.

Complement: A system of proteins in the blood that are important in protecting the body from foreign pathogens. Complement proteins can directly kill foreign invaders or activate other cells that then facilitate their destruction.

Cytokines: Soluble substances produced from many different types of cells (primarily T lymphocytes and macrophages). They have multiple actions, including the mediation of the inflammatory process.

Humoral immune system: The division of the immune system composed of B lymphocytes and plasma cells. This system is the major defense against bacterial infections. The major mediators are antibodies.

Immune complex: A matrix consisting of antigens and antibodies that can aggregate or become trapped in tissues and induce disease through activation of an inflammatory reaction.

Immunoglobulins: The protein products of B lymphocytes produced in five different forms: IgG, IgM, IgA, IgE, and IgD. Each form or class has a specialized function. IgG is the most prevalent class and is responsible for long-lasting immunity. IgM is the immunoglobulin produced on the first encounter with a foreign pathogen. IgA is produced at mucosal surfaces. IgE is important in the allergic response, and IgD is present on the surface of cells.

Macrophages: The scavenger cells of the immune system. They work with T lymphocytes in protecting against viruses, fungi, cancer cells, and intracellular bacteria. They can release cytokines and can directly engulf foreign pathogens.

Opsonization: The process whereby an antibody binds to a microbe and facilitates its destruction by a phagocyte that destroys it.

Phagocytosis: The process of engulfment of a foreign pathogen by a macrophage or neutrophil that can result in the direct killing of the invader.

Plasma cell: This cell represents the terminal differentiation of the B lymphocyte. It is an immunoglobulin factory.

Rheumatoid factor (RF): An autoantibody commonly found in the serum and synovial fluid of patients with RA. It is usually an IgM antibody directed against IgG. The presence or absence of RF can be measured in the clinical laboratory and can assist in the diagnosis of patients with RA.

2

PATHOPHYSIOLOGY OF CARTILAGE AND JOINT STRUCTURES IN RHEUMATIC DISEASE

John H. Bland, MD

In 1948, with the discovery of the rheumatoid factor (RF), the first antibody discovered for rheumatoid arthritis (RA), the field of rheumatology burgeoned into immunology, and many rheumatologic investigators metamorphosed from clinical physicians into immunologists pursuing elegant molecular studies. However, this rapid and clearly important growth overshadowed research into the cell biology and organ physiology of the structures with which rheumatologists and rehabilitation professionals are most concerned: the connective tissue system of joints, synovium, cartilage, ligaments, tendons, muscles, bones, fascia, and joint capsules (Bland, 1988). Unfortunately, physiological studies of joints have mainly been conducted on the knee and hip, usually with the joint at rest. (RF is defined in the glossary in chapter 1 of this volume.)

The aim of this chapter is to present, in dynamic form, current knowledge of the characteristics, physiology, pathophysiology, and cell biology of the connective tissue system, sometimes called the supporting system.

Physiological Concepts of the Connective Tissue System

One can visualize the connective tissue system as a vast "apartment house" of connective tissue—fiber (collagen, reticulin, and elastin) and gel (water and salt-rich carbohydrate polymers such as glycosaminoglycans and proteoglycans)—with a great spectrum of these compounds in varying molecular arrangements and combinations. A joint is a macrocleft in connective tissue, and all other extracellular space is made up of "microclefts" with approximating surfaces that easily glide on one another. Macroclefts and microclefts exhibit relatively little difference in terms of pressure, osmolarity, and hydrogen ion concentration. However, there is a great difference in physiological temperature between the macroclefts and the microclefts. The joint temperature, peculiarly enough, is about 32°C in the joints versus the usual body temperature of 37°C.

Although we speak of joint "spaces" and interstitial "space," there really is no open space, only potential spaces. These spaces resemble a collapsed balloon with a wet, slippery, sliding inner surface. The state of collapse is maintained by a subatmospheric intracavity pressure (i.e., a suction or vacuum pressure). For example, the knee, which is the largest joint space, has an average of

21 ml of synovial fluid or less without demonstrable effusions. The slightest increase in fluid can create an effusion, and the pressure will become positive (Levick, 1983b). Guyton (1963) proved that this negative subatmospheric pressure additionally characterizes the microspaces.

Levick (1983a and 1983b) long studied the mechanism of normal maintenance of subatmospheric pressure in joints as well as in all the microspaces. This pressure differential plays a major role in stabilizing joints. The "suction" of this phenomenon draws articulating surfaces into the best possible fit with one another by guiding the surface contact as the joint moves through its range of motion.

Composition and Organization of Connective Tissue

Bioengineers have educated us in the concepts of the composite materials fiber and gel. Good examples are a swallow's nest (mud and sticks), Fiberglas, reinforced concrete, and connective tissue in animals. All connective tissues are truly composite materials, the two principal elements being collagen (fiber) and proteoglycans (the gel or ground substance). Although there are 12 different types of collagen now identifiable, the principal collagen fibers examined here are types 1 and 2. Elastin supplements the collagen in appropriate tissues such as the ligamentum nuchae at the cervical spine and the aorta. The gel materials are carbohydrate polymers that are very high in molecular weight that bind cations and release them. Innumerable small molecules and ions including albumin and immunoglobulins, are transported in these extracellular spaces between the circulation and the cells (Linn & Sokoloff, 1978).

The physical behavior of connective tissue can be predicted according to the content and organization of fibers and the ground substance. The fibers are in diverse patterns, often in parallel array. In general, the higher the tissue's tensile strength, the more parallel and dense the fibers are. Viidik (1968) characterized connective tissue according to the "tow region" of the tissue in force elongation diagrams. All connective tissues have been shown to have the fibers in an undulating pattern from the origins to their insertions. A short tow region indicates that only a small degree of elongation is needed to straighten the undulating fibers and develop tension in the system. A long tow region indicates that the fibers taking their undulating paths develop tension after a greater degree of elongation. Specific examples of the latter include the inferior portion of the capsule of the shoulder and the posterior aspect of the knee joint (Norris & Okamura, 1996). The straightening process provides the necessary flexibility for joint movement. Each joint has connective tissues of differing characteristics depending on its functional requirements; consequently, the greater the undulating pathway, the greater the flexibility. The process of functional change (from undulating to straight and tense fibers) requires that the fibers glide past one another efficiently, easily, and instantly (Akeson, Woo, Amiel, & Frank, 1984). The freedom for fiber-to-fiber gliding at the critical fiber intercept point is crucial to the extensibility of the system (Figure 1).

When connective tissue is analyzed chemically, little difference is found from one connective tissue to another. The complex and varied physical properties of different connective tissues are accomplished not by altered chemical composition but by varying patterns of fiber and proteoglycan. Thus, a wide functional range of structural connective tissue made of quite identical elements has allowed an ingenious structural economy.

Most of the dry weight is collagen fiber type 1. On a dry-weight basis, the proteoglycans make up only 1% to 2% of the weight, a grossly misleading indication of their functional importance. On a wet-weight basis, 60% to 80% of the total weight is water that is principally bound in the proteoglycan molecules (the gel ground substance). Lubrication, fiber-to-fiber glide, and spacing between fibers is provided by the water. Viscoelastic properties are water dependent.

Temperature in Joints: Clinical Implication

The temperature in healthy joints is 32° to 34°C versus the expected body temperature of 37°C (Hollander & Horvath, 1950; Horvath & Hollander, 1949). For example, the temperature of the resting knee is 32°C (89.6°F). The temperature of the ankle is 29°C (Horvath & Hollander, 1949). The distal finger and toe joints can be even cooler, close to skin temperature. Severe knee synovitis in RA may only raise the intraarticular temperature to 37°C (98.6°F).

Changes in blood flow can alter joint temperature. Joint temperature can be lowered by nicotine (a vasoconstrictor) and by cold. Heat can likewise lower the temperature, but in the presence of severe synovitis, it can increase swelling. Exercise (which increases blood flow to a joint) can increase intra-articular temperature, and stress (which lowers skin temperature) can increase joint temperature severely, which is why inflamed joints must be exercised cautiously. Collagenase, a product of synovitis in rheumatoid arthritis (RA) and osteoarthritis (OA) is maximally active at 37°C and far less active at normal joint temperatures (Hollander, Stoner, & Brown, 1951). Collagenolysis, the breakdown of collagen, has been shown by Harris and McCroskery (1974) to be accelerated by an increase in intraarticular pressure. Effective rehabilitative treatment should be directed toward lowering intraarticular temperatures to more normal levels (32–34°) (Hollander & Horvath, 1950; Horvath & Hollander, 1949). The most effective methods are reducing inflammation through medication, cold modalities, and gentle range of motion (ROM) exercises to prevent the effects of immobilization. However, a word of caution: most physiological studies on joint tissue are conducted in vitro at 37°C, which does not reflect normal joint metabolism. Likewise, studies done on animals

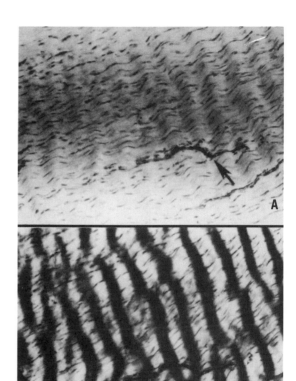

Figure 1. (A, above): Note the undulating pattern of collagen fibers in parallel array in a healthy dog's cruciate ligament. The *arrow* points to a small blood vessel. (B, below): The same cruciate ligament stained with India ink, making the undulating pattern of collagen fibers more graphic; this ligament has a short tow region. *Note.* From "The Chemical Basis of Repair, the Biology of Ligaments," by S.A. Akeson, S.Y. Woo, D. Amiel, & C. B. Frank, In *Rehabilitation of the Injured Knee* (p. 93–209), by C. Y. Hunter & F. J. Frank (Eds.), 1984, St. Louis, MO: Mosby. Copyright 1984 by Mosby. Reprinted with permission.

generally do not reflect the same temperature variables seen in humans. More research is needed on the subject of intra-articular temperature and its variations in the normal state and in inflammatory disease.

Intra-articular Pressure: Clinical Implications

As noted, the pressure in normal joints is clearly subatmospheric, which creates a suction force that is a dynamic stabilizing force for the joint (Werner, Boardman, & Fu, 1996). Müller (1929) was the first to demonstrate pressures of (equal to)–8 cm to–12 cm of water in human knees. This important physical phenomenon has been amply confirmed in experiments extended by McCarty, Phelps, and Pyenson (1966), Jayson and Dixon (1970a and 1972), and Levick (1983). In the shoulder, the humeral head consequently is situated firmly in the glenoid fossa regardless of whether the arm is at rest, lifting, or pulling. The femoral head is held firmly in the acetabulum by a capsule, ligaments, and the negative intrapressure and does not sublux during the swing-through phases of gait. At rest and in motion, the opposing surfaces of articular cartilage are in close proximity at all times as a result of this negative intra-articular pressure. In the normal state, the subatmospheric pressure, or vacuum, increases with activity, weight bearing, or muscle contraction.

This phenomenon is true for all synovial joints, but the functional importance of intra-articular pressure as a stabilizing force varies in relation to static stabilizing forces such as joint geometry and ligamentous restraints. In the shoulder, negative intra-articular pressure plays a critical role in stabilization (Norris & Okamura, 1996). Warner, Deng, Warren, & Torzilli (1992) produced major inferior humeral subluxation by venting the glenohumeral joint to the atmosphere with an 18-gauge needle.

The position of the joint can likewise affect joint pressure. In the presence of an effusion, the intra-articular pressure becomes positive. When an effusion is present in the knee, it is in its most comfortable position at about 30° flexion, the position spontaneously adapted by patients with effusions because it creates the lowest intra-articular pressure. Full joint flexion or extension in the presence of an effusion dramatically increases the intra-articular pressure to 500 to 1000 mmHg. The abnormal tissues of chronic synovitis are less compliant than normal tissue; consequently, inflamed joints in flexion or extension are at risk for rupture. In such instances, one

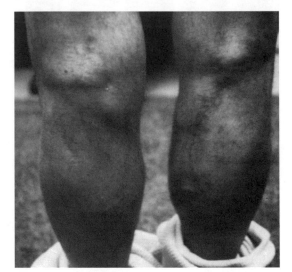

Figure 2. Posterior aspect of the knees of a patient with RA showing massive Baker's cysts that have herniated and dissected down into the calf. A Baker's cyst is a normal bursa for the semimembranosus tendon. When it becomes distended or ruptured, it may produce pseudothrombophlebitis, a syndrome with a positive Homan's sign, tenderness of the calf, and pitting edema of the subcutaneous tissues. This syndrome is frequently misdiagnosed as true thrombophlebitis, a condition rarely seen in RA. More often, the cyst enlarges and may dissect down the calf, sometimes as far down as the ankle, in a massive but unruptured cyst. Reprinted with permission from *Arthritis Care and Research.* Copyright 1988 by The American College of Rheumatology.

may see herniations through the capsule, rupture of the joint, progressive distention, or (in the knee) distention of the bursa for the semimembranosus tendon (a "Baker's cyst" in the popliteal fossa) (Figure 2). Such high pressures are the active forces in the pathogenesis of the geodes or subchondral cysts occurring in RA (Jayson & Dixon, 1970b). A rupture, although generally unusual, is more likely to occur in an acutely produced effusion than in the chronic effusions of RA.

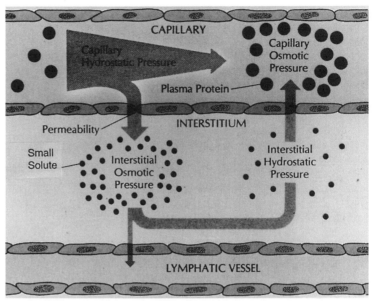

Figure 3. Hydrodynamics of arteriolar–capillary–venule circulation. The capillary hydrostatic pressure is about 25 mm Hg. As this falls, interstial fluid semotic pressure "pulls" fluid into the extravascular spaces. As the venular end of the capillary is reached, the capillary semotic pressure "pulls" fluid back into the capilary and post capillary venule. These vessels are soft and readily compressible. A positive pressure greater than 30 mm Hg compresses the capillaries, compromising delivery of oxygen and consequent hypoxia and anoxia in and around the joint. Reprinted with permission from *Arthritis Care and Research*. Copyright 1988 by the American College of Rheumatology.

Joint effusions can interfere with the blood flow to the joint tissues. According to Starling's Law, the hydrostatic pressure at the arteriolar end of the capillary is about 22 mmHg as it enters the capillary bed. The tissue or interstitial fluid pressure tends to pull fluid out of the capillary, and, at the venular end of the capillary, the colloid osmotic pressure tends to pull fluid into the circulation. Normally, the capillary hydrostatic pressure is about 25 mmHg. As this falls, interstitial fluid osmotic pressure "pulls" fluid into the extravascular spaces. As the venular end of the capillary is reached, the capillary osmotic pressure "pulls back" into the capillary and postcapillary venule. These vessels are soft and readily compressible. A positive pressure of greater than 30 mmHg compresses capillaries, which compromises delivery of oxygen and consequent hypoxia or anoxia in and around the joint. Even small effusions will raise the intra-articular pressure to more than 30 mmHg from its usual subatmospheric levels, which effectively compresses the small vessels and results in hypoxia and, with a large effusion, anoxia. Most large effusions result in hypoxic or anoxic joints (Figure 3). This phenomenon is underappreciated in clinical rheumatology. To apply external heat to such joints may increase the blood flow to a joint that may be getting all the blood it can handle and potentially accentuate and accelerate an already serious degree of hypoxia in all tissues of the joint (Bland, 1988).

A further important and interesting physiological phenomenon occurs when severe distraction of a joint (e.g., the finger) causes the baseline pressure to fall and reach a level at which dissolved gases (nitrogen) come out of solution, thus creating a gas bubble (the process of "knuckle-cracking"). This phenomenon is of more than passing interest (Figure 4). Unsworth, Doneson, and Wright (1971) showed experimentally that, until a force of 10 kg was brought to bear on distracting

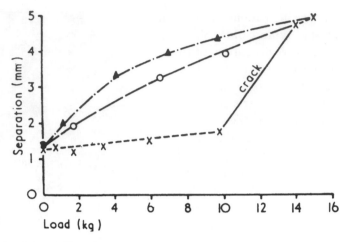

Figure 4. An experiment in knuckle cracking. The ordinate depicts separation of the two surfaces of the middle metacarpophalangeal joint in millimeters measured by X-ray; the abscissa depicts the load or pull on the joint in kilograms. Note the X curve, which shows that 10 kg of force is required before the knuckle cracks (nitrogen appears), and, at that load, the joint space abruptly separates until the bubble of gas appears in the joint and the pressure (negative before that point) becomes positive; ligaments and capsules take up the load. It is suggested that the normal negative pressure (strong vacuum) holds the joint together until the pressure is so negative that nitrogen comes out of solution as a gas and does not return to solution for 20 min. With release of the load, the joint surfaces gradually return to baseline. *Note.* From "Cracking Joints: A Bioengineering Study of Cavitation in the Metacarpophalangeal Joint," by A. Unsworth, D. Doneson, & V. Wright, 1971, *Annals of Rheumatic Disease, 30,* p. 348–358. Copyright 1971 by the BMJ Publishing Group. Reprinted with permission.

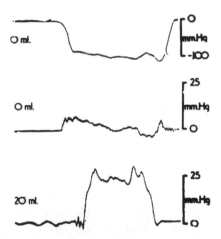

Figure 5. Upper panel: Depicts the intraarticular pressure of the normal human knee at rest with contraction of the quadriceps muscle–in other words, subatmospheric pressure. The muscle contraction results in a marked decrease in pressure to –100 mm Hg. Middle panel: 10 ml of normal saline has been injected and quadriceps muscle contraction caused a mild rise in positive pressure. Lower panel: 20 ml of normal saline has been injected and a rise in intraarticular pressure to 25 mm Hg occurs. This positive pressure will just compress arteriole–capillary–venule. Slightly higher pressure results in hypoxia–anoxia. *Note.* From "Intra-articular pressure in rheumatoid arthritis of the knee: Pressure changes during passive joint distension." by M.I.V. Jayson, & A. St. J. Dixon, 1970, *Annals of Rheumatic Disease,* 30, p. 348–358. Copyright 1970 by the BMJ Publishing Group. Reprinted with permission.

the joint, there was no separation of the surfaces and no "crack" or movement of nitrogen out of solution. At the point of nitrogen coming out of solution, however, the collateral ligaments suddenly take over the force holding the joint together (this force previously having been the subatmospheric pressure). A similar process occurs when an effusion eliminates negative pressure and increases the workload on the ligaments and capsule to hold the joint together (Figure 5). Similar phenomena are seen in intervertebral disks where the "vacuum sign" is well known to radiologists (Figure 6) and in divers who have the "bends."

Intra-Articular Relationships Among Intra-Articular Pressure pH, pO_2, pCO_2, Lactic Acid, and Glucose

With the development of the Clarke electrode in the early 1960s, the ability to measure partial pressures of oxygen (pO_2), carbon dioxide (pCO_2), pH, temperature, lactic acid, and glucose became possible. Treuhoft and McCarty (1971) and Falchuk, Goetzl, and Kulka (1970) independently studied these six parameters. A low synovial fluid pO_2 was found routinely in RA joint

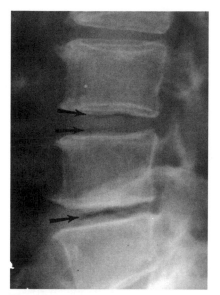

Figure 6. *Arrows* point to bubbles of nitrogen in lumbar intervertebral disc joints. Photo courtesy of John Bland, MD.

fluids, often below 30 mmHg and always accompanied by large decreases in pH and large increases in pCO_2. Simultaneously, concentrations of lactate increased, reflecting the extreme acidotic state of the usual rheumatoid synovial fluid. Much lesser magnitudes of these changes occur in the occasional extreme inflammation of OA. These changes prove that local tissue metabolism has changed from principally aerobic to principally anaerobic or glycolytic. These changes correlate with synovial cell proliferation, focal necrosis, and severe obliterative microangiopathy. Ropes and Bauer (1953) noted an inverse relationship between synovial fluid glucose and lactate levels. Glucose diffuses into cells, binds to phosphate (phosphorylation), and thus is prevented from moving out of the joint space until it is metabolized into pyruvate. Pyruvate is in turn converted into lactate that diffuses out of the cells into the tissue spaces and can be recycled. These data further confirm the grossly abnormal circulatory, pH, and gaseous changes that occur in the presence of joint effusions. The most important clinical implication is that joints with acute inflammation should not be excessively exercised because this would only increase the degree of acidosis, hypoxia, and hypercapnia.

Inflammation and Healing

During inflammation, even the most severe form, from any cause, there is always a parallel healing or tissue repair process actively engaged, even though it may be underappreciated. Although gross inflammation is present, plasma cells make enormous amounts of immunoglobulin (40 mg/day), and billions of lymphocytes die there each day. Macrophages phagocytose debris from inflammation. Angiogenesis, the formation of new capillaries, proceeds rapidly as messenger compounds are produced and thus stimulate capillary proliferation. Fibroblastic synthesis and proliferation is evident, which clearly indicates an actively developed healing process. The clinical goal is to stop the inflammation and allow the normal healing processes to dominate. Healing must occur by itself because drugs are merely ancillary to the natural healing process.

Effects of Movement on Inflammation: Immobilization Effects

Motion in an inflamed joint tends to accelerate the inflammation; rest or immobilization (generally partial) suppresses inflammation. Gault and Spyker (1968) performed studies on splinting in joints. By using a double-blind study, they placed a resting splint on one wrist of a patient with RA. By using the opposite wrist as a control, they carried out a sequential analysis until they reached a significant P value or suppression of inflammation. The splinted wrist showed progressively less inflammation, swelling, and tenderness. Bland and Eddy (1968) showed that patients who have sustained a cerebrovascular accident and subsequently develop OA or RA do not develop inflammatory arthritis on the side of the paralysis. In an experimental model of joint inflammation, McCarty and associates (1966) demonstrated that the degree of inflammation caused by urate crystals injected into dog knees was enhanced by a factor of 10 by simple passive motion of the joint. Some motion, of course, must be maintained to avoid atrophy and contractures, but, in general, during an acute inflammatory process, gentle active ROM exercises are all that is required.

Hyaline Cartilage

This remarkable tissue is avascular, aneural, and alymphatic and caps the ends of bones in joints. Cartilage is hypocellular, with only 5% of the volume occupied by the chondrocytes. Cartilage is 75% to 80% water by weight and is bound primarily in the highly aggregated hydrophilic proteoglycans. This water is vital to nutrition and permits entry of nutrient solutes and exit of waste materials between itself and synovial fluid. Some variation in the water binding occurs with increasing age, probably because of decreasing exercise (Venn, 1978).

Hyaline cartilage is like a water-filled sponge, but major force is required to squeeze water out. Thus, cartilage is a deformable, weeping bearing. DePuky (1935) showed that we are all 0.75 to 1.5 in. shorter at night than in the morning, reflecting the aggregate compression of all hyaline cartilage throughout all joints. During the day, we normally compress all our cartilages, in aggregate, by delivering waste materials to the joint space for pickup by synovial vessel plexuses. With night rest, the cartilage rehydrates by delivering soluble material to the chondrocyte for its metabolic processes (Linn & Sokoloff, 1978).

The surface of hyaline cartilage is almost frictionless, especially at high shear rates. The remarkable frictionless feature in a joint is 50 times less than the friction of ice on ice so that friction is almost, if not actually, nonexistent. Joint lubrication under high-load conditions is due to the film of fluid squeezed out of the cartilage interstitial fluid (weeping lubrication). Under low-load conditions, boundary lubrication from synovial fluid is most important. The matrix comprises a collagenous framework (fibrillary matrix) within which proteoglycan is entrapped. It is the hydrostatic pressure of water bound to proteoglycan, retained and restrained by the collagen meshwork, that gives cartilage its resilience and load-bearing properties.

Chondrocytes are amitotic (they reproduce by direct cell division) unless some pathological change occurs in their microenvironment. These cells conduct their own internal remodeling system and synthesize the collagen and proteoglycan of cartilage as well as the enzymes required for breakdown and turnover. Chondrocytes normally have the longest cell cycle in the body. Because chondrocytes are so few and far between, each cell is quite isolated. Some even say that chondrocytes are lonely. Materials reach and leave the chondrocyte neighborhood by a nutritional double-diffusion barrier—first from capillary to synovium, then from joint space into cartilage. Chondrocyte division proceeds until puberty, after which all mitosis ceases and no new cells appear.

Bursae

Bursae have been paid relatively little attention, although they can hypertrophy along with the other intra- and extra-articular tissues in OA. Bursae are closed sacs lined with synovial membrane, often found about and near joints. They facilitate the gliding of one musculoskeletal structure over another (e.g., skin or tendon over bone). Bywaters (1965) listed 156 known bursae in the body. Tendon sheaths are a specific variety of deep bursae.

Bursae appear early in intrauterine life, at the same time as joints. Motion, pressure, and friction play a major role in their development, as is true with joints. Bursae around joints may have communicating channels into the joint space (e.g., the iliopsoas bursa with the hip joint and the subacromial bursa with the shoulder). So-called "adventitious bursae" (newly developed) may occur at any time over pressure points or bony prominences such as a bunion (hallux valgus) or the exostoses and osteophytes of OA. This ability to produce synovial structures at any time and where needed is an expression of the pluripotentiality of connective tissue cells. In OA, existing normal bursae frequently enlarge, or new bursae develop about the deformed joint with its large osteophytes and altered biomechanics. Such bursae may be the source of symptoms requiring recognition and treatment.

Tendons and Ligaments

Tendons transmit muscle tension to the mobile body part. Tendons have enormous tensile strength, resistance to compression, flexibility, and near-perfect elasticity. These properties result from the highly organized longitudinal arrangement of the collagen structure, similar to that of ligaments and dense fascia. Tendons develop early in intrauterine life and first appear as a condensation of mesenchymal cells followed by collagen deposition. Development of cavitation between flexor tendons and their sheaths occurs by the second month of gestation. Tendons appear even in the absence of muscle, but, without muscle, the tendon rudiments atrophy quickly. Thus, muscle may not be necessary for differentiation, but it is necessary for sustained development. Motion is essential for the development of tendons and is even more important for maintenance of their structure and function.

An adult tendon is 50% to 70% water, but its dry weight is about 75% type 1 collagen with 2% elastin, which are both fibrous proteins imbedded in a proteoglycan or water matrix. Ligaments and capsules are similar to tendons and behave pathologically and metabolically the same. Ligaments are fibrous bands holding bones together. They are necessary to maintain the stability of joints and are required to control posture, but they do not transmit muscle action directly. Ligaments may be mainly collagenous (e.g., cruciate ligaments of the knee) or primarily elastic (e.g., ligamenta flava of the spine plus ligamentous muscles). They may be anatomically classified as intra-articular, extra-articular, or vertebral.

Physiological Consequences of Total Immobilization of a Joint: The Law of Wolff

As a medical student at the University of Berlin in the 1860s, Julius Wolff (1904) became intensely interested in bone and the changes that occur in altering the lines of physical stress. He evolved the Law of Wolff over 35 years. In its simplest form, the law states that bone will alter its size, shape, trabecular pattern, and subchondral, cortical, and trabecular bone according to the lines of physical stress (Wolff, 1904). This implies that the normal size and shape of bone is regulated by normal lines of stress. Unfortunately, Wolff applied the law only to bone, and he did not realize that it really applies to all connective tissues (e.g., ligaments, muscles, bones, joints, cartilage, even fascia).

All connective tissues are dependent on physical stresses for maintenance of their tissue homeostasis. Although physical therapists and occupational therapists may be defeated by flexion contractures and failure of the connective tissues to heal in RA and OA, too often rehabilitative therapy overlooks the normal physiological mechanisms of the connective tissues and physical stresses required to maintain healthy tissue. The recent research documenting the value of exercise

Table 1 Effects of Immobilization (Stress Deprivation) on Synovial Joint Structures

Synovial joint space
- Fibro-fatty tissue proliferation (pannus)

Cartilage
- Fibro-fatty and synovial pannus proliferation over cartilage surface
- Ulceration, pressure contact points, full thickness ulceration

Fibro-fatty and synovial pannus
- Maturation results in adhesions
- Tears at attachment sites: synovium, capsule, and cartilage
- Adhesions result in new planes of motion contrary to normal anatomical planes of motion
- Pannus increases enzymatic degradation (collagenases, proteoglycanases) of surrounding connective tissues

Ligaments
- Increased rate of collagen synthesis
- Loss of parallelism of collagen fibers
- Increasingly random pattern of deposition of collagen
- Marked osteoclastic resorption at the site of ligament–bone attachment
- Collagen fiber continuity is interrupted
- Retained attachment only to periosteum (8 weeks)

Table 2. Summary of Effects of Stress Deprivation and Exercise on Synovial Joints

Stress deprivation
- Increased rates of synthesis of collagen and proteoglycan; increased random deposition of collagen fibril and fiber; rapid, dramatic loss of tensile strength (8–12 weeks)
- Fibro-fatty tissue proliferation over cartilage surface with pannus formation, cartilage ulceration, tissue destruction, adhesion, and flexion contractures
- Osteoclastic destruction of entheses
- Recovery and healing are incomplete at 1 year

Exercise (for recovery)
- Slow increase in tensile strength and hypertrophy of tendons (at least 1 year); ligament change is less so
- Major energy input required for minimal change
- Tendon repair markedly improved by early passive motion, intrinsic repair, rapid increase in tensile strength, no adhesion

and fitness for persons with rheumatoid disease emphasized the importance of joint motion and function (Minor, 1998).

Akeson and colleagues (1984), in a superb review of joint immobilization, noted the protean and grossly destructive effects imposed on any connective tissue by total immobilization. Equally important is the gross disparity between the rapidity of onset and its protracted damage and painfully gradual recovery from the "stress deprivation" that immobilization causes. Table 1 lists, in order, the events that occur in and about joints with total immobilization, all of which are quite predictable. Table 2 summarizes these events and the very slow recovery. The clinical importance is that the damage occurs rapidly, and the repair is extremely slow and less predictable, which is a heavy price to pay.

Curiously, ligaments in and around a totally immobilized joint increase their fibroblastic production of collagen and proteoglycans. However, the tropocollagen synthesized on export to the extracellular space fails to aggregate in parallel array. Instead, the molecules aggregate wholly at random, which results in a disorganized tissue with bonding occurring equally at random. Such a tissue cannot manifest the high tensile strength required for ligamentous function. Figure 7 illustrates the normal parallel array of the anterior cruciate ligament of an exercising rabbit (*left panel*) and a cruciate ligament from the knee of a totally immobilized rabbit showing a random arrangement that lacks normal collagen parallel array (*right panel*).

If total immobilization is so grossly destructive, then it is reasonable to suspect that similar effects result from partial immobilization, a decrease in physical activity, a reluctance to maintain a level of fitness with increasing chronological age, and a general failure to appreciate the dependence on physical stresses for continued functional integrity of all connective tissue.

The principal protection for ordinary joint use is neuromuscular mechanisms, or proprioceptive receptors functioning normally. Hyaline cartilage, although a good absorber of impulsive forces, does not have enough tissue to matter. The bulbousness of the ends of bones allows some absorption, but the great majority of the force protecting joints is that of reflex response. When the reflex is slow or the time between a threatened fall as it relates to

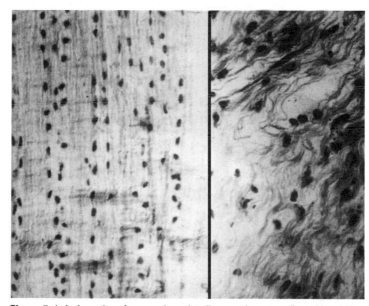

Figure 7. *Left*: A section of a normal cruciate ligament in a normally active rabbit that shows cell nuclei and collagen fibers in parallel array. *Right*: A cruciate ligament from a rabbit's knee immobilized for 10 weeks. Note the random distribution of collagen with loss of parallel array and hence marked changes in the physical properties of the ligament. Akeson, S.A., Woo, S.Y., Amiel, D., & Frank, C.B. (1984). The chemical basis of repair, the biology of ligaments. In C.Y. Hunter & F. J. Frank (Eds.), Rehabilitation of the injured knee (pp. 93–209). St. Louis, MO: Mosby.

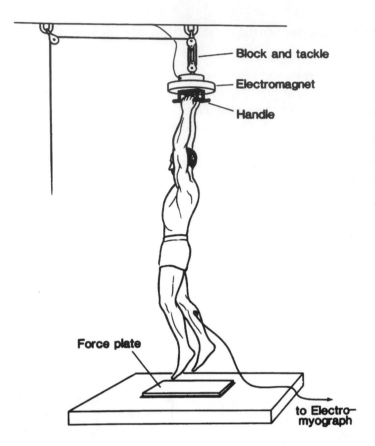

Block and tackle

Electromagnet

Handle

Force plate

to Electro-
myograph

Figure 8. An experiment by Jones and Watt (1971). The subject hangs on handles connected to an electromagnet; a force plate recording pounds per square inch is below him; an electromyograph is connected to his calf to record reflex contraction of the gastrocnemius-soleus muscle. The experiment was designed to study the "functional stretch reflex," a mechanism for landing from unexpected falls. The subject falls but does not know when he will be released. The force plate records the force and time of landing. The electromyogram records the time of muscle contraction, all coordinated. In landing from less than 9 to 13 cm, there was always a painful jolt (i.e., the muscle contracted after the subject hit the force plate, and the reflex failed to protect). Landing from falls 15 to 18 cm and higher were not associated with pain or injury (i.e., the reflex occurred before the subject hit the force plate, which compensated for the impulsive force of the fall). From Jones & Watt (1971)

the integrity of the reflex is too short, injury occurs. Have you ever descended the stairs at night in the dark, thought you were on the last step, and you were not? One can have serious injuries to healthy high tensile strength ligaments and even fractures to healthy bone if protective reflex mechanisms are absent or slow to occur. Figure 8 illustrates an experiment conducted by two physiologists, Jones and Watt (1971), at McGill University.

Conclusion

It is hoped that presentation of the physiological data on joints, muscles, bones, and cartilage related to exercise may favorably influence practice. Any approach to clinical practice should include considerations of temperature, hydrostatic pressure, pH, and partial pressures of oxygen, nitrogen, and carbon dioxide. A rationale has been provided for exercise staging, an approach that considers the presence and degree of joint inflammation in the design of exercise programs. Appropriate exercise prescription in the presence of joint inflammation must carefully balance the need for exercise to maintain connective tissue homeostasis while at the same time avoiding exercises that may undesirably increase intra-articular temperature, intra-articular pressure, and blood flow to already hypoxic joints. An exercise program that begins with gentle active ROM exercise in the acutely inflamed joint and then progresses slowly to isometric and then isotonic resistive exercises as inflammation subsides may strike the balance between too much and too little exercise. Patients must be taught concepts and principles of "good day" and "bad day" exercises so that they may adjust their home exercise programs as necessary.

The issue of physiological differences from one joint to another still must be answered. For example, why is the cervical spine affected in RA but not the thoracic and lumbar spine? Why does psoriatic arthritis affect one proximal interphalangeal joint and not another? Those of us involved in physical therapy, occupational therapy, rheumatology, and orthopedics continue to owe a major debt to Ropes and Bauer (1953), who were among the first to make physiological observations and to review extensively the work that had preceded their studies. Concepts that we still hold regarding how joints work physiologically were established initially by them. Subsequently, relatively few researchers have pursued questions of the physiology of joints and the connective tissue system. Hopefully, the increasing number of researchers will expand our knowledge in this area of science, and this chapter will raise renewed interest and enthusiasm in the organ physiology of joints and their pathophysiology.

References

Akeson, S. A., Woo, S. Y., Amiel, D., & Frank, C. B. (1984). The chemical basis of repair, the biology of ligaments. In C. Y. Hunter & F. J. Frank (Eds.), *Rehabilitation of the injured knee* (pp. 93–209). St. Louis, MO: Mosby.

Bland, J. H. (1988). Joint, muscle and cartilage physiology as related to exercise. *Arthritis Care and Research, 1*, 99–108.

Bland, J. H., & Eddy, W. M. (1968). Hemiplegia and rheumatoid hemiarthritis. *Arthritis and Rheumatism, 11*, 72–78.

Bywaters, F. G. L. (1965). The bursae of the body. *Annals of Rheumatic Disease, 24*, 215–218.

DePuky, P. (1935). The physiological oscillation of the length of the body. *Acta Orthopaedica Scandinavia, 6*, 338–347.

Falchuk, R. H., Goetzl, E. J., & Kulka, J. P. (1970). Respiratory gases of synovial fluids: An approach to synovial tissue circulatory-metabolic imbalance in rheumatoid arthritis. *American Journal of Medicine, 49*, 223–231.

Gault, S. J., & Spyker, J. M. (1968). Beneficial effects of immobilization of joints in rheumatoid and related arthridites: A splint study using sequential analysis. *Arthritis and Rheumatism, 12*, 34-39.

Guyton, A. C. (1963). A concept of negative interstitial pressure based on pressure in implanted perforated capsules. *Circulation Research, 12*, 399–411.

Harris, E. D., Jr., & McCroskery, P. A. (1974). The influence of temperature in fibril stability on degradation of cartilage collagen by rheumatoid synovial collagenase. *New England Journal of Medicine, 290*, 1–6.

Hollander, J. L., & Horvath, S. M. (1950). The influence of physical therapy procedures in the intra-articular temperature of normal and arthritic subjects. *American Journal of Medical Science, 218*, 543–548.

Hollander, J. L., Stoner, E. D., Brown, E. N., Jr. et. al (1951). Joint temperature measurement in the evaluation of anti-arthritic agents. *Journal of Clinical Investigation, 30*, 701–706.

Horvath, S. M., & Hollander, J. L. (1949). Intra-articular temperatures as a measure of joint reaction. *Journal of Clinical Investigation, 28*, 469–473.

Jayson, M. I. V., & Dixon, A. St. J. (1970a). Intra-articular pressure in rheumatoid arthritis of the knee: Pressure changes during passive joint distension. *Annals of Rheumatic Disease, 29*, 261–265.

Jayson, M. I. V., & Dixon, A. St.J. (1970b). Valvular mechanisms in justa-articular cysts. *Annals of Rheumatic Disease, 29*, 415–420.

Jayson, M. I. V., & Dixon, A. St.J. (1972). Unusual geodes (bone cysts) in rheumatoid arthritis. *Annals of Rheumatic Disease, 31*, 124–178.

Jones, M. G., & Watt, D. G. D. (1971). Muscular control of landings from unexpected falls in man. *Journal of Physiology, 219*, 729–737.

Levick, J. R. (1983a). Joint pressure-volume studies: Their importance, design and interpretation. *Journal of Rheumatology, 10*, 353–364.

Levick, J. R. (1983b). Synovial fluid dynamics: The regulation of volume and pressure. In Maraodas and Holborow (Eds.), *Studies in joint disease* (pp. 153–241). London: Pitman.

Linn, F. C., & Sokoloff, L. (1978). Movement and composition of interstitial fluid of cartilage. *Annals of Rheumatic Disease, 37*, 168–174.

McCarty, D. J., Phelps, P., & Pyenson, J. (1966). Crystal induced inflammation in canine joints: An experimental model of quantification of the host response. *Journal of Experimental Medicine, 124*, 99–114.

Minor, M. A. (1998). Exercise for health and fitness. In J. L. Melvin & G. Jensen (Eds.), *Rheumatologic rehabilitation series: Volume 1: Assessment and management* (pp. 351–368). Bethesda, MD: American Occupational Therapy Association.

Müller, W. (1929). Über den negativen luftdruc im Gelenkraum. *Deutsche Zeitschrift für Chirurgie, 218*, 395–401.

Norris, T. R., & Okamura, G. (1996). Anterior and multidirectional shoulder instability. In C. A. Peimer (Ed.), *Surgery of the hand and upper extremity* (pp. 276–277), New York: McGraw-Hill.

Ropes, M. W., & Bauer, W. (1953). *Synovial fluid changes in joint disease*. Boston: Harvard University Press.

Treuhoft, P. S., & McCarty, D. J. (1971). Synovial fluid pH, lactate, oxygen and carbon dioxide partial pressure in various joint diseases. *Arthritis and Rheumatism, 14*, 475–484.

Unsworth, A., Doneson, D., & Wright, V. (1971). Cracking joints: A bioengineering study of cavitation in the metacarpophalangeal joint. *Annals of Rheumatic Disease, 30*, 348–358.

Venn, M. F. (1978). Variation with age of human femoral head cartilage. *Annals of Rheumatic Disease, 37*, 168–174.

Viidik, A. (1968). A rheumatological model for incalcified parallel fibered collagenous tissue. *Journal of Biomechanics, 1*, 3–12.

Warner, J. J. P., Deng, X., Warren, F., & Torzilli, P. A. (1992). Static capsuloligamentous restraints to superior-inferior translation of the glenohumeral joint. *American Journal of Sports Medicine, 20*, 675.

Werner, F. W., Boardman, N. D., & Fu, F. (1996). Principles of musculoskeletal biomechanics: Shoulder. In C. A. Peimer (Ed.), *Surgery of the hand and upper extremity* (pp. 12–14). New York: McGraw-Hill.

Wolff, J. (1904). The law of bone remodeling (P. Macquet & R. Furlong, Trans.). Berlin: Springer-Verlag.

3

DRUG MANAGEMENT OF INFLAMMATION AND RELEVANCE TO REHABILITATION

Eric P. Gall, MD

The pharmacological therapy of rheumatic diseases has a profound influence on the outcome of rehabilitation. Beneficial effects may permit the occupational therapist and physical therapist to have greater success in fulfilling the goals of treatment. The patient with reduced pain, stiffness, and swelling of joints may be both more able and willing to comply with the therapist's prescribed regimen. On the other hand, adverse effects of drugs may interfere or make some procedures dangerous. For example, corticosteroid therapy may cause skin fragility and render splinting difficult at best, and the effects on bone (osteoporosis) can cause fracture with vigorous stretching. The therapist often is in a position to notice side effects of medication that the patient may not reveal to a physician. Communication by the physician and patient to the therapist is essential to know which drugs the patient is taking and what to expect. The therapist should notify the physician of any observation made regarding the effects of such drugs or noncompliance with the medical regimen.

Melvin (1989) stated that "Drug therapy, like painting a picture or rearing a child, is a creative process. There are basic rules that are essential to each activity, but no single method is recommended over all others". The therapist must learn the treatment philosophies of the referring physician and take these into consideration when evaluating and treating patients. Therapy may alter objective measurements of motion and function, and side effects from drugs may interfere with the beneficial effects of therapy.

A knowledge of the major classes of antirheumatic drugs, their properties, and side effects is essential for proper rehabilitation therapy (Ciccone, 1993). Several classes of drugs are discussed in this chapter. Their specific uses in individual diseases are discussed in chapters related to those particular illnesses. The classes of drugs to be discussed include

- nonsteroidal anti-inflammatory drugs (NSAIDs),
- corticosteroids (also anti-inflammatory),
- disease- (or symptom-) modifying anti-rheumatic drugs (DMARDs or SMARDs) (slow-acting or second-line agents),
- biological agents,

- analgesic agents,
- antigout drugs,
- chondroprotective agents, and
- antidepressants.

More than 100 rheumatologic diseases affect approximately 40 million people in the United States and literally hundreds of drugs are available to treat these illnesses. This chapter will discuss only the most commonly used drugs, although brief mention will be made of the author's opinion about the future directions of therapy. The reader is referred to basic textbooks on rheumatic diseases (Kelley, Harris, Ruddy, & Sledge, 1997; Klippel & Dieppe, 1998; Koopman, 1997), pharmacology (Hardman & Limbird, 1996; United States Pharmacopeial Convention, 1996), and rehabilitation (Ciccone, 1993) for in-depth discussions of these agents.

Models of Medication Management of Rheumatoid Arthritis

The preceding list of drugs alluded to two major classes of therapy, NSAIDs and DMARDs (or SMARDs) (Table 1). The concepts regarding the use of these groups of drugs are changing.

Rheumatoid arthritis (RA) is the prototype inflammatory arthritis, and virtually all medications used to treat it are used as primary therapy in the other rheumatic diseases as well. The traditional approach to the treatment of RA has been likened to a pyramid (Smyth, 1972) (Figure 1). The pyramid has been characterized by a firm foundation of diagnosis, rehabilitation therapy, and education coupled with primary therapy that uses NSAIDs to relieve symptoms. Only after these agents failed to relieve pain and the disease progressed (with erosive joint disease radiographically) would more potent DMARD therapy be added to the regimen. NSAIDs would continue to be used to concomitantly, and the least toxic DMARD would be used with serial switching to more potent (and toxic) therapies. In the early 1990s, some researchers criticized this approach as leading to ultimate failure by explaining that patients would eventually switch from one DMARD to

Table 1. Characteristics of Two Major Classes of Antirheumatic Drugs

NSAIDs	DMARDs (or SMARDs)
• Immediate pain and inflammation relief (1–2 days)	• Delayed onset of pain and inflammation relief (2–26 weeks)
• Direct effect on inflammatory response	• Indirect effect on inflammation through immunomodulation or suppression
• Analgesic and antipyretic (reduce fever)	• Nonanalgesic (except secondary) to reduced inflammation or antipyretic
• Little effect on systemic manifestations	• Major amelioration of systemic manifestations
• No radiographic effect on disease progression in RA	• Inhibits radiographic progression
• Primary side effects are gastrointestinal and renal	• Side effects are more complex
• Short-term effect on function	• Long-term effect on function
• Periodic monitoring required	• Frequent monitoring required (specialized knowledge)
• Straightforward pharmacological action	• Complex pharmacological action

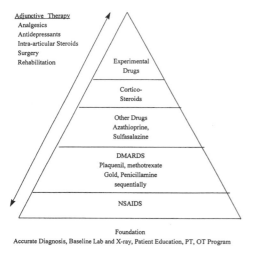

Figure 1. Pyramid approach to therapy for RA.

Early agressive use of DMARD's and combination therapy NSAID's and other Rx adjunctive

Figure 2. Inverted pyramid.

another while the disease progressed relentlessly (Cash & Klippel, 1994; McDuffie, 1990). This has led to the suggestion of "inverting the pyramid" (Katz, Gottlieb, Jaffe et al., 1987; Wilske & Healey, 1989) (Figure 2). In this algorithm, the early aggressive use of DMARD therapy, especially methotrexate, is advocated. Arguments both for and against inverting the pyramid are listed in Table 2. More aggressive treatment, which is still being evaluated, has become increasingly

Table 2. Arguments For and Against the Inverted Pyramid Approach to Treatment of RA

Arguments for this model:	Arguments against this model:
• An immunological trigger (probably within the first 2 years of disease) renders the disease irreversible.	• What is the risk-to-benefit-to-cost ratio of early aggressive therapy?
• Waiting until erosive changes appear on X-ray is too late.	• We cannot accurately predict patients with benign nondestructive disease. Should all patients be put on early DMARD therapy?
• NSAIDs do not prevent erosions.	
• NSAIDs cause toxicity, particularly gastropathy (not benign).	• Life-long (cumulative) toxicity of long-term use of DMARDs is not known; RA is usually a life-long disease.
• Serious toxicity of methotrexate and other DMARDs is overemphasized compared with NSAIDs.	
• Pyramid approach has not led to long-term remission in most patients; many discontinue one after another DMARD secondary to ineffectiveness.	• Cost of drugs and monitoring is high.
	• Compliance is poor when the patient feels well.
• Early use of DMARDs and combinations of drugs may avoid having to try multiple DMARDs.	• Not all patients need to be treated in the same way.
• RA is similar to localized malignancy in its pathological dysfunction; it requires an aggressive approach.	
• DMARDs relieve pain secondarily because of suppression of immune and inflammatory responses.	

popular with rheumatologists not only for RA but also for other inflammatory rheumatic diseases. In addition, combination therapy (using several drugs at the same time) is now common (Felson, Anderson, & Mernan, 1994).

Nonsteroidal Anti-inflammatory Drugs

NSAIDs provide both analgesia and moderate control of inflammation at recommended doses. The analgesic properties of these drugs are present at low doses (commonly seen in over-the-counter preparations of aspirin, ibuprofen, and naproxen), whereas higher doses involve the added suppression of the inflammatory response. NSAIDs have little effect on the progressive destruction caused by RA, even at high doses. Most of the agents work, in part, by blocking prostaglandin and other inflammatory mediators. However, inhibition of neutrophil activation occurs with all NSAIDs and may be equally or more important because it occurs even in NSAIDs that do not inhibit prostaglandins. Although the prostaglandin effect is beneficial, it leads to multiple side effects, particularly gastrointestinal distress and peptic ulcers, renal dys-

Table 3. NSAIDs

I. Carboxylic acids
  A. Salicylates
    1. Acetylated
      a. Aspirin (acetylsalicylic acid)
    2. Nonacetylated
      a. Choline salicylate (Arthropan)
      b. Diflunisal (Dolobid)
      c. Magnesium salicylate
      d. Salicylamide
      e. Salsalate (Disalcid)
      f. Sodium salicylate
      g. Trimagnesium salicylate (Trilisate)
  B. Propionic acids
    1. Ibuprofen (Motrin, others)
    2. Naproxen (Naprosyn)
    3. Naproxen sodium (Anaprox, Aleve)
    4. Flurbiprofen (ANSAID)
    5. Ketoprofen (Orudis, Oruvail)
    6. Oxaprozin (Daypro)
    7. Fenoprofen (Nalfon)
    8. Carprofen
    9. Fenbufen
    10. Suprofen
    11. Tiaprofenic acid
  C. Fenamic (Anthranilic) acids
    1. Meclofenamate sodium (Meclomen)
    2. Mefenamic acid (Ponstel)
    3. Flufenamic acid

  D. Acetic acids
    1. Phenylacetic acids
      a. Diclofenac (Voltaren, Cataflam)
      b. Alclofenac
      c. Fenclofenac
    2. Indolacetic acids
      a. Indomethacin (Indocin)
      b. Sulindac (Clinoril)
      c. Etodolac (Lodine)
    3. Pyrolacetic acids
      a. Tolmetin (Tolectin)
      b. Zomepirac
II. Enolic acid
  A. Pyrazolones
    1. Phenylbutazone (Butazolidin)
    2. Oxyphenylbutazone
  B. Oxicams
    1. Piroxicam (Feldene)
    2. Isoxicam
    3. Tenoxicam
    4. Sudoxicam
III. Nonacidic compounds
  A. Nabumetone (Relafen)
IV. COX-2 inhibitors
  A. Rofecoxib (Vioxx)
  B. Celecoxib (Celebrex)

function, and platelet inhibition (bleeding). There are two major classes of NSAIDs: salicylates and nonsalicylates.

The salicylates may be acetylated (e.g., aspirin) or nonacetylated (e.g., salsalate). The nonsalicylate NSAIDs fall into several major pharmacological clusters (Table 3). More importantly, the nonsalicylates may be either long or short acting (Table 4) or have a particular propensity to have certain side effects (Table 5). The shorter-acting agents have less prolonged effects, and thus toxicity may be less prolonged or less cumulative. On the other hand, short-acting drugs may need to be taken more often and involve more tablets per day, thus leading to decreased compliance. Longer-acting NSAIDs may accumulate in tissues and cause increased toxicity, particularly in the elderly patient who already manifests a decrease in cellular metabolism of drugs. Many long-acting agents, however, only need to be taken once a day, which is convenient.

NSAIDs reduce inflammation by blocking prostaglandin, inhibiting neutrophil activation, stabilizing lysosomal membranes, inhibiting kinins, and causing various other actions. The net results of these pharmacological events are reduced pain, swelling, warmth, and stiffness of joints. In a similar manner, some of the systemic symptoms of RA (e.g., low-grade fever, malaise, fatigue) are improved as well. This obviously makes the patient better suited to participate successfully in a rehabilitation program. With short-acting drugs, the timing of the dose may be critical for an exercise protocol or range of motion evaluation. Taking such an agent 30 min to 1 hr before planned exercise will result in maximal analgesic and anti-inflammatory activity in most cases. Aspirin levels may be measured in the blood to verify therapeutic versus toxic levels. This cannot be done with other NSAIDs.

The major adverse effects of NSAIDs, in addition to problems with overdosage, include gastrointestinal effects (e.g., dyspepsia, gastritis, peptic ulcer, and gastrointestinal bleeding). The patient may complain of heartburn, nausea, or abdominal pain. The vomiting of material resembling coffee grounds indicates bleeding in the stomach or occasionally the duodenum, as does the

Table 4. Long and Short Half-Life NSAIDs

Long Half-Life	**Short Half-Life**
Aspirin (high dose = ≥3,600 mg/day) (30 hr)	Aspirin (low dose = ≤2,400 mg/day) (30 min)
Diflunisal (5–20 hr)	Diclofenac (1–2 hr)
Indomethacin (sustained release)	Fenoprofen (2–3 hr)
Nabumetone (20–25 hr)	Ibuprofen (2 hr)
Naproxen (12–15 hr)	Indomethacin (1 hr)
Oxaprozin (20–25 hr)	Ketoprofen (2 hr)
Phenylbutazone (50–70 hr)	Meclofenamate (3 hr)
Piroxicam (38 hr)	Tolmetin (1–1.5 hr)
Salsalate (16 hr)	
Sulindac (17 hr)	
Etodolac (3.5–11 hr)	
Flurbiprofen (6 hr)	
Celecoxib (11 hr)	
Rofecoxib (17 hr)	

Table 5. Toxicity of Selected NSAIDs: Agents With Increased or Decreased Propensity Effects

Drugs	Marrow Suppression	Platelet Inhibition	Peptic Ulcer	Diarrhea	Liver	CNS	Salt Retention	Renal Toxicity	Asthma Allergy*
Aspirin	—	+++†	+++	—	+	++	—	+	+++
Nonacetylated Salicylates	—	±	±	—	+	+	—	±	±
Diclofenac	—	++	++	—	+	—	+	++	++
Diflunisal	—	+	+	—	±	+	—	+	++
Etodolac	—	++	++	—	±	—	+	++	++
Fenoprofen	—	++	+	—	±	++	—	++	++
Flurbiprofen	—	++	+	—	±	++	+	+	++
Ibuprofen	—	++	+	—	±	++	+	++	++
Indomethacin	—	++	++	+	±	++	++	++	++
Ketoprofen	—	++	+	—	±	—	+	+	++
Meclofenamate	—	++	++	++	±	+	—	++	++
Nabumetone	—	++	+	+	±	+	—	++	++
Naproxen	—	++	+	—	±	+	+	+	++
Oxaprozin	—	++	+	—	±	++	—	++	++
Phenylbutazone	+ (rare)	++	++	+	±	++	++	+	++
Piroxicam	—	++	+	—	±	+	+	+	++
Sulindac	—	++	+	+	±	—	+	++	++
Tolmetin	—	++	+	—	±	—	+	++	++

+ = yes; — = no; + = <1%; ++ = 1-30%; +++ = 3-9%; ++++ = ≤10%.

*Only in sensitive persons; †permanent.

passage of black tarry stools. These signs of bleeding are a medical emergency requiring immediate notification of and evaluation by a physician. Buffering of aspirin may lessen the symptoms but does not protect the gastrointestinal tract. Enteric coating gives partial protection to the stomach, although aspirin is secreted by the gastric mucosa after absorption. Not all patients with serious gastrointestinal toxicity are symptomatic; therefore, close attention to other effects of anemia secondary to blood loss (increased fatigue, shortness of breath) is important. All NSAIDs should be taken with solid food (not on an empty stomach). Antacids that block the H_2 receptor such as cimetidine (Tagamet), ranitidine (Zantac), and famotidine (Pepcid) may relieve symptoms. Misoprostol (Cytotec) will help prevent serious complications of NSAID-induced peptic ulcer disease (Felson et al., 1994). Infection with *Helicobacter pylori* may predispose the patient to peptic ulcer formation caused by NSAIDs (Silverstein, Graham, Sonior, & Wynn Davies, 1995). This may now be easily diagnosed if suspected and treated with antibiotics. NSAIDs and aspirin should not be taken together because side effects may be additive, and therapeutic effects may be reduced as a result of competitive binding. On the other hand, patients taking a single aspirin per day for cardiovascular disease should continue to do so despite NSAID therapy.

Platelet dysfunction caused by NSAIDs may cause ecchymosis bruising or excessive bleeding with accidental trauma sometimes resulting from activities of daily living (ADL), falling, or even prescribed exercise. Nonacetylated salicylates do not inhibit prostaglandin function. Therefore, this class of drugs (salsalate, sodium salicylate, choline salicylate, Trilisate, and others) is less likely to cause bruising, asthma, renal toxicity, sodium retention, and gastrointestinal side effects. These drugs often offer an effective alternative to patients who cannot tolerate aspirin or other NSAIDs.

Aspirin permanently inhibits prostaglandins on the platelet and renders them inactive. This potentially leads to bleeding for up to 7 to 10 days after discontinuation of the drug (until new circulating platelets appear from the marrow). With other NSAIDs, this side effect persists only as long as the drug circulates. Thus, aspirin should be discontinued 7 to 10 days before planned surgery, and other NSAIDs should be stopped 3 to 5 half-lives before the procedure.

Other NSAID side effects include central nervous system (CNS) effects (e.g., tinnitus, impaired hearing, dizziness, psychiatric changes). These side effects are related both to dose and to renal clearance of the drug, particularly in elderly persons. *Such observed side effects should be reported to the physician and are considered drug related, particularly with indomethacin, phenylbutazone, and high-dose aspirin.* Renal toxicity and failure may occur via many mechanisms with most NSAIDs. Patients may present with edema, cloudy sensorium, or muscular twitching and may eventually become comatose, have seizures, develop anuria, or die. Salt retention due to prostaglandin inhibition is not uncommon, particularly with indomethacin. Peripheral edema and shortness of breath due to heart failure may occur in susceptible patients. Hypertension may be caused or exacerbated by certain NSAIDs. Persons with hypertension should only take NSAIDs after their physician considers the risks versus the benefits. Nonacetylated salicylates minimize such side effects.

Some patients have allergic responses to aspirin and other NSAIDs. They may develop severe asthma, anaphylactic shock, or a skin rash. These reactions tend to occur with most or all of the agents. Such reactions usually occur in patients with adult-onset asthma and nasal polyps who require corticosteroid therapy. Drugs should be discontinued, and the physician should be notified.

CNS effects include confusion, lethargy, sleep disorder, and anxiety. Such effects are usually mild but rarely may be severe, particularly with high levels of salicylates with indomethacin and in elderly persons.

NSAIDs may adversely affect pregnancy and prolong labor. The drugs will often interact with other medications, which affects their bioavailability and pharmacology. When used with anticoagulants, NSAIDs may increase the potential for serious hemorrhage.

Thus, NSAIDs are beneficial in controlling pain and inflammation but do not modify the ultimate course of inflammatory arthritis. The therapist and the physician must monitor NSAIDs for both helpful and harmful effects. It is suggested that NSAIDs be placed on a problem list so that the clinician will remember to monitor their use. Often several NSAIDs must be tried (for 2–3 weeks at a time if tolerated) to find the best NSAID from the standpoint of effectiveness with the least side effects.

In osteoarthritis (OA), NSAIDs should be tried only after trying acetaminophen first. If acetaminophen is not effective, one should then try low-dose NSAIDs. Often the larger doses that are required for RA are not necessary for OA.

COX-2 Inhibitors

In early 1999, the marketing of new cyclooxygenase (COX)-2 selective inhibitors began. This is a remarkable story from the discovery of a concept to the marketing of an approved drug within 10 years. Briefly, COX is an enzyme that causes the activation of prostaglandins and thromboxanes, some of which are responsible for inflammation and pain in arthritis and related conditions. Two types of COX were identified. COX-1 is constitutive (appears in normal tissues) and appears to have the physiological functions of protecting gastric mucosa, allowing platelets to aggregate, and having positive effects on vascular tone in the kidney and brain. COX-2, on the other hand, appears in inflammatory sites and is responsible for many of the toxic byproducts in those areas. These "designer drugs" inhibit the "bad" COX-2 without affecting the "good" COX-1. Theoretically and in fact, these agents are much safer to the gastrointestinal tract and cause less (but do not entirely prevent) peptic ulcers and have no adverse effect on platelets predisposed to bleeding. Unfortunately, the drugs do not prevent allergic reactions or effects on kidney function and blood pressure. These drugs are appropriate for the patient who is at risk for ulcers and bleeding.

The agents recently approved include celecoxib (Celebrex) and rofecoxib (Vioxx). The former is approved for RA and OA and is given in a dose of 100 mg twice a day or 200 mg once or twice a day. Rofecoxib is approved for pain control and OA and is given in a dose of 12.5 or 25 mg once a day. The most common side effect is gastrointestinal upset, but the incidence of serious ulcer disease appears to be significantly reduced.

Corticosteroids

Adrenal corticosteroids are potent anti-inflammatory agents that probably do not affect the progression of disease (Hopkins & Morris, 1994), although there is recent controversial information

Table 6. Corticosteroid Side Effects

Glucose intolerance (diabetes)	Hirsutism	Joint pain
Susceptibility to infection	Osteoporosis	Withdrawal when stopped
• Bacterial	Acne	• Abdominal pain
• Viral (i.e., herpes zoster)	Menstrual irregularity,	• Syncope
• Fungal	amenorrhea	• Flare-up of underlying disease
Cataract formation	Avascular necrosis	• Vasculitis
Salt retention	(particularly the hip)	• Vomiting
• Hypertension	Skin fragility	• Hyponatremia
• Congestive heart failure	Hypokalemia	• Circulatory collapse,
• Edema	Pancreatitis	hypotension
Fragile skin	Peptic ulceration or poor healing	• Headaches
Subcutaneous bleeding	of ulcers	• Weakness
(ecchymosis, petechiae)	Increased appetite	• Fever
Psychiatric changes	Insomnia	• Fatigue
• Euphoria, mania	Masking of signs of infection	• Weight loss
• Depression	Leukocytosis	
Cushingoid features	Muscle weakness (myopathy)	

suggesting that they may in some way prevent joint destruction (Fries, Williams, Ramsey, & Bloch, 1988). Certainly their effect on short-term disease activity has led to a markedly decreased prevalence of fused joints and makes it possible to maintain joint range of motion. On the other hand, these drugs are a definite "double-edged sword" because multiple side effects are likely (Table 6). Corticosteroids may be administered orally, intramuscularly, or in intra-articular preparations injected directly into the joint. The therapist must be aware of their potential positive and negative effects.

The systemic (orally or intramuscularly) administration of corticosteroids for more than a few days will interfere with the hypothalamic-pituitary-adrenal axis and render the adrenal gland unable to respond to stress for up to a year after discontinuation of the drug. Patients on chronic corticosteroid therapy should wear an identification bracelet stating that they are at risk under stress from steroid withdrawal. Patients should be given written materials outlining the side effects as well as the risks of altering doses or discontinuing the medication abruptly.

Of the major side effects that most concern therapists, the following should be highlighted. Even low-dose steroids will, over time, cause loss of bone (osteoporosis), which renders an already relatively immobile patient susceptible to fracture from ADL or even vigorous therapeutic exercise. On the other hand, immobility exacerbates the process, and weight-bearing exercise is requisite. The patient may develop sudden increased joint pain that could signal avascular necrosis of bone (particularly in the hip), pathological fracture, or the onset of infection in the joint.

Corticosteroids cause patients to be susceptible to infection and may mask systemic symptoms such as fever. Chronic steroid used frequently causes capillary and skin fragility. The therapist must consider this when splinting or using aids for daily living. Changes in mood and affect (euphoria) are frequent in patients as are the symptoms of depression. Patients may have new or worsening complaints of heart failure and fatigue. Occasionally, with high doses, weakness caused by steroid myopathy may occur. Any recognition of such side effects should be reported to the referring physician. Alternate-day oral doses of steroids are given in an attempt to lessen glucocorticoid side effects. Although this may be partially successful, patients may have withdrawal symptoms and flare-ups of their arthritis on the day they do not take steroids. When patients are taken off steroids, during the weaning process, disease flare-ups frequently occur. Weaning must be a slow process. Symptoms of steroid withdrawal include hypotension, syncope, weakness, fever, joint pain, abdominal pain, and lethargy. Sudden withdrawal can cause circulatory collapse and death.

The intra-articular injection of a depot (long-acting) corticosteroid may benefit patients with inflammatory arthritis or OA. The advantages of such treatments are the relative lack of systemic absorption (and thus side effects) and the ability to handle localized problems. Too-frequent injections (more than two or three per year) may lead to the rapid deterioration of the joint because of increased catabolism (Kirwin & Arthritis Rheumatism Council, 1995). The patient should be cautioned not to overexercise a recently injected joint because of a false sense of well-being. This could lead to damage similar to that seen in neuropathic (Charcot) arthropathy. Occasionally, high doses of steroids are injected into the small joints of the hands under pressure to attempt a medical synovectomy. The hand is then splinted for 3 weeks with a resting splint. Although this may result in remission of the synovitis for 1 to 3 years, skin and subcutaneous atrophy may occur. Tendon rupture may be hastened by this procedure. Finally, injection into an infected joint could cause dramatic worsening of the infection. On the other hand, a joint or soft-tissue injection of steroids properly administered makes beginning an exercise program much easier. Therapists should discuss the proper timing for such injections with the physician.

Disease Modifying Anti-rheumatic Drugs

DMARDs are described in relation to their purported ability to favorably modify the course of RA (Table 7). They certainly are symptom-modifying antirheumatic drugs (SMARDs), but

Table 7. DMARDs

Antimalarial drugs	Cytotoxic agents
• Hydroxychloroquine (Plaquenil)	• Methotrexate (Rheumatrex)
• Chloroquine (Aralen)	• Azathioprine (Imuran)
• Quinacrine	• Cyclophosphamide (Cytoxan)*
Gold salts	• Chlorambucil*
• Oral	• Lefleunimide (Arava)
• Auranofin (Ridaura)	Other drugs
• Parenteral	• Sulfasalazine
• Gold thioglucose (Solganal)	• Cyclosporin A
• Gold thiomalate (Myochrysine)	• Biological and immunomodulator drugs
Penicillamine	• Etanercept (Enbrel)
• D-Pen	• Corticosteroids†
• Cuprimine	

*Not FDA approved; †probably not disease modifying.

whether they cause remission (remittive drugs) is controversial. Perhaps now that they are being used earlier, more aggressively, and in combination with other drugs, there may be a better chance of greatly altering the course of the disease. All DMARDs may be classified as slow-acting drugs in that their effects are not noted for weeks or months after the onset of treatment versus NSAIDs, which have an immediate analgesic and anti-inflammatory effect. All DMARDs alter the immune response, either by generally suppressing it (immunosuppressive) or specifically modifying some of its functions (immunomodulatory). The latter concept can be compared with a radio where one tunes in to a specific station (cell type or cell function) and modulates it (turn it higher or lower). Immunosuppressive agents are less specific and act by killing rapidly turning over cells. These agents suffer from the potential toxicity of injuring normal cells as well. Included in the DMARDs are a group of biological drugs that are under active investigation and will be briefly discussed in a separate section.

Antimalarial Drugs: Hydroxychloroquine (Plaquenil) and Chloroquine (Aralen)

Antimalarial drugs affect cell function, including immune activity and the inflammatory response. The mechanism of action has recently been much better understood. These drugs, although weaker in their effects than some of the other DMARDs, work relatively quickly (6–12 weeks) and are well tolerated. They appear to be effective in early RA and in mild to moderately active synovitis. These drugs are useful for the skin and joint manifestations of systemic lupus erythematosus (SLE) and in some of the spondylarthropathies such as psoriatic arthritis (although occasional exacerbation of the skin manifestations may take place). The drugs usually are used in combination with NSAIDs and often with other DMARDs.

Hydroxychloroquine (Plaquenil), the most commonly used antimalarial drug, is given in a dose of 200 mg once or twice a day. The most important side effect is eye toxicity, which may be manifested by blurred vision, decreased night and color (specifically red) vision, scotoma, or other visual effects. The side effects may be asymptomatic early on. Deposition of the drug in the melanin layer of the retina causes central visual field defects. Color perception, the loss of night vision, and the inability to see the color red are the earliest manifestations of the injury. This destructive effect is exacerbated by exposure to ultraviolet light. Chloroquine and hydroxychloroquine may both cause corneal deposits. These side effects may be lessened greatly by limiting the daily dose. Toxicity is more common with higher doses and is cumulative over time. Ophthalmological follow-up with special studies is necessary every 6 months, even at the onset of therapy. An Amsler grid examination, slit-lamp examination, and other ophthalmological tests are needed. The therapist should check to ensure that patients taking this drug receive this follow-up from an ophthalmologist.

Other side effects of the antimalarial drugs include bitter taste, gastrointestinal upset, skin pigmentation or depigmentation, bleaching of hair, and skin rash (e.g., lichen planus) and more rarely psychosis, hematological problems, cardiological problems, and loss of hearing. All of these effects are rare and usually are not severe. Quinacrine, an uncommonly used antimalarial tablet, can cause yellowish discoloration of the skin that is not related to liver dysfunction.

Immunosuppressive Agents

The anticancer drugs azathioprine (Imuran), methotrexate (Rheumatrex), and cyclophosphamide (Cytoxan) are used to treat many rheumatic diseases. Methotrexate is the most commonly used DMARD in RA, with azathioprine being used less frequently. Both are used in various other rheumatic diseases (e.g., SLE, vasculitis, polymyositis, and scleroderma). Alkylating agents such as cyclophosphamide are not used for ordinary arthritis but may be used for serious complications and various life-threatening manifestations of systemic collagen disease. All of these drugs are cytotoxic and cause cell death of rapidly turning over immunoactive cells. Their toxicity, for the most part, is related to effects on the normal cell population. Immunosuppressive agents may be classified into those present with all of the drugs and those specific to a particular drug (Table 8).

Bone marrow suppression leads to decreased white blood cell (propensity to infection), red blood cell (anemia), or platelet (bleeding) counts. These are usually dose related, and blood counts and symptoms related to decreased individual cell lines should be monitored every 4 to 8 weeks. Unusual bacterial, viral, and fungal infections (e.g., herpes zoster) may appear, and health care professionals should monitor this. Some patients tolerate the drugs poorly in their gastrointestinal tract, which can lead to nausea and vomiting. Pulmonary inflammatory or fibrotic changes are seen in up to 5% of the patients with methotrexate and more rarely with other immunosuppressive drugs. Symptoms may include a nonproductive cough or shortness of breath and should be differentiated from infection, primary lung disease, or congestive heart failure. Hepatic abnormalities are often seen with azathioprine; fibrosis and cirrhosis are feared but extremely uncommon reactions to methotrexate (<0.1%) (United States Pharmacopeial Convention, 1996). Liver function test abnormalities, however, are not uncommon and are monitored regularly to alert the physician to potential toxicity. Methotrexate and

Table 8. Toxicity of Cytotoxic Drugs

	Azathioprine	Chlorambucil	Cyclophosphamide	Methotrexate
Toxicity Shared by All Cytotoxic Agents				
Dose-Related Marrow Suppression	++	++	++	+
Susceptibility to Infection	+	++	++	+
Gastrointestinal Tolerance	++	+	+++	+
Fetal Abnormalities	++	++	++	++
Pulmonary Fibrosis	±	±	±	±
Toxicity Peculiar to Only Some Agents				
Liver				
Enzyme Elevation	+	0	0	++
Cirrhosis and Fibrosis	0	0	0	±
Oral Ulcers	+	±	±	++
Alopecia	0	+	+++	+
Amenorrhea	0	+	+++	+
Azospermia	0	+	+++	0
Cystitis and Hematuria	0	0	+++	0
Allergic Pneumonitis	0	0	0	++
Neoplasia	+	++	++	±

0 = does not occur; ± = slight or rare; + = mild or occasional; ++ = moderate or more common; +++ = severe or common.

azathioprine should not be given to patients who drink alcohol because this predisposes them to hepatotoxicity. Rarely, liver biopsies are required before and during the therapy.

Alopecia (hair loss) may be seen occasionally and may be distressing for the patient taking immunosuppressive agents. Bladder toxicity (bleeding and dysuria) is a side effect peculiar to cyclophosphamide that requires discontinuation of the drug, hydration, and further treatment. Episodes of cystitis caused by cyclophosphamide may predispose patients to bladder carcinoma later on. This side effect is caused by a metabolite, acrolein (Gall & Higby, 1992). Patients should drink large amounts of fluids when taking cyclophosphamide. In rare patients, malignancies may occur with the use of cytotoxic agents, most commonly with cyclophosphamide and less so with azathioprine (relative risk, ~13), and rarely with methotrexate (Clements, 1987). These drugs should not be given with other marrow-suppressive agents. Azathioprine doses must be reduced by approximately two thirds when used with xanthine oxidase inhibitors such as allopurinol; methotrexate should not be used with sulfa trimethoprim (a folate inhibitor). These drugs may be, and usually are, used with NSAIDs. One should be aware of the institution of new drugs in patients with long-term agents.

Methotrexate. This agent is perhaps the best DMARD now approved and available for the treatment of RA. It is used to treat many other rheumatic diseases as well. Methotrexate is a folic acid inhibitor and thus decreases DNA synthesis in the cell.

The drug is given in a single (oral or intramuscular) dose once a week. The patient must be cautioned not to take it daily, and side effects that may be related to the drug should be reported to the treating physician. The therapist should be particularly alert to notice whether the patient is drinking alcohol or using new drugs from another (nonprimary or rheumatic therapy–prescribing) physician. The patient should be aware of the signs of jaundice, edema, shortness of breath, severe nausea, and infection. A peculiar side effect of methotrexate that the therapist may notice is worsening of the rheumatoid nodules, including necrosis and draining material. The reason for this is not clear, but other agents can be used instead of methotrexate when this problem occurs. Pregnancy should be avoided in persons taking any of these cytotoxic agents because the potential for fetal abnormalities is great.

Methotrexate is given orally in doses between 5 and 25 mg once a week. Laboratory follow-up is required every 4 to 12 weeks (more often at the beginning of therapy), and the patient should be examined by his or her primary health care provider regularly. The drug is used to treat psoriatic arthritis, polymyositis, and occasionally other spondylarthropathies, scleroderma, SLE, and various other diseases.

Azathioprine. This drug is usually a second-line drug in RA or a steroid-sparing agent in SLE. It is used in some of the other rheumatic diseases as well. It is given in a dose of 1 to 2 mg/kg body weight/day orally. Toxicity should be regularly monitored by the primary care provider with blood tests performed every 4 to 12 weeks. These specific toxicities have been discussed previously.

Lefleunimide (Arava). This drug was released in 1998 as a new DMARD for treating RA. It is a cytotoxic drug that works by inhibiting pyrimidines. Early use suggests that it is as effective as methotrexate, and its main toxicity is liver function abnormalities. Monitoring is similar to methotrexate. The drug requires a dose loading of 100 mg a day for 3 days followed by a maintenance dose of 20 mg a day. It has a very long half-life, and its action may continue for several weeks after the patient has stopped taking the drug. Cholysteraind resin will hasten the drugs' removal in the case of overdose or toxicity.

Cyclophosphamide (Cytoxan). Cyclophosphamide is one of the most potent of the immunosuppressive drugs mentioned and is the most likely to cause side effects. It is used primarily to treat serious complications of systemic disease, such as necrotizing vasculitis, renal and CNS manifestations of SLE, and resistant progressive collagen diseases. Specialized knowledge is required to use this toxic drug. Long-term sequelae of treatment are not infrequent, and the risks must be carefully weighed against potential benefits.

Cyclophosphamide for rheumatic diseases is given either in oral daily doses of 1 to 2 mg/kg/day or in intermittent intravenous pulses of approximately 750 mg/m^2 every month. Careful monitoring for side effects is necessary, and the effects of marrow suppression, infection, hemorrhage cystitis, or other potential complications must be immediately reported and differentiated from the disease itself, which is a sometimes daunting task.

Gold Salts. This class of drugs, which was originally developed and tested for the treatment of tuberculosis (but was not found to be beneficial), is available in oral and parenteral preparations. During the original trials for treating tuberculosis, gold salts were found to be effective in treating RA. The oral agents are not as potent but have fewer serious side effects. Their use, however, is frequently associated with diarrhea, and rheumatologists often do not prescribe them because of this. In addition, their relative effectiveness is less than that of other agents. Parenteral gold was, for many years, the benchmark DMARD and was considered an effective treatment. The need for intramuscular injection and frequent physician visits (as well as the cost), notable toxicity (leading to discontinuation in up to 30% of patients), the slow onset of action (up to 6 months), and the perception of decreasing effectiveness over time has led to the decreased use of parenteral gold as initial DMARD therapy (Epstein, Hyhke, Yelin, & Katz, 1991). These drawbacks have not compared favorably with the effectiveness and ease of administration of methotrexate.

Parenteral gold still has an important, if limited, place in the treatment of RA. Two parenteral preparations are available, gold thiomalate (aqueous Myochrysine) and gold thioglucose (the oil-based emulsion Solganal). The latter has less toxicity, particularly less of a nitritoid reaction, which causes flushing and dizziness after injection.

Parenteral gold compounds are given by deep intramuscular injection, usually in the buttocks, every 1 to 4 weeks. These compounds are stored in tissues for many years, and both beneficial and toxic side effects may last for months or years. Consequently, close monitoring is needed. There is no correlation with the dose or serum levels to response or toxicity. The initial effects of the drug and ameliorating symptoms take 3 to 6 months before becoming evident. Double-blind studies have shown that gold inhibits the radiographic progression of disease (Sigler, Bluhm, & Duncan, 1974), although these results have been challenged by some authors (Epstein et al., 1991).

Almost one third of patients have side effects requiring discontinuation of the drugs. The most common side effect is a skin rash that may be localized or diffuse and either trivial or severe. Some rashes include a local fixed drug eruption, lichen planus, diffuse maculopapular rash, oral ulceration, or an exfoliative dermatitis that may be life threatening. Any rash should be reported to the physician. The presence of petechiae (tiny 1- to 2-mm hemorrhages in the skin) may indicate a low platelet count and should be immediately reported as well. Hematological complications are one of the most serious concerns. Thrombocytopenia may be sudden and fulminant and not predicted by blood analysis performed even a few days earlier. Thrombocytopenia is usually autoimmune in nature and may lead to bleeding anywhere in the body. Anemia, leukopenia, and thrombocytopenia (pancytopenia) are caused by cumulative direct marrow toxicity and may be slow in developing. Blood tests performed every 1 to 3 months should alert the physician early enough and prevent serious problems with this type of toxicity. Renal toxicity is insidious in its onset. Proteinuria or the presence of formed elements (red cells and casts) in the urine suggest glomerulonephritis and should lead to discontinuation of the drug or a reduction in dose.

Other side effects include a metallic taste, the nitritoid reaction (flushing) previously described, coughing, shortness of breath, diarrhea, and hepatitis. Prolonged gold injections may lead to deposits in the skin that causes a bluish discoloration in the skin that looks like cyanosis or even deposits in the eye that have a glittering appearance on slit-lamp examination.

Penicillamine (Cuprimine, D-Pen)

This is an immunoactive drug that has some anti-inflammatory effects. Penicillamine was used widely in the past but now has much more limited use. It may be particularly effective in patients with severe rheumatoid nodules or vasculitis. In the treatment of RA, penicillamine appears to be less effective than methotrexate and gold and may have more frequent and serious toxicity than either of them.

The most common side effects of penicillamine include loss of taste (dysgeusia), nausea, rash, glomerular nephritis, and marrow toxicity. Serious autoimmune reactions including SLE, Goodpasture's syndrome, myasthenia gravis, and bronchiolitis have been reported. About 10% of patients who are allergic to penicillin will exhibit a cross-allergy to this drug. Penicillamine is poorly absorbed with food and should be taken on an empty stomach. Its toxicity requires careful laboratory and monthly physician monitoring.

Combination Therapy

Patients frequently will take several drugs at a time for RA or SLE. This is similar to treatment for cancer. Chemotherapy drugs used together frequently have a synergistic beneficial effect while lowering the dose of each individual agent, which therefore decreases side effects. On the other hand, some drugs may have cross-reactions, and the literature or a pharmacist should be consulted for those unfamiliar with the pharmacology of the drugs. A patient with RA taking an NSAID, hydroxychloroquine, methotrexate, a low-dose tricyclic antidepressant, and some sort of birth control agent along with vitamins (folic acid) is common. One should be aware of the potential adverse reactions of all of these agents. The goal is to put the patient into remission.

Biological or Immunomodulating Drugs

Many new drugs for the treatment of RA and other immunomodulated diseases are in development. The concept of immunomodulation has been described earlier. Ultimately, the ability to treat rheumatic diseases by being able to target a particular immune abnormality specifically rather than suppressing the entire immune response seems to be a logical approach. In my opinion, diseases like RA are widely variable, and individual patients have specific malfunctions in their immune and inflammatory systems that are best addressed very specifically. Thus, if a particular cell type is overactive (e.g., a CD-4 lymphocyte T-helper cell), it may be suppressed by a monoclonal antibody specific to it. Receptors for cytokines (e.g., interleukin-1) may be blocked by a receptor antagonist. Drugs targeting specific function may be used in combination.

This concept of specific immunotherapy, although attractive, is far from practical at this time. Many biological and immunomodulatory drugs are being studied. Because biological antagonists and intensifiers may interfere with normal biological responses, their ultimate effect on humans is not yet known. Careful guidelines for effectiveness, safety, and long-range toxicity are being developed. The potential, as well as the risk, could be great, and the risk-to-benefit ratio must be defined. The future for this therapy is exciting.

A biological agent close to approval by the U.S. Food and Drug Administration for use in RA is cyclosporin A, a fungal extract. Cyclosporin has a specific effect on T lymphocytes by suppressing the immune response early to an antigenic stimulus (Diasio & LaBuglio, 1996). It is used widely to prevent rejection of tissue transplantation and has had promising results in the treatment of RA and other autoimmune diseases (Yocum et al., 1988).

Despite the drug's effectiveness and lack of cytotoxicity, it has other important toxic side effects, particularly in the kidneys. Kidney abnormalities may be irreversible. Hirsutism (excessive facial and body hair), hypertension, and nausea are not uncommon. Rarely, malignancies may complicate the use of any drug suppressing T lymphocyte function, and such malignancies have been reported with this agent.

Thus, the excitement of new effective treatment with biologically derived immunomodulator noncytotoxic drugs and well-understood effects on immune function must be balanced with the issues of long-term effectiveness, toxicity, and cost. The future has promise, but many barriers must be overcome.

Tumor Necrosis Factor Inhibitor (Etanercept [Enbrel])

Tumor necrosis factor (TNF) is an inflammatory cytokine secreted by macrophages and T lymphocytes responsible for helping regulate cell proliferation, apoptosis (programmed cell death), and the release of other proinflammatory cytokines. It is responsible in part for many of the symptoms experienced by patients suffering from inflammatory diseases (e.g., fatigue, fever, weight loss). Etanercept is the first true biological agent to be marketed for the treatment of RA. It is a designed soluble protein receptor fused to human IgG. The receptor binds two TNF molecules, thus preventing their interaction with TNF receptors on cells and thus blocking the biological activity of the TNF. The result is a potent antirheumatic activity within a few weeks of starting the drug.

Etanercept is administered by subcutaneous injection twice a week and is recommended for patients with severe RA who do not respond to traditional DMARDs. The therapist should be aware of the patient's need to self-inject the drug. The cost is considerable (approaching $1,000 a month). The potential for susceptibility to infection and potentially to malignancy is of concern because the drug blocks a normal biological response to these diseases. These concerns are potential long-term risks and are evaluated over time. Some patients experience a mild inflammation at the site of injection.

Analgesic Agents

Pure analgesic agents (not NSAIDs) such as acetaminophen, narcotic agents (e.g., codeine), and narcotic-like agents (tramadol) are used for arthritis. They have no effect on inflammation or disease progression in RA and only relieve pain. They are useful as adjunctive therapy for RA but are primary agents in the treatment of OA (see below).

Acetaminophen (e.g., Tylenol) may be used for analgesia or to relieve fever. It is useful in patients who cannot take NSAIDs because of peptic ulcer disease or other contraindications. The therapist should be aware that high doses of acetaminophen and its use with major alcohol ingestion can lead to severe liver toxicity and death. Renal toxicity, although uncommon, may occur because acetaminophen and phenacetin are related agents. Narcotics such as codeine and Tylenol 3 contain acetaminophen and can therefore result in the same toxicity.

The narcotic drugs, although occasionally needed for severe pain unresponsive to other therapy, should be used with some caution. The addictive potential of codeine and propoxyphene (Darvon) is low, and that of hydromorphone (Dilaudid) is high. The more addictive agents are more likely to cause tolerance (i.e., the decreasing effectiveness of a given amount of a drug over time that leads to the need for escalating doses) and thus the need for increasing doses to relieve pain. Their effectiveness varies, and patients are left addicted, at risk for side effects, and still in pain. Patients may become psychologically dependent on these drugs without physical addiction and may abuse them. The therapist should report such suspicions to the physician.

Constipation, fatigue, and mental depression are common symptoms that should be monitored with the use of narcotic agents. In persons who are ill or elderly, signs of respiratory system or CNS depression are important signs of impending serious toxicity.

Methadone is sometimes used because it causes less tolerance in patients requiring chronic narcotic use. Nonetheless, other narcotic side effects may be seen with this agent. Tramadol is a new narcotic-like agent that does not have as many of the reported serious narcotic side effects nor the potential for addiction. It has only recently had widespread clinical use. Addiction has not been seen, and constipation and mental depression are rare.

The ethical issue of chronic narcotic prescriptions in patients with chronic arthritic pain is debated and cannot be resolved in this chapter. The therapist should be aware of these issues and of the use and abuse of these drugs. Like cancer, arthritis can sometimes cause debilitating pain that is unresponsive to routine antirheumatic therapy. Health professionals should evaluate the narcotic's side effects (e.g., depression, anxiety, or the amplification of pain) and address these factors before recommending potentially addictive drugs.

Antigout Drugs

Gout and other crystalline diseases may involve both acute attacks of inflammatory arthritis and chronic destructive lesions (Gall, 1993). In the case of gout, the drugs used to treat the disease are

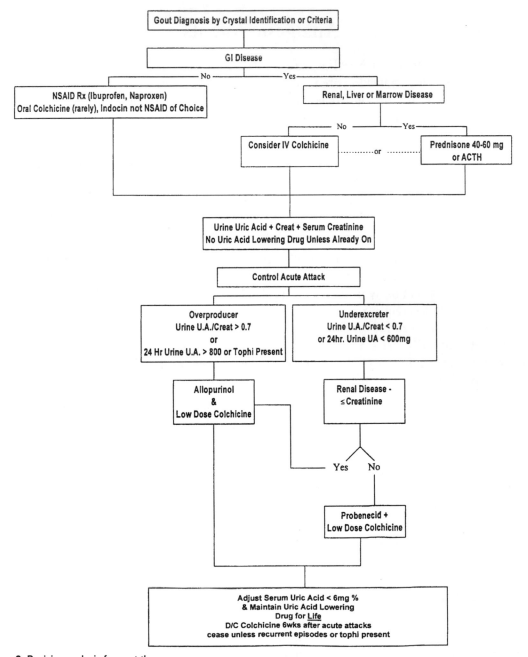

Figure 3. Decision analysis for gout therapy.

similarly classified into those required to treat the acute phase of the disease and those required to lower the circulating levels of uric acid to rid the body of the causative agent. Elevated uric acid levels ultimately cause both the acute and chronic aspects of the disease. An algorithm for the use of these drugs is depicted in Figure 3.

Colchicine

Colchicine functions by inhibiting the inflammatory action of neutrophils. It affects the microtubules, thereby decreasing the secretion of toxic substances from the cell.

The use of colchicine for treating an acute attack of gout has decreased markedly since the advent of modern NSAIDs. The reason for this is the narrow therapeutic-to-toxicity ratio. The drug is given hourly in 0.5- to 0.65-mg doses until the attack is relieved, toxicity occurs, or 10 tablets have been ingested. These endpoints usually occur simultaneously and cause the patient to have moderately severe gastrointestinal distress along with the relief of the acute arthritis. These side effects warn of imminent bone marrow suppression that will occur if the drug is given in excess or continued despite the symptoms. The intravenous use of the drug usually does not have such toxic gastrointestinal side effects and thus eliminates the warning sign for marrow suppression. Intravenous use of colchicine should be supervised by experienced professionals. Extravasation of the drug outside the vein may cause severe soft-tissue necrosis and slough.

NSAIDs are usually equally effective and far less toxic. The most common use of colchicine is in a prophylactic low dose to prevent acute attacks because the uric acid pool is being lowered. One tablet two or three times per day with food will greatly decrease the number and severity of these attacks in patients with gout. Mild to moderate diarrhea is seen in a few patients, even in patients taking low-dose colchicine.

Moderate doses of short-acting NSAIDs (e.g., 800 mg of ibuprofen three or four times a day with food) is preferred to treat the acute attack of arthritis if not contraindicated. Three to five days of treatment is required. Indomethacin and phenylbutazone should be avoided in most patients because of their increased toxicity versus that of other NSAIDs. In patients with a contraindication for NSAIDs (e.g., active peptic ulcer disease), corticosteroids and ACTH may be used for the treatment of an acute attack.

When an acute attack is being treated, a determination is made regarding the patient's renal function and urinary excretion of uric acid. If the patient has normal renal function without a history of urinary calculi, long-term treatment with a uricosuric agent (probenecid) is considered. In patients with high levels of uric acid (>800mg/24 hr), renal compromise, or tophaceous gout, allopurinol (Zyloprim) is given. Both allopurinol and probenecid are titrated to lower the uric acid level to <6.0 mg % (Yocum et al., 1988).

Probenecid

Probenecid lowers uric acid by blocking its reabsorption in the renal tubule. It inhibits the tubular secretion of penicillin and cephelasporin drugs and raises their serum levels. Occasionally (5%), patients will have nausea or a rash. The major side effect at the onset of therapy includes the formation of urinary stones due to the excretion of large amounts of uric acid. This effect may be avoided by hydrating the patient and further avoided, if necessary, by alkalinizing the urine.

Allopurinol

Allopurinol, as previously mentioned, decreases the formation of uric acid. It would be the ideal agent for decreasing uric acid in all patients were it not for allergic reactions, which include rashes in 5% to 10% of patients and a more severe vasculitis.

There is a serious drug interaction of allopurinol with the purine inhibitors 6-mercapto-purine or azathioprine. If the dose of these agents is not reduced by 66% to 75%, fatal marrow suppression may occur when used along with allopurinol.

Once the decision has been made to treat the patient with a drug that lowers uric acid, the patient usually requires life-long therapy and should be counseled by health delivery professionals to take prescribed drugs even though he or she is without symptoms.

Chondroprotective Drugs

In the future, the availability of drugs to protect cartilage from further destruction in OA looks promising. Agents such as antibiotics, cartilage extracts, hyaluronic acid derivatives, and other biological agents are being tested for this possibility. Their purpose is to reduce the enzymatic degradation of cartilage and to promote new cartilage growth and repair of defects. Some of these agents are believed to provide pain relief.

Antidepressants and Muscle Relaxants

Many patients with chronic and painful rheumatic diseases take antidepressants. Patients with fibromyalgia syndrome (FMS) are often given low-dose tricyclic antidepressant drugs. These drugs alter sleep patterns that are known to be deranged and perhaps are causative of FMS (Klippel & Dieppe, 1998). Depression in the chronic rheumatic diseases is both situational and may be an organic consequence of the disease (Bressler, 1992). Treatment of depression may improve function and the patient's ability to cooperate with therapy. Treating depression favorably alters the perception of pain (Bressler, 1992). Drugs (including steroids, NSAIDs, and others) can cause depression. Tricyclic antidepressant drugs are usually used in a single bedtime dose of 10 to 150 mg in such cases. The drugs include nortriptyline, desipramine, amitriptyline, doxepin, and imipramine.

Side effects are most common at the onset of therapy. They include blurred vision, urinary hesitancy, memory problems, tachycardia (rapid heartbeat), tremor, sweating, insomnia, dry mouth, and worsening of glaucoma. In most patients, these side effects will disappear after 3 to 4 weeks of therapy. In some cases, they are intolerable or even severe, and the dose must be lowered or the drug discontinued. On the other hand, when effective, patients often sleep better, awake refreshed, and have a better outlook on their disease. Pain tolerance is improved, and patients are more cooperative with therapy.

Newer agents include trazodone (Desyrel), fluoxetine (Prozac), sertraline (Zoloft), paroxetine (Paxil), and bupropion (Wellbutrin). These agents, although effective, can occasionally have idiosyncratic reactions with increased anxiety and rarely may result in suicide attempts. The patients should be followed from the standpoint of drug side effects, the effects on their disease, and their psychological well-being.

The use of muscle relaxants is controversial in painful spine disorders. Many of them have antihistamine-like side effects, including lethargy, nervousness, dry mouth, and occasionally anxiety. Diazepam (Valium) must be given in such high doses to relax muscle that it may cause somnolence and even severe respiratory and cardiac depression. Muscle relaxants are seldom recommended.

Conclusion

The drugs available for the treatment of arthritis and related diseases are many. Their pharmacology and toxicity is complicated and variable. It behooves physical and occupational therapists and other health professionals to be familiar with the proper and improper use of such drugs. The potential effects and toxicity of the drugs are important to the everyday delivery of care for patients with rheumatic diseases. Often the therapist will be the first to determine noncompliance, the lack of proper monitoring, abuse, toxicity, or drug interactions and is in a good position both to advise the patient and to communicate with the treating physician.

References

Bressler, R. (1992). Depression. In R. Bressler & M. D. Katz (Eds.), *Geriatric pharmacology* (pp. 274–329). New York: McGraw-Hill.

Cash, J. M., & Klippel, J. H. (1994). Second line drug therapy in rheumatoid arthritis. *New England Journal of Medicine, 330,* 1368–1375.

Ciccone, C. D. (1993). Pharmacologic management of rheumatoid and osteoarthritis. In *Pharmacology in rehabilitation* (2nd ed., pp. 213–231). Philadelphia: F. A. Davis.

Clements, P. J. (1987). Cytotoxic immunosuppressive drugs. In H. E. Paulus, D. E. Furst, & S. H. Dromgoole (Eds.), *Drugs for rheumatic disease* (pp. 135–156). New York: Churchill Livingstone.

Diasio, R. B., & LaBuglio, A. F. (1996). Immunomodulators: Immunosuppressive agents and immunostimulants. In J. B. Hardman & L. E. Limbird (Eds.), *Pharmacologic basis of therapeutics* (9th ed., pp. 1291–1308). New York: McGraw-Hill.

Epstein, W., Hyhke, C. J., Yelin, E. H., & Katz, P. P. (1991). Effect of parenterally administered gold therapy on the course of rheumatoid arthritis. *Annals of Internal Medicine, 114,* 437–444.

Felson, D. T., Anderson, J. J., & Meenan, R. F. (1994). The efficacy and toxicity of combination therapy in rheumatoid arthritis. *Arthritis and Rheumatism, 37,* 1487–1491.

Fries, J. F., Williams, C. A., Ramsey, P. R., & Bloch, D. A. (1988). The relative toxicity of disease modifying anti-rheumatic drugs. *Arthritis and Rheumatism, 36,* 297–306.

Gall, E. P. (1993). Hyperuricemia and gout. In H. Greene, W. P. Johnson, & M. J. Maricic (Eds.), *Decision making in internal medicine* (pp. 414–415). St. Louis: Mosby.

Gall, E. P., & Higby, M. (1992). Pharmacologic treatment of rheumatic diseases in the elderly. In M. Katz & R. Bressler (Eds.), *Clinical pharmacology and geriatric therapy* (pp. 467–506). New York: McGraw-Hill.

Hardman, J. G., & Limbird, L. E. (1996). *Goodman and Gilman's the pharmacological bases of therapeutics* (9th ed.). New York: McGraw-Hill.

Hopkins, R. J., & Morris, J. G., Jr. (1994). Helicobacter pylori: The missing link in perspective. *American Journal of Medicine, 97*, 265–277.

Katz, W. A., Gottlieb, N. L., Jaffe, I., et al. (1987). Criteria for initiating disease therapy in rheumatoid arthritis. *Archives of Rheumatology 30*, 561.

Kelley, W. N., Harris, E. D., Jr., Ruddy, S., & Sledge, C. B. (Eds.). (1997). *Textbook of rheumatology* (5th ed.). Philadelphia: Saunders.

Kirwin, J. R., & Arthritis Rheumatism Council. (1995). The effects of glucocorticoids on joint destruction in rheumatoid arthritis. *New England Journal of Medicine, 333*, 142–146.

Klippel, J. H., & Dieppe, P. A. (1998). *Rheumatology* (2nd ed.). St. Louis: Mosby.

Koopman, W. J. (1993). *Arthritis and allied conditions* (13th ed.). Philadelphia: Williams & Wilkins.

McDuffie, F. C. (1990). Conference on therapeutic approaches to rheumatoid arthritis: Challenging the pyramid. *Journal of Rheumatology, 17*(Suppl. 25), 1–44.

Melvin, J. L. (1989). Drug therapy. In J. L. Melvin (Ed.), *Rheumatic disease in the adult and child: Occupational therapy and rehabilitation* (3rd ed., pp. 31–45). Philadelphia: F. A. Davis.

Sigler, J. W., Bluhm, G. B., & Duncan, H. (1974). Gold salts in the treatment of rheumatoid arthritis: A double blind study. *Annals of Internal Medicine, 80*, 21–26.

Silverstein, F. E., Graham, D. Y., Sonior, J. R., & Wynn Davies, H. (1995). Misoprostol reduces the serious gastrointestinal complications in patients with rheumatoid arthritis. *Annals of Internal Medicine, 123*, 241–249.

Smyth, C. J. (1972). Therapy of rheumatoid arthritis: A pyramidal plan. *Postgraduate Medicine, 51*, 31–29.

United States Pharmacopeial Convention. (1996). *Drug information for the health care professional* (Vol. 1, 16th ed.). Rockville, MD: Author.

Wilske, K. R., & Healey, L. A. (1989). Remodeling the pyramid: A concept whose time has come. *Journal of Rheumatology, 16*, 56–57.

Yocum, D. E., Klippel, J. H., Wilder, R. L., Gerber, N. L., Austin, H. A., Wahl, S. M., Lesko, L., Minor, J. R., Preuss, H. G. & Yarbora, C., et. al. (1988). Cyclosporine A in treatment of severe refractory rheumatoid arthritis: A randomized study. *Annals of Internal Medicine, 109*, 863–869.

4

DIAGNOSTIC IMAGING IN THE EVALUATION AND MANAGEMENT OF ARTICULAR DISEASE

Thomas J. Learch, MD, OTR

Diagnostic imaging plays an integral role in the diagnosis and follow-up of patients with articular disorders. Disease processes can be evaluated in early stages, and their progression or remission and response to therapeutic interventions can be systematically followed. The extent and severity of disease can be objectively evaluated. Patients with unclear and confusing presentations may show specific imaging findings that allow for more accurate and timely diagnosis. During the last two decades, advances in imaging technology have been dramatic and offer new insights into diagnosis and progression of various diseases.

For the therapist, diagnostic imaging offers insight into the severity of joint disease, degree of joint destruction, and presence of ankylosis. It aids in determining the degree and type of deformity or subluxation. Imaging helps identify causes of pain so that appropriate intervention can be prescribed.

This chapter will discuss the common arthropathies affecting adults. For purposes of description and clarity, the diseases will be subgrouped into degenerative (osteoarthritis [OA] and diffuse idiopathic skeletal hyperostosis [DISH]), inflammatory (rheumatoid arthritis [RA], ankylosing spondylitis, and psoriatic arthritis), crystal-induced (gout and calcium pyrophosphate dihydrate crystal [CPPD] deposition disease), and collagen-vascular (scleroderma, systemic lupus erythematosus [SLE], dermatomyositis, and polymyositis) disease categories. (There is a glossary of radiographic terms at the end of the chapter.)

Many imaging modalities have been developed to examine various articular pathologies. The most commonly used modalities today are conventional radiography (X-rays or plain films), computed tomography (CT), diagnostic ultrasound, and magnetic resonance imaging (MRI).

Conventional radiographs have long been the mainstay of imaging. They are inexpensive, easily performed, and readily available. Therefore, imaging of articular disorders should start with this modality. Well-performed, high-quality radiographs show osseous and soft-tissue changes that document the severity and extent of disease. They often are sufficient, and no further imaging may be required. Follow-up films allow for evaluation of disease progression or remission.

Advanced imaging modalities such as CT and MRI offer cross-sectional images with improved resolution of anatomical structures, but these tests are much more expensive than plain films. CT, like conventional radiography, uses ionizing radiation. It is especially useful in evaluation of bony details such as fractures or erosions. Multiple images are obtained sequentially in an axial plane. Distal limb structures can be positioned in the scanner to obtain images in other planes. By using computer software, these images can be manipulated to emphasize osseous or soft-tissue detail. Additionally, advanced software can reformat images in other planes (e.g., coronal or sagittal), although these images are less detailed than the images obtained in the original scan plane. Three-dimensional reconstruction of image data is possible, but not all CT scanners have this capability.

MRI is a relatively new modality that uses magnetic forces to obtain diagnostic images. It has been increasingly used for articular disorders (Bollow et al., 1995; Roca, Bermreuter, & Alarcon, 1993; Winalski, Palmer, Rosenthal, & Weissman, 1996). MRI images can be obtained in all planes, and they show precise anatomical detail. They are especially useful in imaging soft-tissue structures such as muscles, tendons, and ligaments. For this reason, MRI has been used in the evaluation of the shoulder rotator cuff and knee menisci. These areas were previously evaluated with arthrography, an invasive procedure that requires intra-articular needle injection of a contrast agent, followed by plain films. MRI accurately evaluates bone marrow; however, cortical bone is less well visualized. Cortical bone is viewed with better detail on CT images.

Diagnostic ultrasound has been increasingly used in musculoskeletal imaging and is gaining wide acceptance (Lund, Nisbet, Valencia, & Roth, 1996). A transducer applied to the skin with a coupling gel sends and receives sound waves to form an image without the use of radiation. These sound waves travel through soft tissues at various speeds but are essentially blocked by bone. This makes ultrasound useful in evaluation of periarticular soft tissues, but it is limited in imaging osseous structures. This modality has been increasingly used to evaluate rotator cuff musculature and tendons. It is especially helpful in viewing cystic structures such as Baker's or popliteal cysts of the knee or synovial cysts in RA.

Because conventional radiography is the most common examination, this chapter will emphasize its use and findings. Radiographic film is placed into a holder called a "cassette" that contains an intensifying screen designed to obtain maximum image resolution of structures with the least amount of radiation. Standard views are obtained, and this allows for easier comparison with previous studies. All films should be appropriately labeled with the patient's name, identification number, date, time, and left and right markers. Films are viewed as if the patient were facing the viewer (i.e., the right side of the patient is on the viewer's left).

The area to be radiographed is positioned under the X-ray beam. The appropriate area and parameters of exposure are determined by the technologist to minimize radiation exposure yet still provide a quality image. The remainder of the body is protected by decreasing the area of exposure or by the use of lead aprons or shields. The X-ray beam is comparable to a small light source. Film views are named after the direction of the beam. If the beam source is anterior to the body part, the film cassette is placed posteriorly. This is called an A-P (anterior to posterior) film. When filming hands, they are placed palm down on the film holder, and the X-ray beam traverses from posterior to anterior (P-A). Generally, two views are obtained, usually an A-P view and a lateral view. Modifications for specific areas and joints are frequently made.

In the hand, P-A and Norgaard (ball catcher's) views are generally obtained. The Norgaard view is a 45° oblique view with the hands positioned as if they are holding a basketball underhand. It allows for early detection of bone erosions in the early stages of RA (Figure 1). Additionally, in this view, the hands are not rigidly positioned against the film cassette. Subluxations and other alignment changes, which may be reduced when the hands are placed flat on a film cassette for the P-A view, are better seen. Hand films are particularly useful in differentiating the various arthropathies and may be the most important set of radiographs obtained.

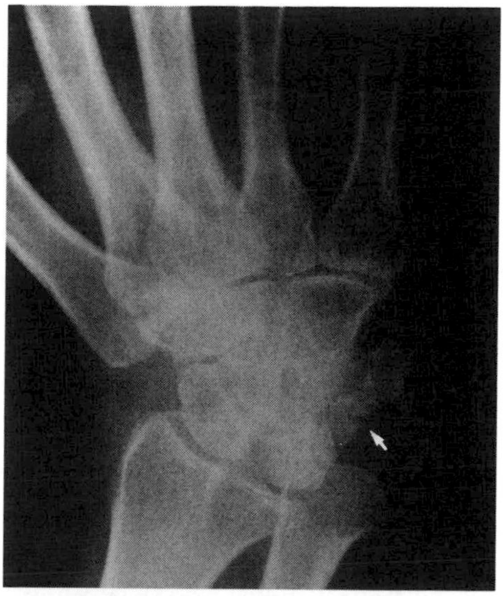

Shoulder films are obtained in an A-P internal and external rotation. These two views adequately show osseous changes and allow for localization of tendon calcifications.

Figure 1. Norgaard radiograph of a hand in a patient with RA showing early erosive change (*arrow*) of the triquetrum.

Knee films are best obtained in an A-P standing position to more accurately view articular cartilage loss. Lateral films are obtained in a nonstanding semiflexed position to view optimally the patellofemoral joint and the suprapatellar bursa for fluid.

Hip joints are best evaluated with an A-P film of the entire pelvis and a "frog-leg" lateral view of the individual hip. The A-P pelvis radiograph is obtained with the hips in internal rotation to elongate the femoral neck. By imaging the entire pelvis, both sacroiliac joints can be evaluated.

In the cervical spine, the lateral flexed view is most important. With this radiograph, alignment is scrutinized, specifically the odontoid and its relationship to the anterior arch of the first cervical vertebra. Excess laxity of the transverse ligament allows abnormal motion and subluxation to occur in this area. This can be seen in posttraumatic conditions, Down's syndrome, and inflammatory arthropathies, and it is especially common in RA.

When viewing plain films, an orderly approach is used so that all areas are examined. Forrester and Brown (1987) suggested using the mnemonic "the ABC's of arthritis."

- A for *alignment*
- B for *bony mineralization*
- C for *cartilage and joint space*
- S for *soft tissues*

This can be expanded to the "ABCD's" with D for *distribution*.

Alignment changes are examined in all radiographs. Their evaluation and description are similar to the occupational therapy and physical therapy evaluation. Additionally, multiple orthopedic and radiographic lines, angles, and measurements have been developed to evaluate posture and deformities. Alignment is particularly important in the evaluation of the wrist and hand, especially in RA.

Bony mineralization refers to the amount of calcium and phosphate present. *Osteoporosis* is the term used when mineralization is decreased. Bony mineralization is usually normal in all arthropathies except RA. Diffuse osteoporosis is commonly seen in the aging process and with RA. It can be seen as a side effect of certain medications such as steroids that are frequently used to treat many arthropathies. Disuse and immobilization likewise lead to osteoporosis. Radiographs underestimate early osteoporosis but are valuable for advanced osteoporosis. Osteoporosis is usually a subjective finding on radiographs and may appear to vary due to technical factors of film exposure. Objective criteria have been described in hand films, where the sum of the widths of the cortices of a metacarpal shaft normally equal the width of the adjacent medullary space (Brower, 1984). In diffuse osteoporosis, the cortices thin, and the ratio is altered (Figure 2). Periarticular demineralization is subjectively evaluated by a decrease in radiographic density in the osseous structures surrounding a joint space. This is a nonspecific finding seen in many disease entities and serves only to confirm pathology.

Cartilage and joint space have the same radiographic density as soft tissues and are therefore not directly visualized on plain films. Normal diarthrodial joints (Drawing 1A) have a uniform covering of cartilage at their articular ends that correlates to the space seen on X-rays between the articular surfaces of adjacent bones. The term *joint space narrowing* is used to describe cartilage thinning. This is a nonspecific finding seen in inflammatory, degenerative, and crystal-induced arthropathies. (Drawing 1B)

Distribution of pathology is an important observation because various arthropathies have characteristic areas of occurrence that are well known to practitioners.

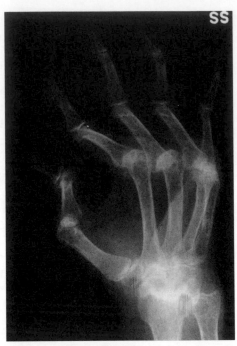

Figure 2. P-A radiograph of the hand of a patient with RA showing thinned cortices of the metacarpal shaft consistent with osteopenia. The second through fifth digits demonstrate typical swan-neck deformities, and the first digit demonstrates a Z or type 1 deformity. The MCP joints are subluxed volarly.

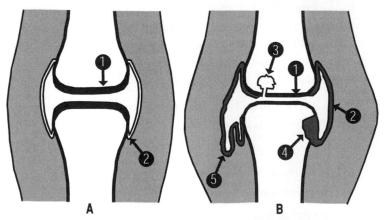

Drawing 1. (A) Normal diarthrodial joint. Normal articular cartilage (1). Note how this thins at peripheral margins, where the normal synovium (2) attaches. This is called the bare area. **(B)** Inflammatory changes in rheumatoid arthritis joint. Articular cartilage (1) is diffusely thinned and a subchondral cyst (3) is present. Inflamed, thickened synovium (2) forms marginal erosion (4) at bare area of joint. A synovial cyst is present (5).

Table 1. Sacroiliac Joint Disease and Distribution

Disease	Bilateral and Symmetrical	Bilateral and Asymmetrical	Unilateral
Ankylosing Spondylitis	+	–	–
Psoriatic Arthritis	+	+	+
RA	–	+	+
OA	+	+	+
Infection	–	–	+

Symmetry, specific joint involvement, and location are important findings, and early changes in these areas may occur before clinical symptoms. Hand films are useful to evaluate distribution and symmetry. Distal joint involvement favors psoriatic arthritis and OA. Proximal joint involvement is seen more with RA. Symmetrical bilateral disease is commonly seen in RA and primary OA.

Large joint involvement favors OA, RA, ankylosing spondylitis, and infection. Sacroiliac joint disease and distribution point to specific disease entities (Resnik & Resnick, 1985) (Table 1).

Soft-tissue changes are easily overlooked on plain films because the eye is naturally drawn toward the more dense osseous structures. To avoid this error, be sure to always first evaluate soft tissues. This may require the use of a hot light to see darker areas of the film. Soft-tissue swelling is a nonspecific finding that signals some type of pathology. The adjacent bones should then be carefully scrutinized.

Degenerative Joint Disease

Osteoarthritis (OA)

OA, or degenerative joint disease, is probably the most common arthropathy seen by radiologists, and it has characteristic imaging findings that allow for confident diagnosis. This includes nonuniform joint space narrowing with subchondral sclerosis and cyst formation and the production of osteophytes. This is present with a background of normal bone mineralization.

Key Findings:
• Joint space narrowing
• Osteophytes
• Sclerosis
• Loose bodies
• Normal bone mineralization
• Unilateral and/or bilateral, asymmetric distribution

Target Sites:
● Very common

In OA, joint space narrowing is not uniform and involves the areas of the joint exposed to the most stress. This contrasts with RA and other inflammatory arthropathies in which the joint space narrowing is diffuse. A good example of this concept is in OA of the hip, where cartilage loss usually involves the superior area of the joint with corresponding migration of the femoral head (Drawing 2). This helps to distinguish OA from inflammatory arthropathies in which diffuse cartilage loss results in axial migration (along the axis of the femoral neck) (Helms, 1989).

Subchondral sclerosis and cyst formation at the areas of stress are common. *Subchondral sclerosis* refers to increased density of bone resulting from cartilage thinning and subsequent articular

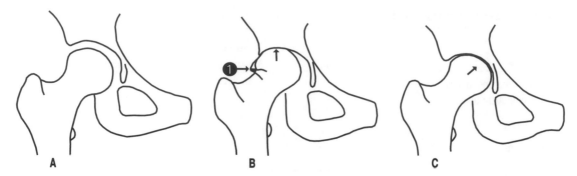

Drawing 2. (A) Normal hip with normal joint space. **(B)** Osteoarthritis of hip with superior joint space narrowing and subsequent superior migration of the femoral head. Note the osteophyte formation (1) at the lateral femoral head-neck junction. **(C)** Inflammatory arthritis of hip with diffuse joint space narrowing migration centrally of the femoral head along the axis of the femoral neck.

bone-on-bone contact. Subchondral cysts, or geodes, are radiographic lucencies underlying articular bone. They are of variable size and measure 2 to 20 mm in diameter. They are thought to occur when synovial fluid is forced through areas of thinned cartilage in weakened subchondral bone, which forms an intraosseous fluid collection. Subchondral cysts can be seen in other arthropathies as well. In OA, they are rarely problematic, but it is important that they not be mistaken for a more aggressive lesion such as metastasis.

Cartilage and subchondral bone degeneration can cause fragmentation of articular areas, which results in intra-articular loose bodies. This is most commonly seen in the knee. If composed solely of cartilage, loose bodies will not be seen on plain films, but when composed of calcium or bone, they are visible. They appear as oval or round smoothly marginated structures in the joint space. Their presence may accelerate the degenerative process if they are not identified and removed. They may cause biomechanical problems by lodging between articular surfaces.

Osteophytes are the most characteristic finding of OA and are easily recognized. They are bony outgrowths continuous with underlying bone that occur at insertions of ligaments near joints. They are covered by a cartilage cap that is not seen on plain films; therefore, their size may be underestimated on X-ray.

OA is broadly categorized into two main types: primary and secondary. Primary OA has a familial pattern that predominantly affects middle-aged women. It is seen in the hands involving the proximal (PIP) and distal (DIP) interphalangeal joints and the base of the thumb (first carpo-metacarpal [CMC] joint) in a bilateral symmetrical manner (Figure 3). Radial subluxation of the first CMC joint is common. Prominent sclerosis and osteophyte formation is present. The osteophyte formation about the PIP and DIP joints gives rise to Bouchard and Heberden nodes that are well known to practitioners. Again, plain films may underestimate their size because only the mineralized osteophyte portion is imaged, and overlying cartilage has a similar radiographic density to surrounding soft tissues.

A subtype of primary OA, called inflammatory or erosive OA, has a similar distribution of joint involvement. In this disease, periodic episodes of inflammation occur that can cause erosions and eventually lead to joint ankylosis.

Secondary OA is related to preexisting afflictions, such as trauma or mechanical deviation, and commonly occurs in the knees, hips, and spine, but it can occur in any joint. The classic findings of nonuniform joint space narrowing, subchondral sclerosis and cyst formation, and osteophytes are typical.

In the hips, superior joint space narrowing with associated subchondral sclerosis and cyst formation and osteophyte formation are present. Osteophytes are most prominent in the lateral acetabulum and femoral head-neck junction, with thickening (buttressing) of the cortex of the medial femoral neck (Figure 4).

The knee is a common site of OA, probably because of its weight-bearing function and susceptibility to injury. Of the three knee compartments (medial, lateral, and

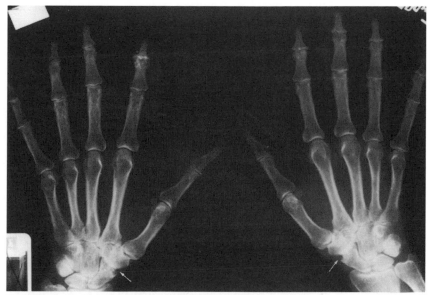

Figure 3. P-A radiograph of the hands of a patient with primary OA. There is joint space narrowing, sclerosis, and osteophytosis about several DIP joints. Additionally, joint space narrowing and subchondral sclerosis is seen symmetrically at the scaphotrapezial joints (*arrows*).

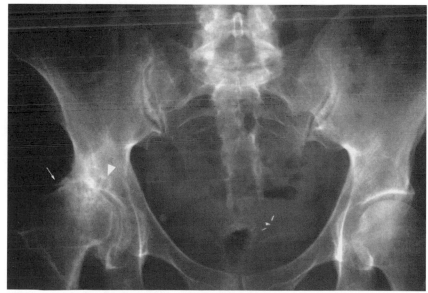

Figure 4. A-P radiograph of the hip in a patient with OA demonstrating right hip superior joint space narrowing with subchondral cyst (*arrowhead*) and osteophyte (*arrow*) formation.

patello-femoral), usually the medial compartment is most severely affected by joint space narrowing (which causes genu varus deformity), subchondral sclerosis and cyst formation, osteophytes, and intra-articular loose bodies (Figures 5A and 5B). Meniscal degeneration and synovial cyst formation occur and are best seen with MRI (Figures 6A and 6B).

In the spine, disc space and facet joint narrowing, end-plate sclerosis, and osteophytes are seen (Figure 7A). Linear gas collections called vacuum phenomena occur in the disc space and are a frequent finding that help to confirm OA and rule out other more serious problems such as disc infection. Because discs are not directly visualized on

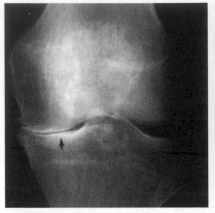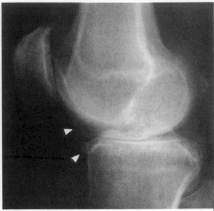

Figure 5. A-P **(A)** and lateral **(B)** radiographs of the knee in a patient with OA show typical findings of medial and patello-femoral compartment narrowing. Subchondral sclerosis (*arrow*) is prominent about the medial tibial plateau. Small osteophytes (*arrowheads*) are seen on the lateral film.

plain films, disc disease is inferred by disc space narrowing. Discs are best seen with MRI (Figure 7B), where they can be directly visualized and their relationship to the thecal sac, spinal cord, and exiting nerve roots can be evaluated.

In other arthropathies, secondary degenerative changes may be seen after the initial insult to the joint from the primary disease process, or the degenerative change can simply be concomitant. The classic findings of OA may be seen to varying degrees. For instance, in RA, secondary OA may be seen with osteophytosis and varying degrees of sclerosis. Due to the underlying osteopenia associated with RA, these findings may be less prominent.

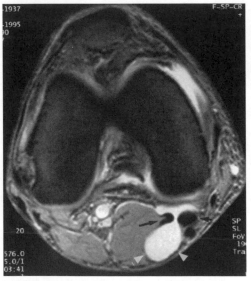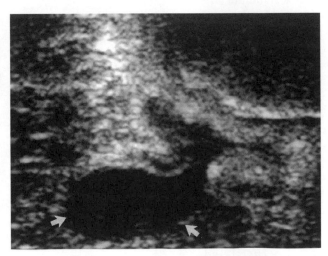

Figure 6. (A): Axial MRI of a knee demonstrating a round, fluid-filled popliteal cyst (*arrowheads*). The fluid has herniated from the knee joint between the tendons of the medial head of the gastrocnemius tendon (*long black arrow*) and the semimembranosus tendon (*short arrow*) to form the cyst. **(B):** Transverse ultrasound image of the same patient as in 6A. The cyst (*arrows*) appears black on ultrasound. Both MRI and ultrasound can easily identify popliteal cysts.

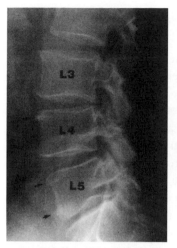 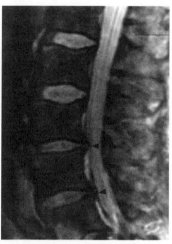 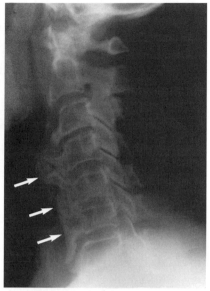

Figure 7. (A): Lateral radiograph of the lumbar spine in a patient with degen-erative spine changes showing disc space narrowing at the L3–L4, L4–L5, and L5–S1 levels. Multiple osteophytes (*arrows*) are present. **(B)**: Sagittal MRI for the same patient as in 7A. The MRI directly visualizes the discs and the amount of their protrusion (*arrowheads*) into the spinal canal.

Figure 8. Lateral radiograph of the cervical spine in a patient with extensive DISH. Note the large protruding osteophytes (arrows) anteriorly at multiple levels that displace the hypopharynx and esophagus, which causes dysphagia.

Diffuse Idiopathic Skeletal Hyperostosis (DISH)

Osteophytes of the spine are seen in DISH, also known as Forestier's disease. This is a common bone-forming disorder seen in 12% of elderly patients in which ossification occurs at the sites of tendinous and ligamen-tous attachments. In the spine, DISH can resemble OA radiographically; however, sclerosis and disc space narrowing are not as prominent. Additionally, in DISH, the osteophytes are at multiple, continuous levels. The lumbar and thoracic spine are the most frequent target sites, followed by the cervical spine. The osteophytes may be quite large, horizontally protuberant, and bridging (Figure 8).

Therapists working with feeding disorders should be familiar with DISH. Dysphagia occurs in up to 20% of patients with DISH when bulky, horizontal osteophytes of the cervical spine encroach on the hypopharynx and esophagus. These osteophytes cause anterior displacement and subsequent narrowing of the structures. Patients complain of feeling that food "gets stuck" in transit during swallowing. This is well visualized during radiographic barium-swallow examinations.

Inflammatory Arthropathies

Rheumatoid Arthritis (RA)

The radiographic hallmarks of RA are alignment abnormalities, periarticular osteoporosis that pro-gresses to generalized osteoporosis, uniform joint space narrowing with marginal erosions, and periarticular soft-tissue swelling with synovial cyst and rheumatoid nodule formation. There is generally a bilateral and symmetrical distribution, especially of the hands, wrists, and feet, where the earliest changes are frequently seen.

Alignment abnormalities are most dramatic in the hands and wrists and tend to be symmetrical. They are caused by the pull of tendons on abnormal joints, which results in the deformities seen on plain films. The abnormal kinetics produce unbalanced forces that result in characteristic deformities of the hand and wrist. On a P-A radiograph, the lunate normally articulates with the medial aspect of the radius. When more than half of the proximal lunate articular surface is medial to the ulnar edge of the distal radius, radial deviation and ulnar translation of the carpus has occurred (Figure 9). Radial deviation of the carpus and ulnar deviation of the fingers is termed the *zig-zag deformity*. Ulnar deviation and palmar subluxation of the metacarpophalangeal (MCP) joints, boutonnière and swan-neck deformities of the fingers, and Z deformities of the thumb (Figures 2 and 9) are determined in a manner similar to occupational therapy and physical therapy evaluations. The relationship between radial deviation of the carpus and ulnar deviation of the fingers must be considered in designing orthoses and in surgical management.

Similar alignment abnormalities occur in the forefoot. Fibular deviation of the toes and dorsolateral subluxation or dislocation of the proximal phalanges at the metatarsal head are common. The fifth toe may be relatively spared.

Key Findings:
- Alignment abnormalities
- Osteoporosis
- Joint space narrowing
- Soft tissue swelling
- Bilateral and symmetric distribution

Target Sites:
- ● Very common
- ▲ Common

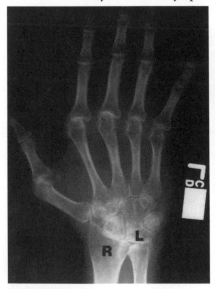

Figure 9. P-A radiograph in a patient with RA. The lunate (L) now has minimal articulation with the radius (R). The entire carpus is radially deviated, and the fingers are ulnarly deviated (zig-zag deformity). The carpal and MCP joints are narrowed.

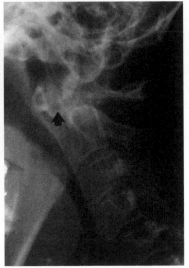

Figure 10. Lateral radiograph of the cervical spine obtained in flexion. There is atlantoaxial subluxation (*arrow*) with widening of the space anterior to the dens. Note the step ladder appearance of the vertebral bodies where there is anterior subluxation at each level.

An important cervical alignment abnormality is atlantoaxial subluxation (Figure 10). This is difficult to discern on physical examination; however, lateral films of the cervical spine obtained in flexion are quite sensitive. In fact, atlantoaxial subluxation can be seen in 33% of patients with RA (Brower, 1988). The distance between the posterior cortex of the anterior arch of C1 and the anterior aspect of the dens of C2 is measured. Normal measurements are less than 3 mm in adults and less than 5 mm in children. This laxity may be quite severe and cause neurological symptoms. Subluxation distances between the odontoid and the atlas measuring more than 8 mm usually require surgical intervention. Lower in the cervical spine, multilevel subluxations are common, which gives a "step-ladder" appearance to the cervical spine on lateral films (Figure 10).

In early RA, periarticular osteopenia is seen adjacent to inflamed joints. Later, this progresses to diffuse osteopenia, which indicates disease progression, medication side effects, or disuse of a painful extremity.

In inflammatory arthropathies, cartilage is diffusely thinned, which results in uniform and pancompartmental joint space. Proliferation of synovium in RA (called *pannus*) spreads over cartilage surfaces and causes irregularities of bone margins and erosions. These erosions begin where the protective cartilage is thinnest, at the so-called "bare areas" of the joint margins. They are called *marginal* or *periarticular erosions*. Initially, these erosions may be quite subtle, but they can progress and lead to marked bone destruction and joint space loss. Radiolucent cysts are seen in the subchondral bone and are formed from the intrusion of pannus or joint fluid. These may collapse and lead to further joint destruction. Bony ankylosis occurs in the wrist and midfoot but is uncommon at other sites.

Soft-tissue swelling occurs about the inflamed joints and results from joint fluid, thickened synovium, and surrounding soft-tissue inflammation. Synovium may herniate along tendon sheaths or between tissue planes to form synovial cysts, which may be quite large (Figure 11B). Additionally, subcutaneous rheumatoid nodules may be seen in up to 20% of rheumatoid patients and usually develop over the elbow and ulna along pressure areas. These soft-tissue changes are generally nonspecific on plain films, which shows homogenous soft-tissue enlargement. MRI offers a more detailed examination of the surrounding anatomy.

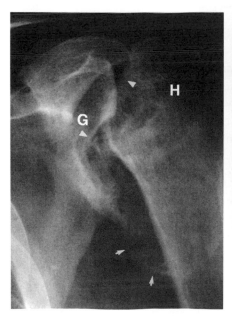
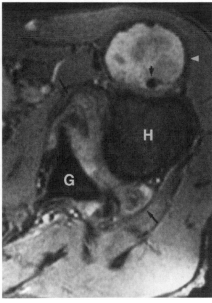

Figure 11. Radiograph and MRI of the shoulder in a patient with RA. **(A):** A-P radiograph of the shoulder shows extensive erosion (*arrowheads*) of the humeral head (H) and inferior glenoid (G). Faint calcific density (*arrows*) outlines a large synovial cyst. **(B):** Axial MRI at the level of the humeral neck. There is a large synovial cyst (*arrowhead*) that surrounds the biceps tendon (*short arrow*). Fluid and pannus (*long arrows*) are present in the glenohumeral joint space.

Generally, there is a bilateral and symmetrical distribution of arthropathy, especially in the small joints of the hands and feet. Large joint involvement of the shoulders, elbows, hips, and knees is frequent in RA, but in these areas, symmetry is less common.

In the shoulder, erosive changes of the acromioclavicular joint with later resorption of the distal clavicle occur. The humeral head is high riding with respect to the glenoid, which indicates rotator cuff atrophy or tear. Erosions may be present about the humeral head (Figure 11A).

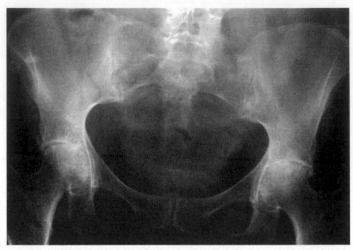

Figure 12. A-P pelvis radiograph of a patient with RA. Note the bilateral uniform hip joint space narrowing.

In the hip, concentric cartilage loss leads to migration of the femoral head centrally along the axis of the femoral neck (Figure 12). In later stages, the joint space becomes obliterated, and the femoral head and acetabulum protrude into the pelvis. This is called *acetabular protrusio.*

The knee is commonly affected with pancompartmental joint space narrowing, erosions, and subchondral cysts. Varus or valgus deformities may be seen. The suprapatellar bursa is engorged by effusion or synovial hypertrophy. Synovial cysts are common, especially in the popliteal area where they are called *Baker's* or *popliteal cysts*, and may be quite large. These are well visualized with MRI and ultrasound (Figures 6A and 6B).

Ankylosing Spondylitis

Ankylosing spondylitis is a chronic inflammatory arthritis of unknown etiology. It is a common cause of low back pain in young men. Unfortunately, it may go undiagnosed for a long time. Early diagnosis is essential for appropriately managing pain, maintaining mobility, and preventing deformity. With appropriate intervention, kyphotic deformities can be avoided.

Key Findings:
• Bony ankylosis
• Proliferative new bone
• Axial skeletal involvement
• Bilateral and symmetric distribution

Target Sites:
● Very common
▲ Common

Ankylosing spondylitis is characterized by bony ankylosis primarily of the axial skeleton, with later secondary involvement of the appendicular skeleton. Erosive disease is infrequent; it occurs early in the disease process at bony insertions of ligaments and tendons (entheses). This progresses to bony proliferation and ankylosis of adjacent bones. When inflammation or calcification occurs at a tendon insertion, it is called *enthesopathy.* Joint ankylosis is the radiographic hallmark and is the most debilitating aspect of the disease. Bone mineralization is normal early on, but as ankylosis occurs, osteopenia is seen.

Sacroiliac joint disease is seen early. There are symmetrical, bilateral changes that begin with small erosions on the iliac side of the joint (Resnick, 1995). The sacral side is protected longer because of a thicker cartilage covering. Reactive bone sclerosis usually accompanies the erosions. Sacroiliac joint disease eventually progresses to fusion and ankylosis with radiographic obliteration of the sacroiliac joints.

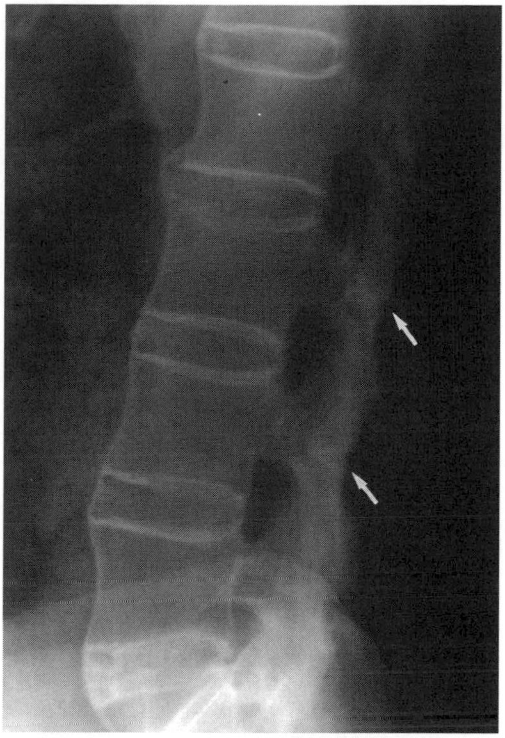

Spine disease usually begins at the thoracolumbar junction or in the lumbar spine. Involvement of the cervical spine is not uncommon. Syndesmophytes are characteristically seen. These are vertically oriented paravertebral body ossifications. In ankylosing spondylitis, syndesmophytes originate at the edge or margin of the vertebral body and extend to the next vertebral body level. They are symmetrical and bilateral and may involve the entire spine, which gives rise to the "bamboo" spine appearance (Figure 13). The apophyseal joints may fuse. At this point, the spine is immobile, and diffuse osteopenia ensues. The disc spaces are usually preserved, although they may calcify.

Figure 13. Lateral radiograph of the lumbar spine in a patient with ankylosing spondylitis. The vertebral bodies are fused with paravertebral ossification, giving rise to a "bamboo" appearance. The facet joints (arrows) are likewise fused.

Ankylosed spines are at high risk for unstable fractures, even from relatively minor trauma. There is a high rate of morbidity associated with these fractures. Weinstein and associates (1982) reported a 12% incidence of fractures in patients with ankylosing spondylitis and an 8% incidence of paralytic spinal cord injuries. The cervical spine is especially vulnerable, usually from hyperextension injuries; neurological compromise and death may result. Fractures of the thoracic and lumbar spine may be less catastrophic and may go clinically unnoticed. Because of the brittle nature of the ankylosed spine, these are referred to as "carrot stick" fractures. They may occur through the vertebral body or commonly through the disc space. At the fracture level, motion returns; therefore, in a patient with an ankylosed spine, new range of motion (ROM) should be evaluated carefully with plain films and advanced imaging as needed.

Hip disease may be seen in up to 50% of patients with ankylosing spondylitis, and it is the most frequently involved joint in the appendicular skeleton. Concentric joint space narrowing is the main feature, with collar-like osteophyte formation at the femoral head–neck junction (Figure 14). Ankylosis may occur, which results in marked disability and subsequent osteopenia secondary to disuse. On the pelvis film, sacroiliac joint fusion helps to confirm the diagnosis of ankylosing spondylitis. The shoulder is the second most common appendicular joint to show involvement. The knee is affected in 30% of patients, and the elbows, hands, and feet are affected in 10% of patients. Joint ankylosis is the classic finding.

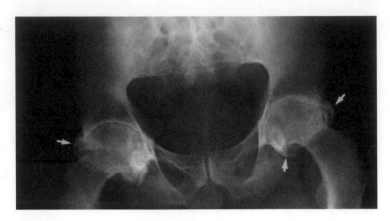

Figure 14. A-P pelvis of a patient with psoriatic arthropathy. Both hip joints are concentrically narrowed, and there is a large amount of surrounding osteophyte formation. Additionally, the sacroiliac joints demonstrate near complete fusion. Similar changes can be seen in ankylosing spondylitis.

Psoriatic Arthritis

Key Findings for patterns 1 and 5:
- Soft tissue swelling
- Joint space loss with marked erosions
- Bone proliferation and ankylosis
- Normal bone mineralization
- Bilateral and asymmetric distribution
- Diffuse digital swelling (dactylitis)
- Bone resorption (mutilans or pencil and cup deformity)

Target Sites:
● Very common
▲ Common

About 5% to 8% of patients with psoriasis develop psoriatic arthritis (Klippel & Dieppe, 1994). Although most patients with psoriatic arthritis have a long history of psoriasis, occasionally the articular manifestations may predate or coincide with the appearance of skin disease. Psoriatic arthritis may be present before or during the appearance of skin disease. The skin disease may not be apparent.

Psoriatic arthritis tends to occur in five clinical patterns (listed in decreasing frequency).

1. Asymmetrical oligoarthritis of the DIP, PIP, and MTP joints that tends to cause ankylosis and may include dactylitis

2. Symmetrical polyarthritis with a similar pattern as RA

3. Symmetrical arthritis and nail involvement confined to the DIP joints of the hands and feet

4. Arthritis mutilans often with sacroiliitis

5. Spondylarthropathy often in association with another pattern (Gladman, 1990; Klippel & Dieppe, 1994; Moll & Wright, 1973)

Radiographic features are often distinctive enough to diagnose the disease in the absence of skin findings. These features include destructive joint space changes with bony proliferation and ankylosis occurring in a bilateral and usually asymmetrical pattern and prominent soft-tissue swelling. Ankylosis is an important feature of psoriatic arthritis and ankylosing spondylitis. It can be seen in primary OA and occasionally in the carpal and tarsal joints in RA. Psoriatic arthritis differs from RA in that the bone mineralization is normal.

Soft-tissue swelling may be the earliest and only radiographic finding. This occurs in periarticular areas of the digits and gives rise to fusiform swelling (spindle digit) or may involve the entire digit, which indicates tenosynovitis and diffuse inflammation (dactylitis) commonly referred to as a "cocktail sausage digit" (Figure 15).

Destructive arthritis of the hands is a common manifestation of psoriatic arthritis (Figure 16). The PIP and DIP joints are most commonly involved; MCP disease and carpal disease are less frequent. Erosive disease begins at the joint margins, then progresses centrally, which results in a conical end to the bone. This can result in mechanical erosion of the distal articular surface and cause a saucerized distortion referred to as *pencil-in-cup deformity* (Figure 16). Bone resorption results in joint instability and shortening of the digit, creating a telescoping of the digit referred to as "opera glass hand" or *arthritis mutilans*. Early detection of mutilans is important because its progression can be halted with surgical fusion (Nalebuff & Garrett, 1976). Tuftal erosions and resorption of terminal phalanges are characteristic. Bone proliferation is another important imaging feature and occurs at the sites of tendon attachments near areas of erosion or along bone shafts, which makes the bone appear abnormally wide. Proliferative bone may cross articular surfaces, which leads to ankylosis.

Similar changes are seen in the feet, although involvement of the MTP joint is seen more frequently than in MCP joint disease. Extensive destructive changes of the first MTP joint are common. Osteolysis of phalanges leads to a strange whittled appearance and arthritis mutilans. Additionally, erosions and bony proliferation may be seen at the Achilles tendon or plantar aponeurosis insertion.

Sacroiliac joint disease may be unilateral or bilateral and is often asymmetrical. Erosions and sclerosis are typical in patients with psoriatic arthritis who complain of low back pain. Ankylosis in sacroiliac joints is much less frequent than with ankylosing spondylitis.

Large joints are usually not affected. The hips may occasionally be involved with concentric joint space narrowing and surrounding osteophyte formation similar to ankylosing spondylitis (Figure 14).

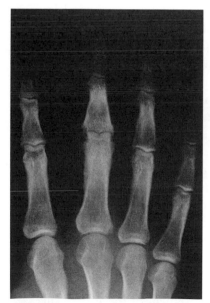

Figure 15. P-A radiograph of the hand in a patient with psoriatic arthritis. The third finger is markedly swollen (dactylitis), and the proximal phalanx is widened by periosteal new bone formation.

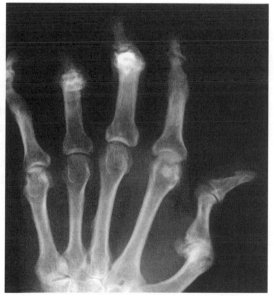

Figure 16. P-A radiograph of the hand of a patient with psoriatic arthritis. There is fusion of multiple joints. The second distal phalange demonstrates a cupping deformity from the mechanical erosion from the middle phalange, an early form of "pencil-in-cup deformity."

In the thoracolumbar spine, bulky, asymmetrical syndesmophyte formations that emanate from the midportion of the vertebral body may be present. These may be difficult to distinguish from degenerative osteophytes or DISH. In the cervical spine, apophyseal joints are frequently affected by narrowing or erosions and sometimes fusion. Atlantoaxial subluxation may be seen.

Crystal-Induced Arthropathies

Gout

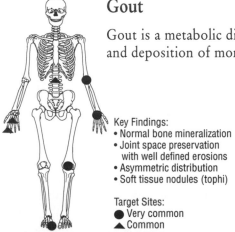

Key Findings:
- Normal bone mineralization
- Joint space preservation with well defined erosions
- Asymmetric distribution
- Soft tissue nodules (tophi)

Target Sites:
- ● Very common
- ▲ Common

Gout is a metabolic disorder resulting in high levels of uric acid in the blood and deposition of monosodium urate crystals in various sites. It mainly affects men (only 5% of cases are in women). When it is seen in women, the patients are usually postmenopausal (Brower, 1988). Most patients are diagnosed and successfully treated before radiographic changes are seen. Only one half of patients with gout will show radiographic evidence of the disease and then only 6 to 8 years after the initial attack (Brower, 1988).

The radiographic findings are characteristic and indicate chronicity of the disease. The earliest finding is reversible soft-tissue swelling adjacent to the symptomatic joint. Urate crystals deposited in the soft tissues give rise to nodules called *tophi*. The crystals are not radiopaque; however, calcium may precipitate with urate crystals in varying amounts and cause changes of the tophi density. If these tophi are adjacent to bone, they may cause pressure erosions. These erosions demonstrate sharply marginated, well-defined sclerotic borders. The presence of an overhanging edge of bone is characteristic of gout (Figure 17). The adjacent bones have normal mineralization, and the joint spaces are not narrowed until late in the destruction process.

The disease classically presents at the first MTP joint; however, involvement of the ankles, knees, hands, and elbows is likewise seen. The tarsometatarsal and CMC joints are frequent target sites. The distribution is asymmetrical.

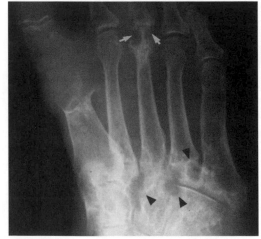

Figure 17. Oblique radiograph of a foot in a patient with longstanding gout. There is marked destructive change of the bones of the first toe from tophaceous deposits. Additionally, erosions with overhanging edges of bone (*arrows*) are present about the distal third metatarsal head. Erosive change is seen in the tarsometatarsal area (*arrowheads*).

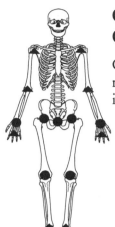

Calcium Pyrophosphate Dihydrate (CPPD) Crystal Deposition Disease

CPPD crystal deposition disease is commonly seen by radiologists who read musculoskeletal films. It is seen more frequently in women, and its incidence increases with age. There is a wide spectrum of both clinical and radiographic findings, and the terminology may be confusing. The following words should be clarified.

Key Findings:
- Normal bone mineralization
- Joint space narrowing and subchondral cyst formation
- Bilateral distribution
- Chondrocalcinosis

Target Sites:
- ● Very common
- ▲ Common

- *Chondrocalcinosis*: calcification of articular cartilage, most frequently from CPPD crystals but in some instances from other types of crystals.

- *CPPD disease*: a general term used to describe a disorder associated with CPPD crystals in or around joints.

- *CPPD arthropathy*: chronic arthritis with a particular pattern of structural joint destruction associated with CPPD crystal deposition.

These terms are used to describe three common presentations of patients with CPPD disease: acute synovitis, chronic arthritis, and incidental radiographic finding. Clinically and radiographically, these entities may overlap (Drawing 3).

Chondrocalcinosis occurs as CPPD crystals precipitate about the joint. When there is a sizeable amount of crystal deposition, chondrocalcinosis is easily visible on radiographs as thin curvilinear densities along cartilage surfaces (Figure 18). The absence of visualization, however, does not exclude its presence. Target sites have been identified, most frequently in the knee, pubic symphysis, and wrist; however, chondrocalcinosis

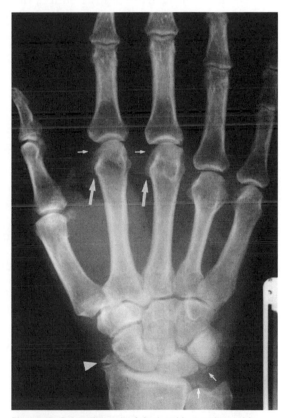

Figure 18. P-A radiograph of the hand in a patient with CPPD arthropathy. Chondrocalcinosis (*short arrows*) is visualized in the carpal joint and the second and third MCP joints. Osteophyte formation (*long arrows*) is present at the second and third metacarpal heads. The fourth metacarpal is shortened from a previous fracture. There is a previous nonunited fracture of the distal radius (*arrowhead*).

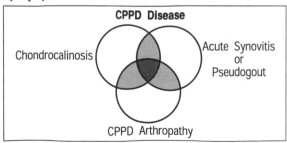

Drawing 3. Diagram of CPPD crystal deposition disease. The radiographic and clinical findings may be grouped into three common categories that have varying degrees of overlap.

can be seen about virtually any articulation. These crystals can be deposited along ligaments, synovium, and bursae. Chondrocalcinosis is a common age-associated phenomenon and may often be an incidental finding on radiographs, especially in elderly women. This radiographic finding must be correlated with the patient's clinical presentation (Klippel & Dieppe, 1994).

CPPD arthropathy is used to describe a particular pattern of structural joint destruction associated with CPPD crystal deposition. These changes may be seen with or without visible chondrocalcinosis. The most common sites are in the knee, wrist, and MCP joints, although the condition may be present in any articulation. Usually involvement is bilateral, but it is not always symmetrical. The radiographic features are similar to OA, with joint space narrowing, subchondral sclerosis and cyst formation, and osteophyte formation. The following radiographic features may help to differentiate CPPD arthropathy from OA:

- Involvement of joints atypical for OA such as the wrist, elbow, and shoulder
- Unusual intra-articular distribution, such as in the lateral compartment of the knee (in OA, the medial compartment is usually more severely involved)
- Prominent subchondral cyst formation
- Variable osteophyte formation, which is not as prominent as seen in OA (Klippel & Dieppe, 1994; Resnick, 1995)

Acute synovitis associated with CPPD disease is the most common cause of an acute monoarticular arthritis in elderly persons. Because it clinically resembles a gout attack, it has been called pseudogout. Radiographs may be normal or demonstrate a spectrum of findings (Figure 18) from chondrocalcinosis to marked CPPD arthropathy. Typically these joints are aspirated to evaluate for crystals and to rule out infection. If the joint space is difficult to aspirate, the radiologist may be asked to assist with image guided aspiration.

Collagen Vascular Diseases

Systemic Lupus Erythematosus (SLE)

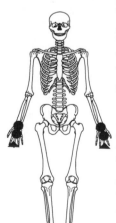

Key Findings:
- Alignment abnormalities of hands
- Periarticular osteopenia
- Uniform joint space narrowing with minimal erosive change
- Soft tissue swelling
- Bilateral and symmetric distribution

Target Sites:
- ● Very common
- ▲ Common

SLE is the most common of the collagen vascular diseases. It affects multiple organ systems with 75% to 90% of patients having arthritic symptoms. The wrist and hand joints are frequently involved, occasionally with a deforming arthritis (Figure 19). Initially, soft-tissue swelling is present, which then leads to atrophy. Like RA, there is periarticular osteopenia that leads to diffuse osteopenia. Lytic lesions in periarticular bone can be seen. Joint spaces are usually not involved.

Reducible subluxations with nonerosive disease are the radiographic hallmarks (Brower, 1988; Weissman et al., 1978). These may not be as obvious with P-A views of the hands, but in the Norgaard views, where the hands are not rigidly positioned on the film cassette, the subluxations become more dramatic. They are similar to those in RA. Typically, there is radial deviation of the carpus and ulnar deviation of the MCP joints. Swan-neck and boutonnière deformities of the fingers and Z deformities of the thumbs are typical. Deforming arthritis of the knees and shoulders may be seen.

Avascular necrosis (AVN) is an unfortunate complication of SLE that can occur in up to 40% of patients. AVN is death of osseous cellular components and marrow occurring as a result of altered blood flow. Other names for this entity include aseptic necrosis, bone infarct, and osteonecrosis.

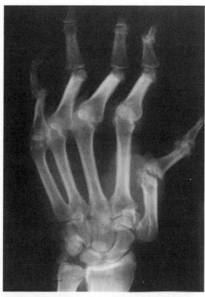

Figure 19. P-A radiograph of the hand in a patient with SLE. Note the swan-neck deformities of the fingers and the Z deformity of the thumb. The base of the first metacarpal is subluxed proximally from the trapezium.

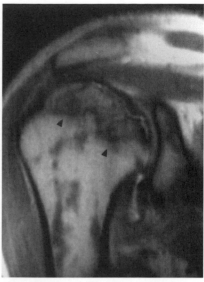

Figure 20. MRI of the shoulder of a patient with AVN. There is a large area of abnormal marrow signal (*arrowheads*) in the humeral head as well as a second patchy area in the proximal humeral shaft, which is consistent with AVN.

AVN is associated with multiple disease processes and predisposing risk factors, the most common of which are probably alcoholism and steroid medication. AVN is seen in patients with RA and SLE as a result of the disease processes themselves or secondary to steroid medication. In 25% of patients, no predisposing factor is found. AVN most commonly involves the femoral head, then the humeral head and talus; however, it may be seen in any bone. Initially, plain films are normal. Early plain film findings begin with subtle mottling or blurring of the bony trabeculae near the articular surface that proceeds to areas of sclerosis. Subchondral fractures may produce curvilinear arcs of radiolucency that are followed by collapse and flattening of bone. Ultimately, osteoarthritic changes in the joint occur. MRI is the most sensitive imaging modality for early disease when plain films may be negative (Figure 20).

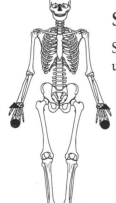

Systemic Sclerosis (Scleroderma)

Scleroderma is a generalized systemic inflammatory connective tissue disease of unknown origin that involves multiple organ systems. It most commonly affects women from 30 to 50 years of age. Soft-tissue and bone changes are commonly seen radiographically, particularly in the hands. The axial skeleton is rarely involved.

Key Findings:
• Normal alignment
• Normal mineralization
• Normal joint spaces
• Symetric atrophy of finger tips with phalangeal tuft erosion

Target Sites:
● Very common
▲ Common

The wrists and hands are commonly affected. Initially, there is soft-tissue resorption of the tufts of the fingers, and this is associated with Raynaud's phenomenon. The distance between the phalange tip and the skin edge decreases, and the fingertips atrophy and become conical

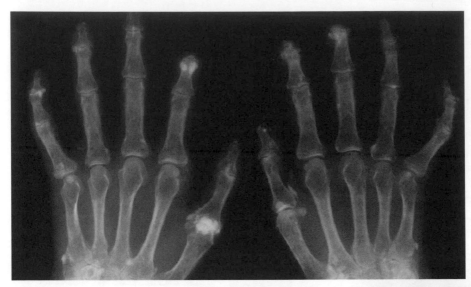

Figure 21. P-A radiograph of both hands in a patient with scleroderma. There is atrophy of the soft tissues of the fingers with erosive change of the terminal tufts. Soft-tissue calcification (*white areas*) is seen at several sites.

in shape. Erosions of the phalangeal tufts are common and result in a pointed appearance (Figure 21).

Amorphous, cloud-like soft-tissue calcifications are often seen. Although the hand is the most frequent site, other areas of the body may be involved. These calcifications may be in subcutaneous tissues, joint capsule, tendons, or ligaments.

Articular disease is occasionally seen with joint space narrowing, deformity, and central and marginal erosions. A frequent target site is the first CMC joint, which is similar to primary OA. However, the presence of globular soft-tissue calcification indicates scleroderma. Other target sites include the interphalangeal joints of the hand and MCP joints.

Dermatomyositis and Polymyositis

Dermatomyositis and polymyositis are disorders of unknown etiology that result in inflammatory and atrophic changes of skeletal muscle. Their imaging findings are similar. The striking radiographic findings of these diseases are seen symmetrically in skeletal musculature of the thorax,

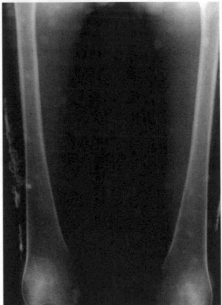

Figure 22. A-P radiograph of both femora in a patient with dermatomyositis. Note atrophic changes of the musculature (light shadow area) with subcutaneous calcification.

upper arm, forearm, thigh, and calf. Initially, inflammatory infiltration results in soft-tissue swelling and increased radiographic density of the muscles. Later, atrophic changes are noted, and dramatic calcification is seen in the subcutaneous tissues, intermuscular fascia, tendons, and fat (Figure 22). The calcifications are linear (along tissue planes), unlike the globular-appearing calcifications of scleroderma. Although joint pain is common, radiographs show little more than soft-tissue swelling and periarticular osteopenia. Destructive joint changes are only occasionally seen.

References

Bollow, M., Braun, J., Hamm, B., Eggens, U., Schilling, A., Konig, H., & Wolf, K. J. (1995). Early sacroiliitis in patients with spondyloarthropathy: Evaluation with dynamic gadolinium-enhanced MR imaging. *Radiology, 194,* 529–536.

Brower, A. C. (1984). The radiographic approach to arthritis. *Medical Clinics of North America, 68,* 1593–1607.

Brower, A. C. (1988). *Arthritis in black and white.* Philadelphia: Saunders.

Forrester, D. M, & Brown, J. C. (1987). *The radiology of joint disease* (3rd ed.). Philadelphia: Saunders.

Gladman, D. D. (1990). Psoriatic arthritis: Ankylosing spondylitis and spondyloarthopathies. *Spine: State of the Art Reviews, 4,* 637–656.

Helms, C. A. (1989). *Fundamentals of skeletal radiology* (1st ed.). Philadelphia: Saunders.

Klippel, J. A., & Dieppe, P. A. (1994). *Rheumatology.* St Louis: Mosby-Year Book.

Lund, P. J., Nisbet, J. K., Valencia, F. G., & Ruth, J. T. (1996). Current sonographic applications in orthopedics. *American Journal of Radiology, 166,* 889–895.

Moll, J. M. H., & Wright, V. (1973). Psoriatic arthritis. *Seminars in Arthritis, 3,* 55–78.

Nalebuff, E. A., & Garrett, J. (1976). Opera-glass hand in rheumatoid arthritis. *Journal of Hand Surgery, 1*(3), 210.

Resnick, D. (1995). *Diagnosis of bone and joint disorders* (3rd ed.). Philadelphia: Saunders.

Resnik, C. S., & Resnick, D. (1985). Radiology of disorders of the sacroiliac joints. *JAMA, 253,* 2863–2866.

Roca, A., Bernreuter, W., & Alarcon, G. (1993). Functional magnetic resonance imaging should be included in the evaluation of cervical spine in patients with rheumatoid arthritis. *Journal of Rheumatology, 20,* 1485–1488.

Weinstein, P. R., Karpman, R. R., Gall, E. P., et al. (1982). Spinal cord injury, spinal fracture, and spinal stenosis in ankylosing spondylitis. *Journal of Neurosurgery, 57,* 609–616.

Weissman, B. N., Rappoport, A. S., Sosman, J. L., & Schur, P. H. (1978). Radiographic findings in the hands in patients with systemic lupus erythematosus. *Radiology, 126,* 313–317.

Winalski, C., Palmer, W., Rosenthal, D., & Weissman, B. (1996). Magnetic resonance imaging of rheumatoid arthritis. *Radiology Clinics of North America, 34,* 243–258.

Glossary

Acetabular protrusio: Medial migration of the femoral head and acetabulum into the pelvis.

Ankylosis: Bony fusion of joint resulting in no motion.

Appendicular skeleton: The portion of the skeleton involving limbs. This includes clavicles, scapulae, and the pelvis.

Arthritis mutilans: The deformity that results from severe osteolysis of the digital bone ends. The digit becomes unstable and shortened with redundant skin, which creates a telescoping appearance.

Atlantoaxial subluxation: Abnormal motion at the first and second cervical vertebrae due to a diseased transverse ligament that normally maintains close apposition of the dens with the anterior arch of C1.

Avascular necrosis: Ischemic death of cellular components of bone and marrow due to altered blood flow. When in articular bone, it can progress to collapse of bone and secondary degenerative change. Also called *aseptic necrosis, bone infarct,* and *osteonecrosis.*

Axial skeleton: The portion of the skeleton that includes the skull, vertebrae, ribs, and sternum.

Baker's cyst: Fluid from the knee joint that enters the gastrocnemius-semimembranosus bursa and forms a cyst of variable size.

Bouchard nodes: Osteophyte formation and soft-tissue swelling around PIP joints (also called *popliteal cyst*).

Boutonnière deformity: Flexion of PIP joint and extension of DIP joint secondary to rupture of the central slip of extensor digitorum communis at the PIP joint.

Cocktail sausage digit: Diffuse soft-tissue swelling of a digit seen in psoriatic arthritis. Now called *dactylitis.*

Enthesopathy: Inflammation or calcification of tendons at their attachments to bone.

Erosion: Focal loss of bone due to adjacent pressure or inflammation.

Heberden nodes: Osteophyte formation and soft-tissue swelling around DIP joints.

Joint space narrowing: Uniform: Loss of entire joint space due to cartilage loss (a sign of inflammatory arthropathy). Nonuniform: Focal loss of joint space due to isolated areas of cartilage loss (a sign of OA).

Loose bodies: Cartilaginous or osseous bodies in the joint space originating from fragmented articular bone.

Mineralization: Calcium and phosphate present in bone. When decreased, osteoporosis is present.

Osteolysis: Destructive changes of bone.

Osteophyte: Bony outgrowth occurring at the insertion of a ligament near a joint (a sign of OA).

Osteoporosis: Decrease in bone mass due to loss of mineralization in bone that is structurally normal.

Pannus: Proliferative synovium seen in RA that can cause erosions.

Pencil-in-cup deformity: Deformity of digits seen in psoriatic arthritis when marginal erosive change of the distal aspect of a phalange produces a pointed appearance. This can then mechanically erode the articular surface of the adjacent bone and cause a saucerized indentation.

Rheumatoid nodule: Soft-tissue accumulation of inflammatory cells forming a distinct mass located near a joint usually on the extensor surface.

Spindle digit: Fusiform swelling of a digit due to PIP joint disease.

Subchondral cyst: Intrusion of fluid or pannus into subchondral bone, giving rise to a lucent area on plain films. This is a nonspecific finding that can be seen in various arthropathies.

Subchondral sclerosis: Increased number and thickness of periarticular bone trabeculae that has a dense, thick, white appearance on plain films and is associated with mechanical changes and cartilage narrowing in OA.

Swan-neck deformity: Flexion of the DIP joint and extension of the PIP joint.

Syndesmophyte: Paravertebral body ligament ossifications that can be seen in ankylosing spondylitis or psoriatic arthritis.

Synovial cyst: Fluid-filled structure adjacent to and frequently continuous with a joint space.

Tophus: Urate crystal deposits that form soft-tissue nodules as seen in gout.

Zig-zag deformity: Radial deviation of carpus with ulnar deviation of fingers.

5

OSTEOARTHRITIS

John H. Bland, MD, Jeanne L. Melvin, MS, OTR, FAOTA, and Scott Hasson, EdD, PT, FACSM

Osteoarthritis (OA) is a disorder of the joints characterized by deterioration of the articular cartilage and secondary new bone formation. Onset is noninflammatory, but secondary inflammation is common. Typically, the disease is slowly progressive, but OA may cease at any point and have remissions and even cartilage regeneration. When inflammation is not present, the term *osteoarthrosis* is often preferred.

Etiology and Population Affected

The etiology of OA, in general terms, is any condition that changes the shape of the articulating surfaces or ligamentous and tendinous supports or alters the tissue matrices of subchondral bone, bone, hyaline cartilage, or surrounding soft tissues. These conditions can alter joint shape beyond normal tolerance or alter remodeling at the bone–cartilage interface and result in OA. The initiating event can be genetic, metabolic, systemic, or traumatic (Table 1).

Joints developing OA may show evidence of hyaline cartilage degeneration in early adulthood. Contrary to currently held views that these areas degenerate secondary to excessive loading, the most interesting and exciting theory is that these areas possibly degenerate because of underuse rather than overuse (Bland, 1997). OA is a disorder of multiple etiologies, and a vigorous search for a single cause of OA is without merit. Abnormal function may begin in any of the structures that make up the joint, but by the time the patient is examined by a clinician, most joint structures are involved.

OA is demonstrable in the knees of 35% of the persons as early as 30 years of age and becomes almost universal with increasing age (i.e., more than 50 years age) (Heine, 1926). At least 85% of persons 70 to 79 years of age have diagnosable OA (Cooper, 1994; Roberts & Burch, 1938).

Associations are well established between OA and diabetes mellitus, high blood pressure, and hyperuricemia independent of obesity. The inheritance of an oddly shaped joint may result in OA. Childhood hip disorders, Legg-Calve-Perthes disease, slipped capital femoral epiphysis, and congenital dislocation of the hip lead to early hip OA, as do milder degrees of acetabular dysplasia.

Table 1. Classification of Osteoarthritis

```
Primary (idiopathic)
    Localized
        Hands and feet
        Knee
        Hip
        Spine
        Other
    Generalized
        Three or more joint areas
        Erosive form
Secondary
    Posttraumatic
    Congenital and developmental
        Localized
            Hip diseases (e.g., Legg-Calve-Perthes disease)
            Mechanical and local factors
                (e.g., obesity, hypermobility, valgus, and varus)
        Generalized
            Bone dysplasias
            Metabolic diseases
    Calcium deposition diseases
        Calcium pyrophosphate desposition disease (CPPD)
        Hydroxyapatite arthropathy
        Destructive arthropathies
        Secondary to other bone and joint disorders
            (e.g., avascular necrosis, RA, Paget's disease)
    Miscellaneous other diseases
        (e.g., endocrine, neuropathy)
```

Occupation and repetitive use of certain joint groups have been associated with OA, particularly in the hands. Because sports are associated with risks of joint damage, OA is common in athletes.

Geographical area, ethnic group, or climate does not influence OA prevalence in a population. Men and women are equally affected. Men have a higher incidence before 45 years of age, and women have a higher incidence after 45 years of age (Kellgren & Lawrence, 1957; van Saase, van Romunde, Cats, Vandenbroucke, & Valkenburg, 1989). Severe disease more commonly affects women than men (22% vs. 19%) in patients with primary generalized OA (Kellgren & Moore, 1952; Lawrence, Bremner, & Bier, 1966).

Epidemiology

Evaluating the prevalence of clinical or symptomatic OA is difficult. Epidemiological data is based on radiological changes. Most persons more than 55 years of age manifest the structural changes of OA (Kellgren & Lawrence, 1958). Population studies do not identify the prevalence of clinically significant OA because, at a given time, the radiographic lesions may not be associated with pain or disability (Cobb, Merchant, & Rubin, 1957; Dieppe, 1994). One survey demonstrated clinical complaints in only 25% of a group of coal miners, all of whom had definite and sometimes extensive radiological evidence of OA in their knees. In the United Kingdom, it is estimated that there is 1 case of symptomatic OA for every 18 cases of radiological OA (Badley, Thompson, & Wood, 1978; van Saase et al., 1989; Wood, 1976). A 10% incidence of radiological OA has been shown in persons 15 to 24 years of age (Lawrence et al., 1966).

OA and Disability

OA probably has the highest morbidity of all illnesses of humankind and is a major health problem in the developed world. In western countries, OA is an extremely common cause of disability. It is the most frequent cause of rheumatic symptoms and results in the greatest loss of time from work (Cooper, 1994; Hadler, 1985; Kramer, Yelin, & Epstein, 1983). The disease has an enormous socioeconomic effect and is a great monetary loss for all over the world. Although elderly patients have the highest incidence of the disease, OA causes more absenteeism than any other joint disease in persons who are gainfully employed in industry as well as in the armed forces (Brown & Lingg, 1961; Short, 1947).

Obesity, Osteoporosis, and Hypermobility

OA can reasonably be viewed as occurring through two major mechanisms: 1) factors influencing a genetic predisposition to the condition and 2) factors resulting in abnormal biomechanical loading at specific joint sites. Obesity is closely associated with OA of the small joints of the hands and the knees and less so with OA of the hip. Obese persons have between a four- and sevenfold greater risk of developing OA of the knee (Leach , Baumgard, & Broom, 1973). It is not entirely clear whether obesity precedes or even perhaps causes OA or whether it results from the sedentary lifestyle of patients with OA. If obesity is an aggravating factor, diet planning must be reinforced. If the patient lacks nutritional knowledge, referral to a dietitian or community weight control program is necessary.

Heredity clearly plays a role in generalized OA and in the development of osteophytes in the distal (DIP) and proximal (PIP) interphalangeal (IP) joints (Heberden's and Bouchard's nodes). Women have a much greater incidence of polyarticular OA than men do, which suggests some hormonal mediation. OA has a reverse association with osteoporosis, which is demonstrated by hip joint studies that consistently report that elderly patients with hip OA are at lower risk for sustaining femoral neck fractures (Cooper, 1994).

Generalized ligamentous laxity with consequent joint hypermobility, albeit within the range of normal, affects a substantial portion of healthy persons. Such hypermobility diminishes throughout childhood and continues to do so more slowly in later years. Women are more mobile than men are, and Asians are more mobile than whites. Generalized joint laxity is a feature of several rare inherited disorders of collagen (e.g., Ehlers-Danlos syndrome). Hypermobility without identifiable collagen gene defects may result in various overuse lesions and certainly OA. This has been documented in OA of the basal thumb joint (Jonsson & Valtysdottir, 1995).

Aging and OA

Common misconceptions about OA are listed in Box 1. There is nearly universal evidence of some cartilage damage in persons more than 65 years of age. Subchondral bony reaction and osteophytes were noted in the knees of 60% of men and 70% of women who died in the seventh and eighth decades of life, most of whom had no symptoms (Stankovic, Mitrovic, & Ryckewaert, 1980). Figure 1 illustrates the relationship of age with OA joint involvement. Age is a major determinant in the prevalence of OA at the following sites: the DIP and PIP joints of the hands, first carpometacarpal (CMC) joint of the thumb, cervical spine, lumbar spine, hip, knee, and first metatarsophalangeal (MTP) joint. The most frequently involved joint sites in older persons are the DIP joints of the hands followed by the first MTP joint of the foot; the knee and hip are much less frequently involved. Table 2 lists characteristics of OA versus the aging process.

Box 1
OA Myths and Reality

Myths and Misconceptions

- OA is a consequence of chronological age.
- OA is secondary to wear and tear.
- Cartilage cannot heal and repair itself.
- Chondrocytes are effete cells that cannot replicate or change rates of synthesis and degradation of cartilage macromolecules.

Reality

Aging

Although OA is a disease of increasing prevalence with advancing years, a cause-and-effect relationship cannot be assumed; in fact, the concept of aging is an elusive one. One idea is that aging is, in effect, a disease caused by the cumulative acquisition of injuries to tissues that ultimately leads to loss of structure and later function. Another belief is that aging is a genetically determined process by which all living materials, at varying rates, deteriorate with time. A third notion is that aging is some combination of both mechanisms. Table 2 lists characteristics of aging compared with those of OA, with few features in common.

Wear and Tear

In the strictest sense, OA is not a wear-and-tear phenomenon. Mammalian joints, if initially normal and not subjected to grossly excessive loads or other damaging circumstances, cannot be worn out. The lubrication is so efficient that there is almost no shearing force. Wear cannot occur unless there are shearing forces operating between two surfaces. The coefficient of friction is that of

ice on ice, or fivefold lower than the lowest coefficient of friction devised by lubrication engineers with ball bearings and oil. The joint is an efficient piece of machinery.

Cartilage Cannot Heal Itself

Although poorly responsive to trauma, there is hard evidence that healing of cartilage lesions can and does occur. The new cartilage may be a mix of fibrocartilage and hyaline cartilage. The distal end of the bone has increased turnover, and even the uninvolved contralateral bone has increased metabolism. With the burgeoning knowledge of hyaline cartilage physiology and cell biology, how to arrest and reverse the process is better understood.

Chondrocyte Microbiology

The chondrocyte is sometimes thought of as an effete cell. The chondrocyte is anything but effete because it is metabolically active and responds to mechanical, endocrine, biochemical, and microenvironmental stimuli with increased rates of synthesis of proteoglycans, type 2 collagen, and degradative enzymes. Chondrocytes do not normally divide after puberty, but with appropriate stimuli such as a change in the microenvironment or OA, the cells form clones or brood clusters (OA). One could say that chondrocytes have no sex after Bar Mitzvah.

OA Is Thought To Be Inexorably Progressive

The course of OA frequently remits spontaneously. With careful surgical planning, OA of the hip can be arrested and at least partially reversed.

Pathogenesis

The most prominent early (although not necessarily the first) change is seen in the articular cartilage and is characterized by a decrease in both proteoglycan content and state of aggregation and an increase in water content. There is a decrease in chondroitin sulfate chain links and a change in glycosaminoglycan composition. At the cellular level, the chondrocyte, a normally amitotic cell, divides to form clones (brood clusters) of cells (Figures 2a and 2b). The chondrocyte increases its normal synthesis of proteoglycans and type 2 collagen by two- to fourfold in an apparent attempt to reverse the matrix depletion. There is augmented DNA–RNA turnover and increased enzyme synthesis. The increased

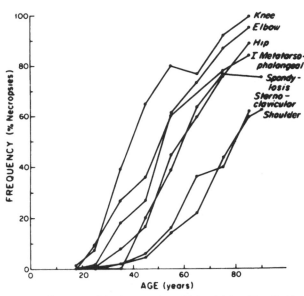

Figure 1. Note the striking increase in multiple OA joints identified by a pathologist appearing as early as 15 years of age and becoming universal after 60 years of age. Figure courtesy of John Bland, MD.

chondrocyte synthesis of matrix elements continues as the disease progresses until a stage is reached where tissue changes are advanced and synthesis fails. At the tissue level, the cartilage loses its smooth texture, becomes fibrillated, and develops clefts and crevices at first tangential to the surface and later vertical to it that extend down to and through the subchondral bone (Sledge, Sternberg, & Tsukamoto, 1981). Joint surfaces lose their congruity (Figure 3).

Before, during, or after the changes in articular cartilage, the subchondral bone undergoes a proliferative process. The bony proliferation occurs primarily at the joint margins and floor of the cartilage lesions. The proliferation appears to be an attempt to increase the area available for load bearing, but it has the undesirable effects of decreasing compliance and increasing the stiffness of

Table 2. Osteoarthritis Versus Aging

Osteoarthritis	Aging
Highly anabolic and synthetic process	Normal metabolism
Enzymatic destruction of hard tissue	Normal enzymatic remodeling
Remodeling of all tissues joints (articular and periarticular)	Cartilage changes only
Chondrocyte mitosis	No mitosis
Intense increased synthesis (collagen)	Normal rates of synthesis (collagen and proteoglycan)
Increased water content in cartilage	No change
Fibrillation is focal and progressive (non–weight-bearing sites)	Fibrillation is not progressive (weight-bearing sites)
Eburnation (ivory-like)	No eburnation
Osteophytes occur with other changes	Osteophytes occur only with excessive use
No increased collagen X link	Increased collagen X link
Inflammation	No inflammation
No pigment (cartilage)	Pigment (cartilage)

Box 2
Osteoarthritis in Phylogenesis and Evolution

Evidently, OA has accompanied humankind throughout its evolutionary history, and a similar, if not precisely the same, process occurs in other animals that fuse their epiphyses as they reach adulthood (Hutton, 1987). The process of OA has been shown to occur in reptiles, in many bird species, whales, dinosaurs, rodents, many domestic animals (dogs, livestock) and wild animals (foxes, wolves, lions, and tigers). Strangely enough, two animals that hang upside down, bats and sloths, do not develop OA (Sokoloff, 1969). (No therapeutic implications should be deduced from this.) The paleopathology of joint disease has intrigued researchers since 1895 when Virchow described spinal osteophytosis and other skeletal abnormalities in the cave bears of Bonn (as cited in Kaiser, 1962). As far as we know, OA has not been identified in invertebrate animals, but we should remain prepared for a surprise some day.

This phylogenetic preservation, absence of symptoms and structural change, biosynthetic activity (at the tissue level, chondrocyte, osteocyte, and synoviocyte activities increase at certain phases of the process, and cell division and biosynthesis are marked), and most commonly a satisfactory clinical outcome strongly suggest that OA is indicative of an inherent, genetically determined repair process of synovial joints. In most cases, this metabolically active process keeps pace with various triggering insults and is not progressive; this capability of healing can be quite marked and clinically impressive (Bland, 1997; Bland & Cooper, 1984).

Of course, sometimes there is a failure to compensate that results in joint failure or perhaps so-called "decompensated OA," with definite symptoms and disability. Such interpretation, at least in some part, explains the marked heterogeneity of OA, which involves a wide variety of insults triggering a repair reaction (OA) with each resulting in a different pattern of involvement. As with comparable biological processes, many constitutional or intrinsic and environmental factors may operate to modify the response, which results in a variable outcome. Factors related to initiation and progression of OA may differ, different factors operate at different joint sites, and complex interaction between factors is probable (Doherty, 1994).

For example, a total lateral meniscectomy grossly changes normal knee biomechanics and is a predictable well-recognized predisposing factor for OA of the knee. However, not all patients develop postmeniscectomy OA even with such a severe mechanical insult. Thus, this seems to be an insufficient cause of OA. A higher frequency and severity of postmeniscectomy OA in persons predisposed to the (genetic) development of generalized OA supports interaction between local or mechanical factors and systems or constitutional factors in its development (Doherty, Watt, & Dieppe, 1983).

Another illustrative interaction is noted in Blount's disease, in which only a small number of patients develop knee OA in later life, even though they have severe bilateral varus deformities (Zayer, 1980). There are seemingly myriad studies investigating occupational and recreational trauma,

continued on next page

the subchondral bone. The more brittle subchondral bone is, the more prone it is to develop microfractures. This results in new callus formation and more microfractures. Osteophytes develop, and subluxations and joint instability follow (Figure 4).

Synovial proliferation and active synovitis appear. Synovial cells at the periphery become metaplastic and, in some instances, produce osteophytes (a mix of bone covered with hyaline-like cartilage and fibrocartilage). All local elements in and about the joint hypertrophy, including capsule, ligaments, tendons, muscles, bursae, and bones. Figure 5 demonstrates extensive remodeling of the bone end and the connective tissues about it.

The clinical correlates to this are pain, stiffness, and restricted motion. The inflammatory components result in heat, redness, and swelling and may exaggerate bony prolifera-

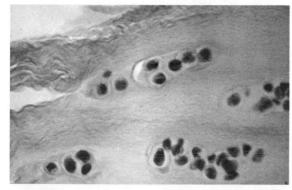

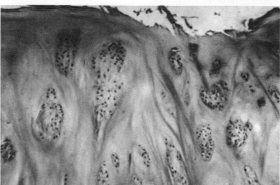

Figure 2. (A): Brood clusters or clones formed as chondrocytes begin mitotic activity in OA. Note the shredding of the hyaline cartilage. (B): The cartilage surface has lost its smooth surface texture, becomes fibrillated, and develops clefts and fissures. The cloning is somewhat more advanced than that in 2A. Photos courtesy of John Bland, MD.

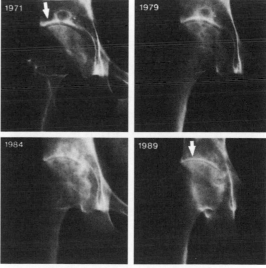

Figure 3. OA of the right hip in a male runner 34 years of age. Note the increased density of subchondral bone (*arrow*, 1971) and a well-formed subchondral cyst. The patient was in a vigorous treatment program, improved materially from 1971 to 1989, and continued with active exercise but changed his sport from marathons to race walking. Photo courtesy of John Bland, MD.

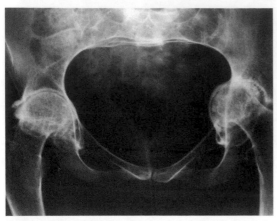

Figure 4. Bilateral OA of both hips in a woman 63 years of age. Marked osteophytes have developed, joint space is narrow, and unfortunately the femurs are pushing the acetabulum into the pelvic cavity (acetabular protrusio) with medial migration of both femoral heads (an unusual but not rare event). Photo courtesy of John Bland, MD.

tion and cartilage erosion. Joint destruction is the endpoint. Table 3 lists the four steps in the pathophysiology of OA.

In OA, the forces of synthesis and degradation obviously are operating in tandem. Unchecked, the process proceeds to an imbalance of these forces and joint destruction. The keys to arresting or reversing the process are the usual slow rate of progression and the evidence that the tissues involved are capable of repair. In fact, OA seems to be a manifestation of repair processes. Much of the pathophysiology is the result of this vigorous, although inadequate, attempt at repair. The goal is to ablate, arrest, or reverse the metabolic cascade responsible for joint destruction without adversely compromising other cellular functions.

This summary of the molecular and tissue cellular events in OA represents a current formulation of pathophysiology. It is important to recognize that, regardless of the initiating or primary event, the joint undergoes changes that result in a characteristic endpoint, which we have operationally and clinically defined as OA. The precise sequence of the changes and their relationship to one another is subject to debate. We must emphasize that the course may arrest at any point, may continue on to gross joint destruction, or may reverse itself at least to some measurable degree. The earlier that therapy is begun, the greater the chance for reversal by the mechanisms of normal pathophysiology.

Diagnosis

Because OA resembles more a process that can be triggered by many constitutional and environmental factors than a disease, attempts to define and classify OA as a single disease entity have not been useful. Modern trends have been to separate OA into more homogeneous groupings or subsets, to define etiological factors, and to determine natural history and prognosis.

Table 3. Four Steps in the Pathophysiology of Osteoarthritis

> 1. The microenvironment of the chondrocyte changes: chondrocytes mitose and produce clones that increase rates of all export products, proteoglycans, collagen, and enzymes.
>
> 2. Subchondral bone osteoblasts increase rates of synthesis, density of subchondral bone increases, stiffness increases, and microfractures follow.
>
> 3. Osteophytes form at the periphery of the joint (metaplastic synovial cells), and there is active inflammatory process and synovitis.
>
> 4. Pseudocysts form in trabecular bone below subchondral bone; there is increased volume and density in all articular and periarticular structures, capsules, tendons, ligaments, and bones.

First, patients should be classified by their disease subset (Table 1) (Altman, 1995) to identify patients with primary (idiopathic) OA versus patients with OA related to or secondary to another disease. Second, criteria must be applied to separate this group of patients from those with other forms of arthritis (Table 4) (Altman, 1995; Altman et. al., 1986). The differential diagnoses for OA include gout, calcium pyrophosphate deposition disease (CPPD) (pseudogout), low-grade sepsis, seronegative RA, metabolic disorders, hydroxyapatite crystal diseases, and cholesterol crystal deposition. (Figure 6) Osteophytes alone, without structural or joint space changes, do not indicate OA; they appear to be part of normal aging and are without clinical importance. Patterns of joint involvement are the same all over the world and have shown little or no change since observers began to subdivide causes of arthritis (Simkin, 1995; Van de Putte, 1995).

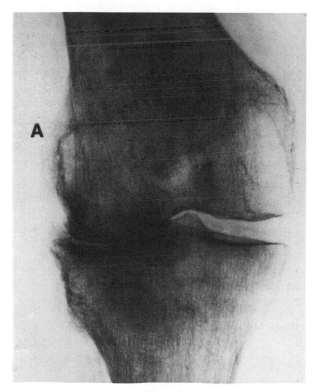

Figure 5. OA of the knee involving only the medial compartment with striking joint space narrowing and extensive remodeling of all surrounding tissues. Photo courtesy of John Bland, MD

Table 4. Classification of Osteoarthritis of the Knee, Hip, and Hand Based on Clinical Examination With Radiographs (Altmanetal, 1986)

Knee

Knee (articular and not periarticular or referred) pain for most days of the previous month

plus

Radiographic osteophytes at tibiofemoral joint margins

or

Synovial fluid (two of three of the following: clear, viscous, white blood cell count less than 2,000 cells/mm [more than 40 years of age counts as one criteria if synovial fluid is not available])

Morning stiffness of the knee for >30 min

Crepitus on active motion of the knee

Hip

Hip (articular and not periarticular or referred) pain for most days of the previous month

plus

At least two of the following three:

- ESR 20 mm/hr
- Radiographic femoral or acetabular osteophytes
- Radiographic hip joint space narrowing

Hand

Hand pain, aching, or stiffness

and

3 or 4 of the following features:

Hard-tissue enlargement of 2 or more of 10 selected joints

Hard-tissue enlargement of 2 or more DIP joints

Fewer than 3 swollen MCP joints†

Deformity of at least 1 of 10 selected joints*

---

*Second and third DIP joints, second and third PIP joints, and first CMC (trapeziometacarpal) joint in both hands.

†MCP joint swelling must be consistent with other OA findings.

Note: ESR=erythrocyte sedimentation rate, MCP=metacarpophalangeal, DIP=distal interphalangeal, PIP=proximal interphalangeal

Primary Versus Secondary OA

The term *primary OA* refers to the classic, localized idiopathic involvement of the finger DIP and PIP joints and to a condition of generalized primary OA that occurs in the hands and weight-bearing joints at the same time. Although it is possible to develop primary OA of the hips, knees, and spine, this distinction is usually not made because, by the time a patient seeks treatment, it is not possible to discern whether it is primary or secondary to altered alignment or other factors.

Course and Prognosis

Clinicians often mistakenly regard OA as a common (indeed universal) slowly progressive disorder occurring in mid to later life that primarily affects weight-bearing, peripheral, and axial joints and is clinically characterized by pain, deformity, limitation of motion, and inexorable progressive disability. Until recently, reversal or even arrest of the process was rarely considered. Currently, prognosis includes a broad spectrum from the disappearance of symptoms, to partial reversal, to simply reaching an asymptomatic state without much change in clinical and radiological characteristics.

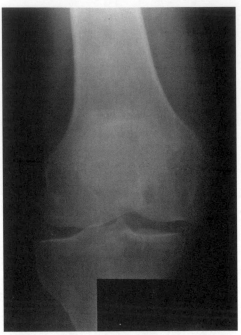

Figure 6. An example of osteoarthritis developing secondary to calcium pyrophosphate dihydrate crystal deposition in the hyaline cartilage of the knee; note densities of the crystals in both compartments.

Joint Immobilization Effects: Partial and Total

An immobilized healthy joint will develop cartilage changes similar to those of OA and is referred to as an *immobilization arthropathy* (Akeson, Woo, Amiel, & Frank 1984). In both OA and immobilization arthropathies, the cartilage shows fibrillation, flaking, fissuring, and overall thinning. In OA, however, the chondrocytes proliferate in clones or brood clusters and overproduce their macromolecules. In an immobilized joint, the chondrocytes degenerate and die within a relatively short time, which suggests that they require mechanical stimulation to survive. OA develops over years, whereas immobilization arthropathy is characterized by an acute onset, presumably due to the abrupt alteration of joint function. Immobilization arthropathies are most likely a consequence of nutritional failure. Avascular cartilage, which behaves like a water-filled sponge, releases fluid on compression and reabsorbs it on release of pressure. Alternating compression and reexpansion allows the supply of nutrients and the removal of metabolic waste products. Thus, immobilization and mobility (relative or absolute) profoundly affect the health and well-being of the hyaline cartilage and the chondrocyte.

These physiological data may be effectively applied clinically. The immobilized joint, even for relatively short periods, shows a proliferation of fibro-fatty tissue that fills the joint and grows over the cartilage surface. This tissue has some of the same characteristics of the pannus of RA and ultimately erodes the cartilage by enzymatic degradation. Even slight movement of the joint will slow the process. Compression, in addition to immobilization, accelerates the process. The rate of synthesis of proteoglycan markedly decreases in 3 weeks in immobilized dog knees (Akeson et al., 1984). The proteoglycan aggregates (with hyaluronate) are no longer formed in the cartilage and do not aggregate normally with exogenous hyaluronate. On return to use and weight bearing, proteoglycan aggregation returns to normal, which is an important clinical point. However, increased water content and loss of aggregability of proteoglycans did not return to normal when the animals were subjected to vigorous exercise versus normal weight bearing. Vigorous treadmill exercise resulted in continued thinning of cartilage, decreased uronic acid content, and abnormal Safranin O staining, even though net proteoglycan synthesis increased. This suggests that immobilized cartilage is vulnerable to loading and that excessive exercise at that point could accelerate the OA sequence (Akeson et al., 1984).

Drug Therapy

Pain is the primary reason that patients with OA seek treatment. The common use of nonsteroidal anti-inflammatory drugs (NSAIDs) for OA is now considered a mistake. The American College of Rheumatology (ACR) guidelines for management of OA recommend adequate doses of analgesics such as acetaminophen (Tylenol) as the first drug of choice (Hochberg et al., 1995). OA symptoms often are episodic, and if NSAIDs are used, their use should be evaluated routinely, particularly in elderly patients. There is no convincing evidence that these drugs alter the progression of OA in humans. In fact, a hastening of progression, especially by indomethacin, has been suggested. A new line of NSAIDs has been introduced called cyclooxygenase-2 (COX-2) inhibitors (e.g., Celebrex), which selectively inhibit only the prostaglandins that mediate inflammation and do not affect the prostaglandins that protect the stomach lining and kidneys. These may offer new options for patients at risk for gastrointestinal ulcers with typical NSAIDs.

OA is not a simple wear-and-tear phenomenon; rather, it is an active process that is part of the reparative response to injury. Thus, it is reasonable to postulate that such a process may be manipulated to produce beneficial or detrimental effects on joint function and symptoms. This concept has developed into an interest in *chondroprotective* and *chondrodestructive* agents that may beneficially or adversely affect the OA process. Use of "chondro" to describe such agents reflects the current emphasis on cartilage, which may not be totally appropriate. Joints are complex organs, and their successful function is not simply the consequence of a single tissue but rather of all tissues about the joint. Perhaps "arthroprotective" would be more descriptive.

Intra-articular corticosteroid therapy is considered an adjunctive measure, a component modality that may be included in a comprehensive management program. Indications for its use include the following.

- To provide pain relief and suppress the inflammatory synovitis
- Provide adjunctive therapy for one or two joints that are not responsive to other systemic therapy

- To facilitate a rehabilitation program or orthopedic procedure
- To prevent capsular and ligamentous laxity (e.g., in a large joint effusion)
- To bring about a medical synovectomy
- To treat acute effusions occurring with associated crystal deposition disease

Physical or occupational therapists may refer the patient back to the physician if a physician's judgment is needed in one or more of these indications.

Psychosocial Factors and Patient Adherence

In most textbooks and patient publications, OA is often distinguished from RA as the "noncrippling" form of arthritis. In fact, many persons (especially elderly patients) are profoundly disabled by OA. In a 1972 study, OA was the second most common condition (after ischemic heart disease) qualifying persons for Social Security disability insurance (Weinberger, Tierney, & Booher, 1989). Loss of mobility, function, and independence has an effect on the person's personality, self-esteem, identity, and role in society.

Gross (1981) described how patients with OA react to their losses, similar to cancer patients, in the stages identified by Kubler-Ross, including denial, anger, bargaining, depression, and acceptance. However, patients with OA differ from terminally ill patients in that the fluidity between the stages is more marked. If OA progresses and its effect on function increases, the sense of loss continues. The stages of emotional adjustment to loss may be repeated and extend for many years.

Patients' emotional responses to OA can certainly influence their desire to know more about the disease and to follow through with medications, exercise, use of a cane, or joint protection techniques. The challenge is to evaluate the patient's response to OA, tailor the therapeutic intervention to meet his or her needs, and help the patient move closer to positive instead of passive acceptance. One way is to include a global inquiry in the initial evaluation such as "How has the OA affected your life? Has it affected your relationship with your spouse or other people?" This offers patients an opportunity to talk about the effects of OA on their lives. The response provides the clinician with an opportunity to evaluate how well the patient is handling the condition both psychologically and physically.

There is increased interest in the role of psychosocial variables and how they alter pain perception and reporting in patients with OA, especially because severity of pain correlates only weakly with radiographic evidence. These variables may explain why coping skills training and self-management training programs are often as effective or more effective in reducing the symptoms of OA than pharmacological intervention (Creamer & Hochberg, 1998).

Several studies have demonstrated that self-report, when implemented in a nonthreatening manner, can provide a valid estimate of noncompliance (Morisky, Green, & Levine, 1986; Weinberger et al., 1989). When patients do not follow through with appointments, home exercise, or other treatment recommendations, the clinician should explore psychological factors such as denial, depression, and anger (either passive-aggressive or overt) and address them. Sometimes a patient's emotional reactions can cause "selective hearing," and he or she may have distorted the instructions. Instructing the patient in a manner that puts the patient in control often improves compliance and functional outcome. Keefe and associates (1987) evaluated the effectiveness of teaching pain coping skills to persons with OA of the knee and found that patients who demonstrated a sense of control over their pain and a rational thinking style experienced less functional impairment.

Calfas, Kaplan, and Ingram (1992) compared the effectiveness of 10-week courses of cognitive behavioral intervention with didactic OA education in improving function, quality of life, and depression. For a 1-year period, the two approaches were found to be equivalent. Memory and retention are closely related to attention. If patients are restless from sitting too long or are uncomfortable or distracted by clinic activities, give them a break to stretch or a glass of water or move them to a more comfortable chair or a quieter part of the clinic. Try to get their full attention before teaching them their home program, and give them a written version of the home program.

Sometimes it helps patients to identify their anger toward OA and how they may be turning it against themselves by not complying with treatment. It is hard to be good to your joints if you hate your arthritis. One technique that may be helpful is to point out that part of the body is working to control and eliminate the inflammation and that they should nurture and support these healthy parts of their bodies. This offers them a paradigm for fighting the arthritis but not fighting their bodies.

Clinical Features

General Symptoms

Some symptoms are common to all forms of OA and may occur in any combination. They include

- joint pain particularly with functional use, secondary muscle aching, spasm, or muscle inhibition;
- aching in the joints during cold weather (considered a response to changes in barometric pressure);
- stiffness after prolonged (15–30 min) static positioning (referred to as "gelling" or "gel phenomenon");
- crepitation on motion;
- limited joint motion and joint deformity due to osteophyte formation or cartilage loss;
- muscle weakness and atrophy as a result of disuse; and
- joint inflammation effusions, which even if minimal can cause impairment (Bland & Stulberg, 1985; Dieppe, 1994).

The most probable causes of joint stiffness include low-grade inflammation, effusion, synovial thickening, muscle shortening, or spasm. Some patients misinterpret limited range of motion (ROM) secondary to osteophytes as stiffness.

Pain in OA

In OA, the process of the cartilage degeneration and osteophytosis may cause mild stiffness or decreased ROM but generally is painless. Pain is primarily associated with inflammation even if there are no obvious signs such as swelling, redness, or warmth. Even mild effusions can cause disproportionate disability. Pain can result from impingement or stretching of the sensitive capsule over a sharp osteophyte. Weight bearing on thin cartilage can transfer pressure to sensory nerves in the subchondral bone. Pain may originate from periostitis, the sites of bony remodeling, subchondral microfractures, periarticular muscle spasm, bone angina due to decreased blood flow, and elevated intraosseus pressure (Altman & Dean, 1989). For many patients, pain amplification from fibromyalgia, depression, anxiety, or poor sleep plays a major role in their experience of pain (Dieppe, 1994; Moldofsky, Lue, & Saskin, 1987).

Rehabilitation

The purpose of occupational therapy and physical therapy is to evaluate functional performance and to teach patients how to self-manage their OA. Self-management includes eliminating aggravating factors; reducing stiffness, pain, and inflammation; maintaining ROM; maintaining or increasing muscle strength; restoring muscle balance; reducing joint stress; and increasing functional independence. The goal is that, when patients leave therapy, they will know how to manage pain and symptoms and prevent reoccurrences when possible (Boutaugh & Brady, 1998). In addition, it is important that patients are aware of community resources that are available to help them maintain or achieve goals (Haralson-Ferrell, 1998) (Box 3).

Hand Involvement

In the past, OA was described as typically affecting the IP joints and thumb trapezial-metacarpal (or CMC) joint. These are the joints that tend to be the most symptomatic. But osteophytosis can occur at the metacarpophalangeal (MCP) joints (where they can contribute to flexor tendon triggering), in the wrist and intercarpal joints (where they cause limited motion and pain with wrist motion), and over the volar aspect of the thumb (Buckland-Wright, Macfarlane, & Lynch, 1991; Moratz, Muncie, & Miranda-Walsh, 1986). Several studies on hand involvement have shown that women often have greater symptoms, more DIP involvement, and more generalized OA than men (Carmen, 1989; Moratz et al., 1986).

In the hand, osteophytes at the DIP joint are named after a British physician and are termed *Heberden's nodes*. At the PIP joint, osteophytes are named after a French physician and are termed *Bouchard's nodes*. Osteophytes are characteristic of OA at these joints and therefore correlate with cartilage loss and are diagnostic of primary OA.

OA in the joints of the thumb may be either primary or secondary. OA most commonly occurs in the CMC joint, and it may be the first or the only symptomatic joint. OA can affect the three other trapezial joints, and this is referred to as *pantrapezial arthritis* or *STT* (scaphoid-trapezium-trapezoid) *arthritis*. It is possible to have pantrapezial arthritis with only the CMC joint symptomatic. Inflammation and pain secondary to functional use can occur in adults at any age,

---

Box 3
Resources

Organization Resources

The Arthritis Foundation
1330 West Peachtree Street
Atlanta, GA 30309
404-872-7100 or 1-800-283-7800
Internet address: www.arthritis.org

This organization provides an excellent booklet on OA, self-management techniques, and specific medications at no charge; aquatic and land-based exercise classes and the Arthritis Self-Management Course nationwide; and a free health video lending library in some chapters. The Arthritis Foundation can refer patients to rheumatologists.

The Arthritis Society
National Office
250 Bloor Street East
Suite 901
Toronto, ON M4W 3P2 Canada
416-967-1414 or 416-967-7171(fax)
Internet address: www.arthritis.ca

This organization offers specialized patient care programs, recreational exercise programs, resource libraries, and consumer education materials.

Internet Resources

Searching "osteoarthritis" on the Internet brings up an extensive array of resources and sales pitches, unproven remedies, and misinformation (11,262 listings). "HOTBOT" is one of the best search directories for information on diseases.

- Arthritis Foundation and The Arthritis Society both have Web sites (see addresses above).

- The Amazon Bookstore (www.amazon.com) is the easiest online bookseller to search. There are five current self-help books on OA.

- Abledata is a national database for adaptive equipment and assistive devices (www.abledata.com).

- One Step Ahead News (www.osanews.com) is the Web's online news magazine for persons with disabilities and provides excellent links to other sites related to coping with disabilities, including one on Americans With Disabilities Act (www.osanews.com/Links/ada.htm).

Product Resources

Aris Isotoner Gloves
11 Cayadutta Street
Gloversville, NY 12078

Beiersdorf, Inc. (formerly Futuro, Inc.)
P.O. Box 5529
Norwalk, CT 06856-5529
1-800-933-0214

3M Company (Minnesota Mining & Manufacturing Company)
3M General Office
Mail Stop 224-5M-38
St. Paul, MN 55144
1-800-328-1063, 1-612-737-9587, or 1-800-446-4516

but OA in the CMC joint tends to occur in women more than 40 years of age who have joint laxity and often a shallow dorsal radial facet of the trapezium (Dray & Jablon, 1987; Jonsson & Valtysdottir, 1995).

Anticipation and apprehension of hand pain during functional activities can result in muscular guarding that extends up the entire extremity into the neck. About one third of the patients referred to one author (J.M.) for CMC joint splints have demonstrated cervical tension or pain secondary to muscular guarding of the limb to protect the thumb.

Erosive OA is a less frequent generalized subset of OA characterized by aggressive synovitis, joint erosion, and ankylosis typically of the DIP and PIP joints. Radiographic changes are more similar to RA than to primary OA; however, these patients test negative for Rh factor and have normal sedimentation rates. Often this form of OA tends to subside over months or years and leaves residual deformity (Cooper, 1994).

In the hand, the most common symptoms are pain, stiffness, and tenderness, and the classic signs are bony enlargement, limited motion, or deformity. Pain typically results from inflammation, capsule irritation over an osteophyte, instability, and strain on a capsule. Another source of pain in the digit joints is mucous cysts that appear as a soft mass over the dorsum of the joint and connect to the joint through a pedicle. They can become inflamed and exacerbate osteophyte formation (Dieppe, 1994).

Deformity takes several forms in the hand.

- Bony enlargement of the joints
- Angulation deformity resulting from asymmetrical cartilage degeneration or asymmetrical osteophytosis
- Mallet finger deformity resulting from attrition of the distal attachment of the extensor communis tendon over osteophytes
- Classic thumb deformity of CMC joint adduction, MCP hyperextension (or lateral deviation), and IP joint flexion. First metacarpal adduction produces a characteristic "squaring" of the joint (Swanson & de Groot-Swanson, 1985).
- Loss of digit flexion results from volar joint osteophytosis, and lost of extension results from dorsal osteophytosis. Wrist ROM may likewise be limited (Moratz et al., 1986). This is generally considered a limitation rather than a deformity.

Early signs and symptoms of CMC joint inflammation include tenderness, aching, throbbing, and crepitation. If inflammation is moderate to severe, swelling, redness, and warmth may be present. Pain can radiate distally down the thumb or proximally up the forearm similar to deQuervain's tenosynovitis. Symptoms of CMC joint arthritis are aggravated by repetitive pinch, grasp, or twisting prehension activities and nonprehension application of force with the heel of the hand or thenar area (e.g., stapling paper or squeezing oranges).

Evaluation

Evaluation of the hand with OA should include both active and passive ROM. Affected joints with a hard "endfeel" at the end of range indicate that motion is limited by osteophytes or bony blockage. If there is a lag or difference between active and passive ROM, the cause must be ascertained and treated.

The main differential diagnosis for CMC joint OA is deQuervain's tenosynovitis of the first dorsal compartment because of the similarities of pain patterns. There are two assessments that can distinguish the difference between these two conditions. The grind test (metacarpal compression and rotation) is a specific test for localizing pain or crepitus to the CMC joint, and the Finklestein test (full thumb flexion and wrist ulnar deviation) is a specific test for localizing pain in the first dorsal tendon compartment. It is critical to differentiate between these two conditions because the design and function of prescribed hand splints is different for each condition. (See volume 4, chapter 8, of this series for a description of the these tests.)

In only one study of OA in the hands were the patients systematically evaluated by an occupational therapist (Moratz et al., 1986). This evaluation of 77 patients revealed that 39% had complaints related to tendon involvement including crepitus (32%), triggering (12%), and locking (4%). In addition, wrist ROM was limited in all planes: 60% in flexion, 44% in extension, 49% in ulnar deviation, and 32% in radial deviation.

Evaluation of the OA hand should include evaluation of pain during ROM and strength testing, at rest, with motion, with palpation, and during function; swelling and inflammation; tendon pain, lag, triggering, and crepitus; stiffness; ROM (active, passive, and lag); grind test; Finklestein test; function and disability; and current self-management strategies.

Treatment of Inflammation and Pain

Moratz et al. (1986) reported that disability was associated more with pain than limited motion or strength, and this corroborates experience in the clinic. The focus of hand therapy for OA is the reduction of pain, inflammation, and stiffness and the adaptation or compensation for loss of ROM to maintain function.

If a DIP joint becomes so painful that it interferes with hand function, a rigid, custom-molded thermoplastic cylinder orthosis or a tripoint splint that blocks flexion (made from 1/16-in. material) can effectively reduce pain and improve overall hand function by allowing the patient to use the hands without fear of pain or trauma. For the PIP joint, rigid immobilization can be used for severe pain, but this is generally not an acceptable option for the patient because it limits hand function and can result in shortening of the collateral ligaments, which increases PIP joint stiffness.

For the CMC joint, a custom-fitted immobilization thermoplastic splint that provides a C-bar to stabilize the CMC joint in abduction but allows full thumb IP joint and wrist mobility can be effective in reducing inflammation. In a 3-month follow-up study of 28 patients who used this type of splint, 4 patients became pain-free after treatment, another 24 reported a notable reduction in pain, 7 were able to reduce or discontinue use of NSAIDs, and 24 (68%) used the orthosis to reduce pain during specific activities (Colditz & Melvin, in press; Melvin, 1989a). Any orthosis without a C-bar allows too much motion in the CMC joint. Pantrapezial OA requires a splint that immobilizes both the CMC joint and the wrist. Because splints of this type are designed to protect the joints, it is important to teach patients to relax during activities and let the splint do the work.

For inflammation of the CMC joint, cold modalities can be effective in reducing symptoms and are the recommended modality, but generally patients with inflammation of the PIP and DIP joints do not tolerate cold and prefer heat or no modality at all.

Corticosteroid injections may be indicated for acute inflammation. For the CMC joint, many hand surgeons and orthopedists believe that the best resolution of inflammation may be achieved with a combination of an injection and splint immobilization.

In the presence of major inflammation, swelling, or pain, a patient may not use the joint through full ROM, which results in a contracture of the collateral ligaments or capsule. Patients should be taught early that, if they lose mobility during a flare-up, they should see a practitioner to regain mobility when the inflammation subsides. Strengthening and muscle rebalancing should be delayed until the acute inflammation is resolved.

Joint protection for OA of the hand focuses on evaluating the daily activities that aggravate the joint and providing instruction in adaptive methods or assistive devices that can reduce pain and stress to the joint. For the CMC joint, the most stressful activities require a strong pinch and applying pressure with the heel of the hand (e.g., stapling).

The force and tension with which an activity is performed, rather than the activity itself, may be the primary aggravating factor. Some persons hold a pen lightly, and some hold it firmly, but all write. Many patients, especially women with CMC joint arthritis, may need to learn how to perform their activities with a lighter touch.

Many patients believe they have two options: give in to the arthritis or suffer through the pain. They must be taught that pain aggravates the arthritis, and performing activities without pain helps the arthritis. It is important to teach patients how to problem solve ways to reduce pain during activities. Have patients make a list of all the daily activities that cause pain and create solutions to those problems after they are taught the basic principles. (Joint protection, assistive technology, and adaptive methods specifically for the hand are discussed in volume 4 of this series.)

Treatment of Stiffness

For stiffness or mild inflammation in the PIP and DIP joints, there are some soft splint options. Seemless stretch-cotton tubular tan digit sleeves (medium size) that can be cut to length are comfortable, keep the joint warm, increase circulation, and can reduce pain and stiffness. They allow full motion but remind the person to use the digit carefully and are excellent to use at night because they can reduce nocturnal swelling and stiffness and are not as confining as gloves. Self-adhesive tape, such as Coban (3M Company, St. Paul, MN) can be used because it restricts motion slightly and reminds the patient to be cautious of the joint. The only drawback is that the tape becomes dirty after a few hours of wear. Another option (especially at night) is to wrap an inch-wide strip of plastic food wrap (4-in. long) firmly but not tightly around the joint. It self-adheres and keeps the joint warm, which increases comfort.

If excessive stiffness limits functional ability, use of Beiersdorf (formerly Futuro) thermoelastic gloves or Isotoner gloves (Box 3) at night has been shown to reduce morning stiffness (Culic,

Battaglia, Wichman, & Schmid, 1979; McKnight & Kwoh, 1992). Because OA usually is a bilateral condition, the patient can apply the above treatments to one hand and use the other as a control. This way, patients can determine whether the treatment actually works. Squeezing a soft foam ball in warm water in the morning can be quite helpful in decreasing stiffness. Self-evaluation with a visual analog scale can be helpful for evaluating and reporting the effectiveness of these interventions (e.g., "The patient rated PIP pain 9/10 without a sleeve and 5/10 with a sleeve").

One study (Garfinkel, Schumacher, Hsain, Levy, & Reshetar, 1994) demonstrated that a yoga regimen combined with patient education for 10 weekly sessions was effective for reducing pain and tenderness and improving ROM in the hands of patients with symptomatic OA. Patients in a control group did not receive treatment other than medication and showed no notable improvement.

Compensation for Limited ROM

For persons with limited finger flexion, reducing pain during activities is often accomplished by building up handles so that the person can exert force within available ROM. Patients with thumb adduction contractures may need handles narrowed to fit their limited web space.

Surgery

For DIP or thumb IP joints with chronic pain or with severe flexion or angulation deformity, surgical arthrodesis in about 5° of flexion provides an effective functional and cosmetic solution and eliminates the problem of mucoidal cysts. Arthroplasty may be appropriate for selected cases but generally is not recommended for the DIP joints. For PIP joints with severe pain or deformity of one or two digits, an implant arthroplasty is a possible solution. If a person performs hard physical work, arthrodesis of the index finger PIP joint in 20° to 40° flexion may be the preferred operation with an implant arthroplasty of the remaining PIP joints.

For the CMC joint that is persistently painful despite conservative measures, or if deformity limits function, surgical options include resection arthroplasty of the CMC joint with or without a condylar implant or resection arthroplasty of the entire trapezium with a trapezium implant or "anchovy" tendon spacer (Swanson & de Groot-Swanson, 1985).

Lower-Extremity Joint Involvement

The knee is the most commonly affected weight-bearing joint, with the hip joint a close second. The first MTP joint is commonly involved. The hindfoot joints can be affected. The ankle joint is rarely involved except after trauma. Secondary OA of the knee joint usually occurs after injury to the medial collateral and anterior cruciate ligaments and the medial and lateral meniscal cartilage (Noyes, Matthews, Mooar, & Grood, 1983). However, persons with postural malalignment, ligamentous instability, and abnormal joint movement (hypermobility) that is not injury related are candidates for premature OA of the knee joint (Cooke, Dwosh, & Cossairt, 1983; Howell, Woessner, Jimenez, Seda, & Schumacher, 1979; McDermott & Freyne, 1983).

OA of the hip frequently results from abnormal hip joint alignment that alters the wear on the articular cartilage and produces incongruent surfaces with cartilage thinning and abnormal bone growth (Jerring, 1980). Other causes of secondary OA (Table 1) may occur in persons in their twenties who had hip dysplasia during childhood or avascular necrosis of the femoral epiphyses (Legg-Calve-Perthes disease). Slipped capital femoral epiphysis can occur in children 10 to 15 years of age and result in secondary OA in the fifth or sixth decades (Catterall, 1981).

OA of the ankle is similar to that of the knee (i.e., in most cases, the degenerative process occurs after severe joint injury with ligamentous damage). Sports associated with an increased incidence of knee, hip, and ankle OA are noncontact sports such as ballet (Washington, 1978), gymnastics (Murray & Duncan, 1971), and running (Lane, Bloch, Jones, Marshall, & Wood, 1986) and contact sports such as football (Vincelette, Laurin, & Levesque, 1972), rugby (Hughston, 1962), and soccer (Klunder, Rud, & Hansen, 1980). A study of 350 college football players found a 90% incidence of foot and ankle OA versus only 4% to 5% for age-matched control subjects (Vincelette et al., 1972).

The first MTP joint is a prime site for OA that may contribute to hallux valgus and hallux rigidus, or OA may result secondary to these two conditions. Volar osteophytes may cause irritation to the sesamoid bones (sesamoiditis). OA can develop in the other MTP joints and in the IP joints in association with OA of the hand. OA of the subtalar joint is more common than in the ankle joint but is seldom a clinical problem. Osteophyte formation on the talonavicular, calcaneocuboid, and midtarsal joints may be associated with discomfort and stiffness around the hindfoot, which impairs gait and balance on uneven surfaces (Dieppe, 1994).

Symptoms

As ambulation and other activities involving weight bearing become painful, patient activity decreases (Hampson, Glasgow, & Zeiss, 1996). Inactivity and continuous afferent transmission of signals may lead to weakness of the quadricep, gastrocnemius, hip flexor, and gluteal muscles and a concomitant shortening of the hamstring, calf, and adductor muscles. In the early phase of lower-extremity OA, there is typically a decrease in muscle strength and dynamic balance that reduces a person's ability to perform functional activities such arising from a chair; getting out of a bed, bathtub, or car; going up and down steps and stairs; squatting to pick up objects; and walking a quarter mile and beyond (Felson, Naimark, & Anderson, 1987). In addition, falls may be more prevalent in patients with lower-extremity OA (Ekdahl & Andersson, 1989; Ekdahl, Jarnlo, & Andersson, 1989; Mathias, Nayak, & Isaacs, 1986).

In the knee joint, severe deformity primarily affecting the medial compartment can result in a varus or "bowlegged" appearance. Valgus or "knock-knee" deformities can occur but are more often seen in RA. In the hip joint, pain may become much greater because osteophyte growth limits joint motion. Hip joint extension contractures can result in the inability to flex the hips to 90°, thus limiting the ability to sit straight in a chair and consequently increasing strain on the back. Hip adduction contractures can result in the inability to separate the legs, thus interfering with the ability to urinate, perform hygiene, ambulate, or have sexual intercourse. Finally, hip flexion contractures can prevent the person from standing erect and result in knee flexion when standing. This impairs gait and encourages flexion contractures of the knee joint and the development of OA in the knee.

In the ankle, joint ROM declines, especially in dorsiflexion, and at the subtalar joint, eversion is frequently reduced. However, no soft-tissue deformities have been reported in the literature.

Surgery may be indicated when function is limited and the patient is unable to negotiate home, work, or community environments without a great deal of assistance because of pain or deformity. Options include osteotomy, total joint arthroplasty at the hip or knee, and fusion of the ankle joint. In addition, arthroscopic surgery can remove loose bodies and shave osteophytes that limit motion and cause pain in the knee and ankle with less risk and faster recovery than open surgery. (See volume 5, chapters 5–7, on hip, knee, and ankle

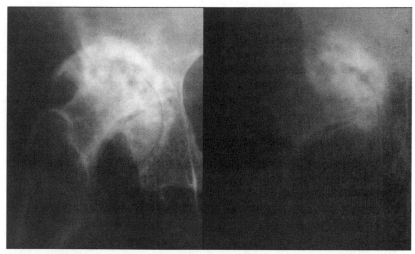

Figure 7. (Right) 1972: 72-year-old woman. Severe unilateral osteoarthritis of the hip, lateral subluxation, osteophytosis, large subchondral cysts, increased subchondral bone density, narrow joint space and complete loss of sphericity. Pain and limited motion main complaint. (Left) 1975: Large lateral acetabluar shelf has remodeled, sphericity regained, joint space reappeared, osteophytes remodeled out, bone density increased throughout femoral neck, head, and acetabulum. Treatment program: rest alternating with exercise; extensive active and passive range of motion and both active and passive stretching, weight-bearing to tolerance over 3 years. A tribute to Wolff's law. Pain diminished to acceptable level. No current interest in total hip replacement. Photo courtesy of John Bland, MD.

surgery in this series.) Surgery can cause a further decline in muscle strength and power unless a specific muscle strengthening program is undertaken. Preoperative rehabilitation can assist in a better postsurgical outcome by improving the patient's function and overall fitness level (McNeal, 1990).

Evaluation

The lower-extremity evaluation should include both objective and self-report measures. Objective measures include evaluation of strength, ROM, balance, gait, and cardiovascular endurance. In addition, timed measures of sit-to-stand "get up and go" (Mathias et al., 1986) and walking a specific distance may provide additional information on patient function in typical daily tasks. Self-report measures include a visual analog scale for pain and standardized questionnaires such as the Arthritis Impact Measurement of Health Status (AIMS and AIMS2; Meenan, Mason, Anderson, 1992), the Health Assessment Questionnaire (Fries, Spitz, Kraines, & Holman, 1980), and the Short Form-36 (SF-36) (Ware & Sherbourne, 1992). It has been suggested that the SF-36 be administered in combination with the AIMS2 to obtain information on the quality of life of the patient (Chewning, Bell, & Nowlin, 1994).

Treatment

A comprehensive occupational therapy and physical therapy program for patients with lower-extremity OA should focus on teaching the patient the skills needed for self-management. OA self-management skills include pain and symptom management; flexibility exercises of the muscles in the lower extremity and trunk; joint mobilization and reduction of soft-tissue contractures; strength training of the quadriceps, gluteal, hip abductor, and other lower-extremity muscles; endurance training for lower-extremity muscles and the cardiovascular system; functional training to improve balance, gait, transfer ability, activities of daily living (ADL), and recreational activities; and patient education for self-management, appropriate progression of exercises, and ambulation aids if necessary.

Pain and Symptom Management

Numerous thermal modalities are available to reduce OA pain. Cold packs and ice massage reduce swelling and can temporarily decrease joint pain, especially in the presence of acute swelling. Because the ankle joint is a surface distal structure, the use of cryotherapy such as ice, ice massage, or contrast baths often effectively reduce swelling and pain. Most persons with OA prefer heat and will gain temporarily relief from heat applications. Thermal modalities of heat and cold usually are less effective in the hip joint because the joint structure is much deeper than that of the knee and ankle joints. ROM and muscle stretching exercises may be performed during heat or cold applications.

For the foot, a metatarsal pad can help reduce weight-bearing pressure on the joint. A custom orthosis can reduce pain by redistributing pressure, and a rocker sole can facilitate push-off for patients with limited MTP dorsiflexion.

Behavioral methods to reduce pain and inflammation include joint protection techniques and ambulation aids. Exercises to increase joint ROM, reduce contractures, and strengthen muscles may reduce pain caused by tight soft-tissue structures, joint malalignment, and unstable joints. Teaching patients to create a "flare-up management plan" and put it into writing can facilitate effective self-management after clinic treatment.

Flexibility Training, Joint Mobilization, and Contracture Reduction

A well-designed comprehensive flexibility exercise program is necessary for persons with lower-extremity OA. Gentle active ROM should be performed for all involved joints. Active muscle stretching can be performed during walking, cycling, and other activities, but because these activities tend to use single-plane motions and do not include abduction and adduction or internal and external rotation and extension of the hip and inversion and eversion of the ankle joint, additional stretching exercises should be included to address ROM limitations in these joints. Passive muscle stretching and static stretching with prolonged positioning up to several minutes may be necessary to fully stretch some muscles.

Stiffness and muscle shortening can be treated by first using surface heat or cold on the joint or target muscles followed by muscle stretching, appropriate positioning, and joint mobilization. Joint mobilization is usually more effective on smaller joints such as the ankle and the knee, but active ROM exercise within the pain-free range is highly recommended for all lower-extremity joints. Joint mobilization may effectively reduce severe acute pain when the joint is subluxed, and the home program should include patient self-mobilization and stretching techniques (Levoska & Keinanen-Kiukaanniemi, 1993). The preferred mobilization technique usually involves distraction and gentle anterior and posterior glides that may effectively liberate the ankle or knee joint.

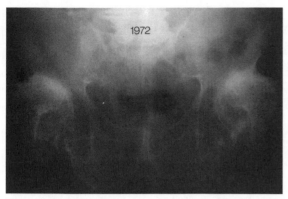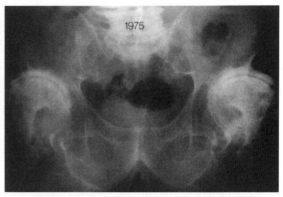

Figure 8. (A) 1972: 85-year-old man, retired professor of German, former athlete. Bed and chair patient. Bilateral osteoarthritis of hips with little motion, active or passive, in either hip. (B) 1975: In three years of vigorous active and passive exercises, intense education, strong family and physical therapy support, patient is able to walk one mile twice daily with Canadian crutches until his death at age 94. Photo courtesy of John Bland, MD.

After a patient is able to handle active and non–weight-bearing exercise, partial weight bearing may be considered. Special devices have been developed to stretch and strengthen the muscles about the ankle joint. One device that is often used in the clinic to improve ankle joint mobility is the BAPS wobble board (Spectrum Therapy Products, Jasper, MI), which allows ankle movement in multiple planes. The ankle can be exercised in the home setting with partial weight bearing when sitting or standing with partial upper-extremity support. Patients with stiff ankles may benefit from a rocker sole on their shoes to facilitate push-off and a custom orthoses designed to evenly distribute weight-bearing forces.

Patients with hip flexion or knee flexion contractures should be instructed in prone lying for 30 min daily to stretch contractures. Use of an abduction pillow while prone lying is beneficial for patients with adduction contractures.

Training for Endurance and Strength

Improving function usually requires increasing endurance (Box 4) and muscle strength (Box 5). Additionally, muscle and joint proprioception reeducation may facilitate the performance of specific tasks such as walking and getting up and down from a seat (Minor, 1996). Strength and endurance exercise may potentially increase pain and inflammation, and the exercise prescription should reduce this risk. Positioning during exercise must consider leverage and applied forces and be appropriate for the patient's joint status. Isometric and short-arc exercises for muscle strengthening usually are recommended. However, low-load resistance exercise for patients with OA and RA has been shown to improve lower-extremity strength, sit-to-stand time, and lower-extremity muscular endurance without negatively affecting joint count and number of painful joints (Komatireddy, Leitch, Cella, Browning, & Minor, 1997). Patients should be instructed in resistance exercises that consider joint integrity and degree of inflammation as well as muscle strength grade. Patients must be taught to increase resistance gradually and to adjust the amount of resistance as the joint and muscle status changes and the disease course varies.

Aerobic exercises have been shown to be highly beneficial for persons with rheumatic diseases and can reduce symptoms in all joints, including the hands (Minor, 1996; Minor, 1998; Minor,

---

Box 4
Aerobic Exercise Guidelines in Rheumatic Disease

Components of the Program

Warm-Up

The warm-up occurs before the aerobic exercise and may involve stretching and gentle active movements of the trunk and extremities. The warm-up period should last 5 to 10 min.

Aerobic Activity Prescription

Intensity. The intensity or workload of the exercise must be at a level that causes an increase in the heart rate of 20 to 40 beats/min (target heart rates for persons 50–70 years of age are 110–130 beats/min) and be perceived as somewhat difficult.

Duration. The goal is to eventually exercise for at least 30 min continuously. Initially, the patient may only be able to sustain exercise for 5 to 10 min before having symptoms of joint pain or shortness of breath.

When this occurs, the exercise must be given in blocks of 5 to 10 min with rest periods in between to build to 30 min per exercise session.

Frequency. Exercising 3 to 4 times per week is adequate to improve overall fitness and health. Nevertheless, exercise should be a daily endeavor, and patients should be encouraged to perform some type of exercise (especially ROM exercises) daily.

Mode. Exercise should involve a low load but must involve large muscles to stimulate the cardiovascular system. In addition, exercises can be chosen that are functional activities such as walking. Exercise should be enjoyed.

Cool-Down

The cool-down occurs after the aerobic exercise and may involve stretching and gentle active movements of the trunk and extremities. The cool-down period should last 5 to 10 min.

Hewett, Webel, Anderson, & Kay, 1989). Low-impact exercise at low to moderate intensity is recommended, and stationary cycling, treadmill, brisk walking, dance, and aquatic exercise have all been shown to increase endurance in patients with OA (Minor et al., 1989; Suomi & Lindauer, 1997). The exercise prescription should consider patient preference and convenience to enhance adherence to the regimen.

Water exercise. Aquatic aerobic exercise is especially beneficial for persons with lower-extremity OA because it reduces weight-bearing forces on the trunk and lower-extremity joints (Box 4). Water jogging and walking are excellent aerobic activities, and swimming encourages endurance and strength development. Strength training can easily be accomplished in an aquatic environment because the water provides resistance as the body or body part moves through the water (Box 5). To increase resistance, a fin or paddle can be applied to the hand or foot. To improve muscular flexibility, endurance, strength, and cardiovascular conditioning before surgery, aquatic exercise in the home or community environment may be recommended several weeks to several months

---

Box 5
Resistance Exercise Guidelines for a Strengthening Program

Components of the Program

Warm-Up

The warm-up occurs before the resistance exercise and should include gentle stretching of the muscles that are to be trained during the resistance phase of the exercise program. The warm-up period should last 5 to 10 min.

Resistance Exercise Prescription

Intensity. Exercise should involve a moderate load (using weights, machine resistance, or body segment), and the patient should be able to complete 6 to 10 repetitions before the muscle feels fatigued. However, any movement (resisted or not) that causes sharp joint pain should be avoided.

Duration. The duration will vary depending on the number of muscle groups exercised.

A total workout that includes 4 to 6 specific exercises for the major muscle groups should last 30 to 45 min.

Frequency. Exercise 3 to 4 times per week (exercise upper extremities 2 times per week alternating with lower extremities 2 times per week).

Mode. Exercise should involve a moderate load and can involve large groups or specific muscles. Weights, aquatic exercise, elastic bands, or machine exercise can be used. Exercise should be enjoyed.

Cool-Down

The cool-down occurs after the resistance exercise and may involve gentle stretching of the exercised muscles or walking. The cool-down period should last 5 to 10 min.

---

beforehand (Suomi & Lindauer, 1997). The Arthritis Foundation sponsors aquatic exercise programs for persons with arthritis throughout the United States (Box 3).

Home exercise programs must be customized for the water because the force of buoyancy is opposite that of gravity. Water provides numerous benefits for persons with arthritis when exercise programs consider this phenomenon.

Cycling. Stationary cycling reduces weight-bearing forces on lower-extremity joints and has proven successful in conditioning the cardiovascular system and improving lower-extremity endurance in patients with OA and RA (Hasson, Henderson, Daniels, & Schieb, 1991; Lyngberg, Danneskiold-Samsoe, & Halskov, 1988). Often a patient initially tolerates cycling for less than 10 min at a very low workload. Short-interval workouts that gradually increase in duration allow the patient to gain cardiovascular and muscular endurance. A patient can cycle longer than 30 min in a single continuous work session after just a few weeks of training. Cycling at a workload to attain a heart rate of 110 to 130 beats/min 3 times a week for 30 to 45 min will result in dramatic improvements in muscular and cardiovascular endurance (Box 4). The target heart rate must be modified to accommodate for age, fitness level, other medical conditions, and medication use.

Cycling usually is recommended primarily for patients with mild to moderate hip or knee OA or who are deconditioned. Cycling is generally not recommended for patients with severe hip OA or who have undergone recent total hip arthroplasty and should not be used if it causes pain.

Walking. Walking is the most commonly prescribed conditioning exercise for patients with lower-extremity OA (Minor et al., 1989; Nordemar, Ekblom, Zachrisson, & Lundquist, 1981). During walking, the ground reaction force is approximately the same as the person's body weight, and the more compliant the surface or the footwear, the more this force is reduced. A clinical gait analysis and evaluation of the need for corrective footwear or orthoses should be part of a comprehensive lower-extremity evaluation in patients with OA, especially if walking is recommended as a primary method for maintaining fitness.

Patients should be educated regarding the components of appropriate footwear and given advice regarding selection. Athletic shoes for running may be recommended versus athletic shoes for walking because running shoes generally have a better shock-absorbing sole. (See the Appendix at the end of this volume for guidelines on how to select appropriate footwear.) Additionally, the effect of walking surfaces and posture on gait should be discussed with the patient. Leg-length discrepancy can be an aggravating factor for OA of the knee. The discrepancy should be corrected with shoe lifts.

Altering the forces on the lower extremities may require changing the way a person walks rather than limiting his or her walking. Patients may need to use assistive gait devices such as a cane or walker to reduce lower-extremity weight bearing and correct an antalgic gait. Even if a patient is severely deconditioned or uses an assistive device, they should be encouraged to walk short distances and gradually increase the distance as they are able.

Patients initially may experience fatigue or increased joint pain when starting a walking program and may only be able to walk 5 to 10 min or a short distance. Joint pain should begin to diminish if the patient walks daily for short sessions (5–10 min) while working toward a goal of 20 to 30 min each day. After 4 to 6 weeks, many patients should be able to walk continuously for 30 min or longer. A walking regimen should be part of each patient's home exercise and activity program because it is a necessary functional activity.

Functional Training To Improve Balance, Gait, Transfers, ADL, and Recreation

Functional performance of persons with OA frequently is reduced. Tools have been developed to assist clinicians in determining the extent of limitations. Rejeski and associates (1995) evaluated the functional performance of 440 persons with OA of the knee and found that they had difficulty with many functional activities, including walking one quarter of a mile; going up and down steps; getting into and out of a bathtub, car, or bed; standing up from a chair; lifting and carrying groceries; bending down and picking up clothes; running errands; and doing light chores compared with control subjects. Brooks, Callahan, and Pincus (1988) evaluated the effectiveness of a self-report ADL questionnaire in detecting functional improvement after 4 weeks of rehabilitation for OA of the knee. They found the questionnaire to be as sensitive and valid as traditional observer-reported measures for detecting change in clinical status.

The incorporation of work simplification methods to minimize painful motion and the use of elevated chairs and joint protection principles to minimize stress and pain are priority treatment objectives for OA of the lower extremities (Cordery & Rocchi, 1998; McCloy, 1982; Neumann, 1989; Robinson, 1985). Patient education is extremely important because many persons have misconceptions about what to do for their arthritis (Boutaugh & Brady, 1998). The classic example of this is the patient with OA of the knees who continues, by choice, to live in an apartment above the ground floor because he or she believes that climbing the stairs several times a day (even though it is painful) will keep his legs strong. For some patients, this may further wear down the cartilage and increase inflammation. There are non–weight-bearing, nonpainful ways (e.g., isometric exercise or aquatic exercise) to keep leg muscles strong. However, patients who can climb stairs without increased pain may benefit from the process.

Patients who have difficulty ambulating or who must use ambulation aids should be counseled on how to adapt their homes to reduce architectural barriers and reduce safety hazards (Bates, 1994; Carter, Campbell, Sanson-Fisher, Redman, & Gillespie, 1997; Chandler & Duncan, 1993).

If there is a decrease in ambulation status and the patient needs to use a crutch, walker, or wheelchair, it is important that the patient receive training in how to do ADL with the required ambulation aids. Additionally, patients with limited finger flexion may need a padded handle on the ambulation aid, whereas those with thumb adduction contractures may require a narrowed handle to prevent thumb pain or allow a secure grip.

Shoulder Involvement

OA of the shoulder joint accounts for only 5% of all patients with painful shoulder conditions (Caillet, 1981). The major causes of shoulder disability are the result of periarticular involvement (e.g., tendonitis, bursitis, rotator cuff tears, myofascial shoulder pain, and adhesive capsulitis). However, OA of the glenohumeral joint can result from overuse, joint laxity, limited motion, or physical trauma.

OA secondary to overuse and joint laxity can begin at a young age and result from participation in activities such as baseball pitching and gymnastics (Aubergie, Zenny, Duvallet, Godefroy, & Horreard, 1984; Hansen, 1982) and, for persons with disabilities, from participation in wheelchair sports. These activities usually involve high repetitive forces about the shoulder joint. In gymnastics, the entire upper extremity becomes a weight-bearing appendage, and all upper-extremity joints act as shock absorbers for many skills in the floor exercise, the vault, and the balance beam. In a study by Aubergie and associates (1984), more than 70% of high-school gymnasts had delayed bone maturation and articular changes that may be a precursor to OA. Persons with paraplegia must bear weight through their upper extremities, and elite wheelchair athletes from the 1970s are beginning to report shoulder and elbow difficulties, including the development of OA (Gellman, Sie, & Waters, 1988). OA from immobilization or simply limited ROM of the shoulder joint after injury or surgery (including mastectomy) can become severe enough to warrant a total shoulder arthroplasty. Limited motion appears to hasten articular degeneration and may result in adhesive capsulitis ("frozen shoulder syndrome") or biceps muscle contracture. Bony changes of the articular joint surface can cause a corresponding loss of joint motion, and osteophyte growth can limit joint motion further in specific planes. In non–weight-bearing joints, it is believed that movement of the joint and some weight bearing through the long bones may be critical in providing nutrition to the articular cartilage. (See chapter 2 in this volume for a review on how immobilization can alter joints.)

Symptoms associated with shoulder OA include pain and joint laxity and occur later in the disease process. Early problems that a patient may develop can be related directly to periarticular problems from repetitive overuse as described above. Physiological changes that occur from periarticular involvement and with upper-extremity OA include pain, stiffness, and decreased shoulder ROM and arm and forearm muscle strength. Depending on the severity of the periarticular involvement or OA, functional activities may or may not be compromised, but recreational and work activities requiring specific movement patterns and joint loading frequently are affected. (Differential diagnosis of shoulder pain is discussed in volume 1, chapters 6 and 7, of this series.)

Patients may not have pain if they limit their activity, but they are likely to develop adhesive capsulitis and muscle contractures. Adhesive capsulitis should be suspected when the patient is unable to reach overhead without pain or is unable to reach normal end ROM because of bony blockage or joint adhesion. If limited function and pain are severe, then corticosteroid injections or surgery may be indicated.

Surgical options depend on the periarticular problem, status of joint laxity, and condition of the joint surfaces. Options include arthroscopic repair of a rotator cuff tendon, surgical manipulation of a joint, joint tightening, or a total joint arthroplasty. (See volume 5, chapter 3, of this series.)

Evaluation

Objective measures include evaluation of pain, inflammation, stiffness, strength, ROM, ADL, and posture. Self-report measures are the same as those for the lower extremity.

Treatment

A comprehensive exercise program for a patient with OA or periarticular involvement of the shoulder joint should include pain and inflammation management, flexibility and ROM exercises for the shoulder and shoulder girdle musculature, posture training, instruction in joint protection and adaptive ADL methods to reduce stress to the shoulder, muscle endurance and strength training for upper-extremity and posture muscles, and patient education for appropriate progression of exercises and self-management.

Pain Management

Joint protection methods and adaptive equipment designed to eliminate unnecessary shoulder motion and stress or to improve posture are helpful in reducing pain and inflammation, but they must be combined with exercises to maintain ROM of the shoulder complex.

Using a cold pack or ice massage may reduce joint swelling and temporarily decrease joint pain. Heat may reduce stiffness and pain. Studies on small numbers of patients have shown that electrical stimulation and pulsed ultrasound may be used as adjuncts for pain relief (Hasson, Mundorf, Barnes, Williams, & Fujii, 1990; Hasson, Wible, Reich, Barnes, & Williams, 1992). These are usually only used in a clinic setting, however, and patients should be taught pain relief interventions that they may use at home.

Use of an arm sling may be helpful in cases of severe pain, but slings increase the risk of adhesive capsulitis and biceps contracture. The sling should only be used for short periods and in conjunction with anti-inflammatory measures and ROM exercises to promote shoulder joint motion in all planes.

Exercise

Patients always should be instructed in ROM exercises, especially in the acute stages, to avoid shortening of the inferior aspect of the capsule and development of frozen shoulder syndrome. Gentle active exercise that emphasizes rotation, flexion, and abduction is important to maintain or increase ROM. Correct posture should be emphasized because patients frequently develop protective postures to reduce pain, and exercises to improve strength and flexibility of the shoulder girdle and posture musculature should be included as appropriate.

Exercises such as wall walking and finger ladder climbing may be contraindicated if the patient has subacromial bursitis because active flexion or abduction against gravity only causes greater impingement of the subacromion bursa. Exercising in a gravity-eliminated position or active assisted exercise with gentle distraction of the joint or Codman's (pendulum) exercises may be preferable. Codman's exercises are particularly recommended if the patient has acute pain or severely limited motion (Bland, Merrit, & Boushey, 1977). Cane exercises may be appropriate for some patients, but the applied force to the shoulder joint due to the long lever arm may increase pain. Shoulder ROM with the elbow flexed reduces the lever force and may be less painful for patients.

Patients can perform various shoulder mobilization exercises with the elbow in contact with a bed or plinth (Caillet, 1981). However, for joint capsule adhesions, passive joint mobilization is the most effective method of reducing adhesions. Mobilization can be provided with specific anterior, posterior, or rotatory forces applied to stretch the shoulder joint capsule.

Joint stiffness and muscle shortening can be treated with surface heat on the joint and friction massage to the joint followed by muscle stretching and joint mobilization. Friction massage can be provided directly to musculotendinous regions with the force applied transversely to the tendon's insertion.

Muscular strength and endurance of the elbow, shoulder, and shoulder girdle muscles is an important component of the treatment program. A program beginning with isometrics and progressing to short-arc exercise with low-grade resistance is usually recommended. Performing resistance or muscular endurance training in a painful range is not advisable, and full-arc exercise with resistance or use of equipment such as an upper-body bicycle ergometer generally is not recommended until the patient tolerates low-grade exercise satisfactorily. Hold–relax and contract–relax exercises are particularly effective techniques to increase ROM and strength as long as they are applied in the pain-free range.

Strengthening exercises should be included in the patient's home exercise program. Isometric exercises, short-arc exercises, and elastic bands such as Theraband™ (Hygenic Corp, Akron, OH) can be used to allow the patient to exercise almost any muscle group at different resistance loads and in different positions at home. Pulley systems can be used to improve muscular endurance and strength for the upper extremity. Pulleys normally use a low load to increase flexibility but can be used to increase strength by simply increasing the load. Aquatic exercise offers the advantage of warm water and reduced forces at the joint and is an excellent exercise to increase both flexibility and strength. The shoulder should be submerged to take advantage of the buoyancy of the water. If patients choose to swim, they must be reminded to observe good postural guidelines and to avoid developing protective postures and positions while swimming.

Cardiovascular endurance should be considered in a comprehensive program. Aerobic activity that does not irritate the shoulder joint such as a walking or an aquatic program is recommended. (See Box 4 for aerobic exercise guidelines.) Patients should be carefully monitored and cautioned to progress slowly.

One potential concern for the elbow and shoulder joints is the development of hypertrophic bone secondary to overuse with exercise. As with all exercise programs, increasing the frequency, workload, and duration of an existing program should be undertaken cautiously, and patients should be monitored frequently.

Spinal Involvement

OA of the spine involves two distinct articular systems: the hyaline cartilage of the apophyseal joints (spinal OA) and the fibrocartilage of the discs (spondylosis). OA in the apophyseal joints of the spine is similar to the peripheral diarthrodial joints and includes cartilage degeneration, fibrosis, and abnormal bone growth. The result may be narrowing of the neural foramina with nerve root compression. This can be painful or painless with muscle weakness and sensory changes as the only symptoms. Degeneration of the disc results in narrowing, which reduces the distance between vertebrae, decreases spinal flexibility, and results in a diminished ability to respond to physical stress. In addition, osteophytes can be produced around the body of the vertebrae and can further hinder spinal flexibility.

Involvement of spinal OA and spondylosis occurs most commonly in the lower cervical, mid-to-lower thoracic, and lower lumbar spine regions. This is most commonly found in middle-age and elderly persons. However, persons with ligamentous instability and idiopathic hypermobility or restricted mobility are candidates for development of premature OA of the spine. Sports activities associated with an increased incidence of spinal OA include noncontact activities such as ballet and gymnastics; weight lifting, where compressive forces that are applied to the spine are very high; and contact sports such as football, soccer, and wrestling, where trauma to the spine is quite common (Panush & Brown, 1987).

Symptoms associated with spinal OA include stiffness, muscle spasms, and pain. These initial symptoms can occur early in the disease process in some persons, whereas other persons may be asymptomatic for many years. Decreased ROM and decreased trunk and neck strength occur in the early phase. When symptoms are present, this often leads to decreased activity. Inactivity for several weeks to years may lead to muscle weakness of the back and abdomen and tightness of trunk musculature.

Later in the disease process, pain, muscle spasm, and osteophyte growth can severely limit trunk or neck motion. The patient may be unable to bend over and may develop "disc signs" with radicular pain into the buttocks and lower limb while in a flexed position (e.g., sitting). The patient may be unable to flex and rotate the neck and may demonstrate disc signs with radicular pain into the shoulder girdle and upper extremity, or muscle weakness and sensory loss without pain may be evident.

Surgery may be indicated when function is limited, pain is unrelenting, and further signs of nerve root compression such as numbness and tingling are present. Options include decompression and laminectomy.

Evaluation

Objective measures include evaluation of trunk or neck strength, ROM, sensation, balance, gait, posture, and cardiovascular endurance. In addition, timed measures of trunk flexion and walking a specific distance may give further information about the level of patient function in more normal day-to-day tasks. To detect cervical nerve compression, the most distal ulnar and median hand muscle should be tested as well as hand sensation (Bland, 1995). Subjective measurements are the same as those used for the lower extremities.

Evaluation of ADL specifically should include the following:

- Occupational use that aggravates the involved area
- Posture during reading, writing, driving, watching television, work, and recreation
- Muscular tension or emotional stress during an activity that may contribute to pain and muscle spasm
- Sleep posture and type of pillow and mattress used

Inquiring about whether the patient's lumbar or cervical pain is worse at night, on awakening in the morning, or in the afternoon can be informative. Pain that is greater at night or on awakening may indicate that the mattress, pillow, or positioning could contribute to the pain, or it may reveal that stiffness from prolonged positioning is a major problem. Pain that is greater in the afternoon may indicate that daytime activities, positioning, or weight-bearing activities on the lower extremities are contributing to the problem.

Treatment

The optimal therapy and home exercise program for a patient with spinal arthritis should incorporate education about pain and symptom management (including relaxation training), flexibility and ROM exercises for the trunk and neck, posture training, education about joint protection and work simplification, strengthening the trunk and cervical musculature, and fitness and cardiovascular conditioning. For patients who work in relatively fixed positions such as at a computer or who have jobs in which positioning aggravates symptoms, an occupational therapy or physical therapy ergonomics evaluation and training program to reduce symptoms at work may help the person remain employed.

Pain and Symptom Management

OA of the spine is either a chronic or episodic condition. Treatment should focus on teaching patients self-management principles for pain, spasm, and stiffness (the problems that first brought them to therapy) and how to minimize reoccurrences and manage flare-ups.

Box 6
Why One Joint and Not Another?

A question that the clinician may ask is why is this joint involved and not that joint, or why are joints involved at all in certain diseases? Seeming preferential localization of pathology in one or a few tissues or organs characterizes many disease states and frequently aids in diagnosis. Localization of pathology may determine treatment or prognosis. Disappointingly, little is known about factors that determine organ localization in diseases. Why is the diarthrodial joint one of the most common sites of chronic inflammation in humankind? Most rheumatic diseases, certainly including OA, have preferential joint locations, whereas many other joints are spared completely. Surely joint susceptibility must reflect patterns of joint structure and function as well as biomechanics. Perhaps we can learn more from joints spared than from joints involved.

Patient education should include an explanation of the pain-spasm cycle so patients understand how interventions work. Heat applications are commonly used to relax back and neck musculature and are often the first modality tried because they are soothing. If heat does not relieve muscle spasm, a cold pack or ice massage is likely to be effective. This should be applied in conjunction with positioning and conscious relaxation techniques to encourage relaxation of the spinal muscles. Caffeine and the acid in coffee can increase muscle tightness and should be avoided when muscle spasm is a problem. Nicotine is likewise a stimulant and vasoconstrictor. Some persons benefit from electrical stimulation (transcutaneous electrical nerve stimulation [TENS]) but should not become dependent on it and neglect more the lasting pain-relief measures of good posture, correct body mechanics, and exercise. Pain management may include immobilization of the cervical or lumbar area with a cervical collar or back brace. Neck collars and back braces used for prolonged periods without concomitant ROM exercises can encourage muscle shortening secondary to immobility. In one author's (J.M.) experience, soft cervical collars can be beneficial in gently correcting faulty cervical and thoracic postures by encouraging correct alignment while the muscles are warm from the foam. The collar can be used to train patients how to position themselves for proper neck alignment.

Muscle relaxants, although not administered solely to relieve pain, may be used in conjunction with pain relievers to reduce muscle spasms. Corticosteroid injections into facet joints or muscle trigger points can likewise decrease pain.

Exercise

Exercises to increase trunk or cervical flexibility, increase strength, and promote good posture may decrease pain, especially the pain caused by poor posture and adaptive positioning. The loss of flexibility and strength may be slow and insidious, and patients may not be aware that they have greatly decreased ROM. Joint and muscle stiffness can be treated with superficial heat, massage, stretching, and joint mobilization. Gentle ROM exercises may be performed in front of a mirror so that the patient may observe and correct postural deviations. Various massage techniques can be provided directly to soft-tissue regions followed by joint mobilization and muscle stretching (Sprague, 1983). The patient can perform various trunk and neck mobilization exercises, which are well illustrated by Twomey and Taylor (1987).

Strengthening exercises for patients with cervical or lumbar spondylosis can include isometric exercises for patients with greatly limited mobility or pain during motion and isotonic exercises when the patient has no pain during nearly full active ROM. Strengthening and muscle endurance training should include teaching patients to find their "neutral" spine. This is a position in which the normal curves of the neck and back are maintained. The patient should maintain this position when lying, sitting, standing, lifting, and walking. The position becomes increasingly challenging to maintain when upper- and lower-extremity movements are added (Saal, 1990). The patient should be taught how to maintain the neutral spine position while performing functional activities and working.

Patients with spinal OA, especially with lumbar spondylosis, can be deconditioned and benefit from cardiovascular endurance training. A walking or cycling home program or water exercise can be highly beneficial for the patient (Box 3). The patient should chose an aerobic activity that does not cause pain in the joints.

Positioning and Joint Protection for the Spine

Bed and leisure positioning. Sleeping positions, the mattress, and the type of pillow that a patient uses at night can strongly influence neck and back pain and stiffness. Patients with cervical arthritis should not sleep in the prone position because it requires prolonged positioning at the extreme of lateral neck rotation. Patients with lumbar arthritis should adapt prone lying to keep the spine in neutral. If a patient complains of greater neck pain at night or on awakening than experienced during the day, this may be due to the type of pillow used. A regular pillow props up the occipital area and flattens the normal lordotic curve of the cervical spine, which places stress on the cervical joints and ligaments. A pillow that supports the neck in a normal lordotic curve can effectively reduce muscle spasm and associated pain and stiffness (Jackson, 1978; Melvin, 1981).

Joint protection. Cordery and Rocchi (1998) expanded joint protection principles for the treatment of OA. "For OA, protection is directed to strengthening the muscular support and shock absorption for a joint; reducing total load on the joint in activities by using different techniques or devices; managing inflammation; avoiding pain (which inhibits muscle strength and function); and getting physically fit so as to reduce muscle tiredness and fatigue." These authors reviewed a wide range of methods for incorporating these principles into ADL.

Specifically for the spine, joint protections include maintaining proper support and posture during activities that maintain the spine in neutral alignment versus keeping the spine "straight" or flattening the lumbar spine (a neutral spine reduces the demand and strain on the spinal muscles) (Mackenzie, 1981), learning how to consciously relax neck and back muscles, avoiding staying in one position for long periods, using a supportive mattress and pillow, and wearing soft or cushioned soled shoes to reduce shock to the spine. Athletic shoes designed for running provide the greatest shock absorption.

Instruction in basic body mechanics and relaxation techniques are essential to achieve these goals for the spine. For many patients, learning how to incorporate these measures into daily activities requires practice and experience with the activity. Helping patients learn to sit, walk, and work with the spine relaxed is a major challenge in back and neck treatment.

Conclusion

OA once was regarded as an inevitable consequence of aging, a wear-and-tear phenomenon, or a consequence of abnormal joint mechanics. This is no longer the case. New formulations of etiology and pathogenesis as related to management have been proposed. When management and therapy can be closely related to etiology, and the pathogenic steps are identified in a disease process, arrest or reversal becomes possible. The stakes are high because this disorder is universal in humans. Rehabilitation must focus on self-management training rather than encouraging dependence on clinic-based treatment. OA is a multifactorial process, perhaps not a disease but rather an ancient Paleozoic mechanism of repair of dense tissues developing in vertebrate animals.

References

Akeson, S. H., Woo, S. L. Y., Amiel, D., & Frank, C. B. (1984). The biology of ligaments. In L. U. Hunter & F. J. Funk, Jr. (Eds.), *Rehabilitation of the injured knee: The chemical basis of tissue repair* (pp. 93–209). St. Louis, MO: Mosby.

Altman, R. D. (1995). The classification of osteoarthritis. *Journal of Rheumatology, 22*(1, Suppl. 43), 42–43.

Altman, R., Asch, E., Bloch, D., Bole, G., Borenstein, D., Brandt, K., Christy, W., Cooke, T. D., Greenwald, R., Hochberg, M., et al. (1986.). Development of criteria for the classification and reporting of osteoarthritis: Classification of osteoarthritis of the knee. *Arthritis and Rheumatism, 29*(8), 1039–1049.

Altman, R. D., & Dean, D. (Eds.). (1989). Pain in osteoarthritis. *Seminars in Arthritis and Rheumatism, 189*(Suppl. 2), 1–4.

Aubergie, T., Zenny, J., Duvallet, A., Godefroy, D., & Horreard, P. (1984). Bone maturation and osteoarticular lesions in top level sportsmen. *Journal of Radiology, 65*, 555–561.

Badley, E. M., Thompson, R. P., & Wood, P. H. N. (1978). The prevalence and severity of major disabling conditions: A reappraisal of the government social survey on the handicapped and impaired in Great Britain. *International Journal of Epidemiology, 7*, 145–151.

Bates, P. S. (1994). The self-care environment: Issues of space and furnishing. In C. Christiansen (Ed.), *Ways of living: Self-care strategies for special needs*. Bethesda, MD: American Occupational Therapy Association.

Bland, J. H. (1995) *Disorders of the cervical spine* (2nd ed.). Philadelphia: Saunders.

Bland, J. H. (in press). On the occasional arrest and reversibility of osteoarthritis of hips and knees. *Arthritis Care and Research.*

Bland, J. H., & Cooper, S. M. (1984). Osteoarthritis: A review of the cell biology involved and evidence for reversibility: Management rationally related to known genesis and pathophysiology. *Seminars in Arthritis and Rheumatism, 14*(2), 106–133.

Bland, J. H., Merrit, J. A., & Boushey, D. R. (1977). The painful shoulder. *Seminars in Arthritis and Rheumatism, 7*(1), 21.

Bland, J. H., & Stulberg, S. D. (1985). Osteoarthritis: Pathology and clinical patterns. In W. N. Kelley, E. D. Harris, S. Ruddy, & C. B. Sledge (Eds.), *Textbook of rheumatology* (2nd ed.). Philadelphia: Saunders.

Boutaugh, M. L., & Brady, T. (1998). Patient education for self-management. In J. L. Melvin & G. Jensen (Eds.), *Rheumatologic rehabilitation series: Volume 1: Assessment and management* (pp. 219–258). Bethesda, MD: American Occupational Therapy Association.

Brooks, R. H., Callahan, L. F., & Pincus, T. (1988). Use of self-report activities of daily living questionnaires in osteoarthritis. *Arthritis Care and Research, 1*(1), 23–32.

Brown, W. R., & Lingg, C. (1961). Musculoskeletal complaints in an industry, annual complaint rate and diagnosis, absenteeism and economic loss. *Arthritis and Rheumatism, 4*, 283–302.

Buckland-Wright, J. C., Macfarlane, D. G., & Lynch, J. A. (1991). Osteophytes in the osteoarthritic hand: Their incidence, size, distribution, and progression. *Annals of Rheumatic Diseases, 50*, 627–630.

Caillet, R. (1981). Musculoskeletal pain. In *Shoulder pain* (2nd ed., pp. 38–73). Philadelphia: F. A. Davis.

Calfas, K. J., Kaplan, R. M., & Ingram, R. E. (1992). One-year evaluation of cognitive behavioral intervention in osteoarthritis. *Arthritis Care and Research, 5*(4), 202–209.

Carmen, W. J. (1989). Factors associated with pain and osteoarthritis in the Tecumseh community health study. *Seminars in Arthritis and Rheumatism, 18*(4), 10–13.

Carter, S. E., Campbell, E. M., Sanson-Fisher, R. W., Redman, S., & Gillespie, W. J. (1997). Environmental hazards in the homes of older people. *Age and Aging, 26*(3), 195–202 .

Catterall, A. (1981). Legg-Calve-Perthes' syndrome. *Clinical Orthopedics and Related Research, 158*, 41–52.

Chandler, J. M., & Duncan, P. W. (1993). Balance and falls in the elderly: Issues in evaluation and treatment. In A. A. Guccione (Ed.), *Geriatric physical therapy*. St. Louis, MO: Mosby.

Chewning, B., Bell, C., & Nowlin, N. (1994). A comparison of AIMS2 and SF-36 health quality of life measures. *Arthritis and Rheumatism, 37*(Suppl.), S225.

Cobb, S., Merchant, W. R., & Rubin, T. (1957). The relation of symptoms to osteoarthritis. *Journal of Chronic Disease, 5*, 197–204.

Colditz, J. C., & Melvin, J. L. (In press). Orthotic treatment for arthritis of the hand. In J. L. Melvin & E. A. Nalebuff (Eds.), *Rheumatologic rehabilitation series: Volume 4: The hand: Evaluation, therapy, and surgery*. Bethesda, MD: American Occupational Therapy Association.

Cooke, T., Dwosh, I., & Cossairt, J. (1983). Clinical pathologic osteoarthritis workshop. *Journal of Rheumatology, 10*(Suppl. 9), 1–118.

Cooper, C. (1994). Osteoarthritis: Epidemiology. In J. H. Klippel & P. Dieppe (Eds.), *Rheumatology* (p. 7.3.2). St. Louis: Mosby Year-Book.

Cordery, J. C., & Rocchi, M. (1998). Joint protection and fatigue management. In J. L. Melvin & G. Jensen (Eds.), *Rheumatologic rehabilitation series: Volume 1: Assessment and management* (pp. 279–322). Bethesda, MD: American Occupational Therapy Association.

Creamer, P., & Hochberg, M. C. (1998). The relationship between psychosocial variables and pain reporting in osteoarthritis of the knee. *Arthritis Care and Research , 11*(1), 60–65.

Culic, D. D., Battaglia, M. C., Wichman, C., & Schmid, F. R. (1979). Efficacy of compression gloves in rheumatoid arthritis. *American Journal of Physical Medicine, 58*(6), 278–284.

Dieppe, P. (1994). Osteoarthritis: Clinical features and diagnostic problems. In J. H. Klippel & P. Dieppe (Eds.), *Rheumatology* (pp. 7.4.1–7.4.16). St. Louis: Mosby Year-Book.

Doherty, M. (1994). *Color atlas and text of osteoarthritis*. St. Louis: Mosby Yearbook.

Doherty, M., Watt, I., & Dieppe, P. (1983). Influence of primary generalized osteoarthritis on development of secondary osteoarthritis. *Lancet, 2*, 8–11.

Dray, G. J., & Jablon, M. (1987). Clinical and radiologic features of primary osteoarthritis of the hand. *Hand Clinics, 3*(3), 351–369.

Ekdahl, C., & Andersson, S. (1989). Standing balance in arthritis. *Scandinavian Journal of Rheumatism, 18,* 33–42.

Ekdahl, C., Jarnlo, G., & Andersson, S. (1989). Standing balance in healthy subjects. *Scandinavian Journal of Rehabilitation Medicine, 21,* 187–195.

Felson, D., Naimark, A., & Anderson, J. (1987). The prevalence of knee osteoarthritis in the elderly: The Framingham osteoarthritis study. *Arthritis and Rheumatism, 30,* 914–918.

Fries, J. F., Spitz, P., Kraines, R. G., & Holman, H. R. (1980). Measurement of patient outcome in arthritis. *Arthritis and Rheumatism, 23,* 137–145.

Garfinkel, M. S., Schumacher, H. R., Hsain, A., Levy, M., & Reshetar, R. A. (1994). Evaluation of a yoga based regimen for treatment of osteoarthritis of the hands. *Journal of Rheumatology, 21*(12), 2341–2343.

Gellman, H., Sie, I., & Waters, R. (1988). Late complications of the weight-bearing upper extremity in the paraplegic patient. *Clinical Orthopedics and Related Research, 233,* 132–135.

Gross, M. (1981). Psychosocial aspects of osteoarthritis: helping patients cope. *Health and Social Work, 6*(3), 40–46.

Hadler, H. (1985). Osteoarthritis as a public health problem. *Clinics in Rheumatic Disease, 11,* 175–185.

Hadler, N. M., Gillings, D. B., Imbus, J. R., Levitin, P. M., Makvec, D., Utsinger, P. D., Yount, W. J., Slasser, D., & Moskovitz, N. (1978). Hand structure and function in an industrial setting: Influence of three patterns of stereotyped repetitive usage. *Arthritis and Rheumatism, 21,* 210–220.

Hampson, S., Glasgow, R., & Zeiss, A. (1996). Coping with osteoarthritis by older adults. *Arthritis Care and Research, 9,* 133–141.

Hansen, N. (1982). Epiphyseal changes in the proximal humerus of an adolescent baseball pitcher. *American Journal Sports Medicine, 10,* 380–384.

Haralson-Ferrell, K. M. (1998). Community resources in comprehensive rehabilitation. In J. L. Melvin & G. Jensen (Eds.), *Rheumatologic rehabilitation series: Volume 1: Assessment and management* (pp. 393–408). Bethesda, MD: American Occupational Therapy Association.

Hasson, S., Henderson, G., Daniels, J., & Schieb, D. (1991). Exercise training and dexamethasone iontophoresis in rheumatoid arthritis. *Physiotherapy Canada, 43,* 11–14.

Hasson, S., Mundorf, R., Barnes, W., Williams, J., & Fujii, M. (1990). Effect of pulsed ultrasound versus placebo on muscle soreness perception and muscular performance. *Scandinavian Journal of Rehabilitation Medicine, 22,* 199–205.

Hasson, S., Wible, C., Reich, M., Barnes, W., & Williams, J. (1992). Dexamethasone iontophoresis: Effect on delayed muscle soreness and muscle function. *Canadian Journal of Sports Science, 17,* 8–13.

Heine, J. (1926). Uberdie arthritis deformans. *Virchow Arch, 260,* 521–663.

Hochberg, M. C., Altman, R. D., Brandt, K. D., Clark, B. M., Dieppe, P. A., Griffin, M. R., Moskowitz, R. W., & Schnitzer, T. J. (1995). Guidelines for the medical management of osteoarthritis: Part II: Osteoarthritis of the knee: American College of Rheumatology. *Arthritis and Rheumatism, 38*(11), 1541–1546.

Howell, D. S., Woessner, J. F., Jimenez, S., Seda, H., & Schumacher, H. R. (1979). A view on the pathogenesis of osteoarthritis. *Bulletin on the Rheumatic Diseases, 29,* 996–1001.

Hughston, J. (1962). Acute knee injuries in athletes. *Clinical Orthopedics and Related Research, 3,* 31–35.

Hutton, C. (1987). Generalized osteoarthritis: An evolutionary problem. *Lancet, 2,* 1463–1465.

Jackson, R. (1978). *The cervical syndrome* (4th ed.). Springfield, IL: Charles C. Thomas.

Jerring, K. (1980). Osteoarthritis of the hip: Epidemiology and clinical role. *Acta Orthopaedica Scandinavia 51,* 523–530.

Jonsson, H., & Valtysdottir, S. T. (1995). Hypermobility features in patients with hand osteoarthritis. *Osteoarthritis and cartilage, 3*(1), 1–5.

Kaiser, H. E. (1962). Untersuchingen zur vergleichender Knochen-ind Gelenkdpatholiogie fossiler und rezenter. *Tiere Frank Path, 72,* 276–292.

Keefe, F. J., Caldwell, D. S., Queen, K., Gil, K. M., Martinez, S., Crisson, J. E., Ogden, W., & Nunley, J. (1987). Osteoarthritic knee pain: A behavioral analysis. *Pain, 28*(13), 309–321.

Kellgren, J. G., & Lawrence, J. S. (1957). Osteoarthrosis and disc degeneration in an urban population. *Annals of Rheumatic Diseases, 17,* 388–397.

Kellgren, J. H., & Lawrence, J. S. (1958). Radiological assessment of osteoarthrosis. *Annals of Rheumatic Disease, 16,* 494–502.

Kellgren, J. H., & Moore, R. I. (1952). Generalized osteoarthritis and Heberden's nodes. *British Medical Journal, 1,* 181–187.

Klunder, K., Rud, B., & Hansen, J. (1980). Osteoarthritis of the hip and knee joints in retired football players. *Acta Orthopaedica Scandinavia, 51,* 925–927.

Komatireddy, G. R., Leitch, R. W., Cella, K., Browning, G., & Minor, M. (1997). Efficacy of low load resistive muscle training in patients with rheumatoid arthritis functional class II and III. *Journal of Rheumatology, 24,* 1531–1539.

Kramer, J. S., Yelin, E. H., & Epstein, W. V. (1983). Social and economic impact of four musculoskeletal conditions: A study using national community based data. *Arthritis and Rheumatism, 26,* 901 907.

Lane, N., Bloch, D., Jones, H., Marshall, W., & Wood, P. (1986). Long-distance running, bone density and osteoarthritis. *JAMA, 255,* 1147–1151.

Lawrence, J. S., Bremner, J. M., & Bier, F. (1966). Osteoarthrosis: Prevalence in the population and relationship between symptoms and x-ray changes. *Annals of Rheumatic Disease, 25,* 1–24.

Leach, R. E., Baumgard, S., & Broom, J. (1973). Obesity: Its relationship to osteoarthritis of the knee. *Clinical Orthopaedics, 93,* 271–273.

Levoska, S., & Keinanen-Kiukaanniemi, S. (1993). Active or passive physiotherapy for occupational cervicobrachial disorders? A comparison of two treatment methods with a 1 year follow-up. *Archives of Physical Medicine and Rehabilitation, 74*(4), 425–430.

Lyngberg, K., Danneskiold-Samsoe, B., & Halskov, O. (1988). The effect of physical training on patients with rheumatoid arthritis: Changes in disease activity, muscle strength and aerobic capacity: A clinically controlled minimized cross-over study. *Journal Clinical and Experimental Rheumatology, 6,* 253–260.

Mackenzie, R. A. (1981). *The lumbar spine: Mechanical diagnosis and therapy.* Waikanae, New Zealand: Apinnal.

Mathias, S., Nayak, U., & Isaacs, B. (1986). Balance in elderly patients: The "get up and go" test. *Archives of Physical Medicine and Rehabilitation, 67,* 387–389.

McCloy, L. (1982). The biomechanical basis for joint protection in osteoarthritis. *Canadian Journal of Occupational Therapy, 49*(3), 85–87.

McDermott, M., & Freyne, P. (1983). Osteoarthritis in runners with knee pain. *British Journal of Sports Medicine, 17,* 84–87.

McKnight, P. T., & Kwoh, C. K. (1992). Randomized, controlled trial of compression gloves in rheumatoid arthritis. *Arthritis Care Research, 5*(4), 223–227.

McNeal, R. (1990). Aquatic therapy for patients with rheumatic disease. *Rheumatic Disease Clinics of North America, 16*, 915–929.

Meenan, R., Mason, J., & Anderson, J. (1992). The content and properties of a revised and expanded Arthritis Impact Measurement Health Status Questionnaire. *Arthritis and Rheumatism, 35*, 1–10.

Melvin, J. L. (1981). *Cervical support pillow to reduce neck pain: Follow-up survey of patient response.* Arthritis Health Professions Association Conference, San Antonio, TX.

Melvin, J. L. (1989a). Orthotic treatment for osteoarthritis of the thumb carpometacarpal joint: Evaluation of efficacy and compliance: AHPA Scientific Meeting, Cincinnati, Ohio. *Arthritis Care and Research, 2*(1), S10.

Melvin, J. L. (1989b). *Rheumatic disease in the adult and child* (3rd ed.). Philadelphia: F. A. Davis.

Minor, M. (1996). Arthritis and exercise: The times they are a-changin'. *Arthritis Care and Research, 9*, 79–81.

Minor, M. (1998). Exercise for health and fitness. In J. L. Melvin & G. Jensen (Eds.), *Rheumatologic rehabilitation series: Volume 1: Assessment and management* (pp. 351–386). Bethesda, MD: American Occupational Therapy Association.

Minor, M., Hewett, J., Webel, R., Anderson, S., & Kay, D. (1989). Efficacy of physical conditioning exercise in rheumatoid arthritis and osteoarthritis. *Arthritis and Rheumatism, 32*, 1396–1405.

Moldofsky, H., Lue, F. A., & Saskin, P. (1987). Sleep and morning pain in primary osteoarthritis. *Journal of Rheumatology, 14*(1), 124–128.

Moratz, V., Muncie, H. L., Jr., & Miranda-Walsh, H. (1986). Occupational management in the multidisciplinary assessment and management of osteoarthritis. *Clinical Therapeutics, 9*(Suppl. B), 24–29.

Morisky, D. E., Green, L. W., & Levine, D. M. (1986). Concurrent and predictive validity of a self reported measure of medication adherence. *Medical Care, 24*, 67–74.

Murray, R., & Duncan, C. (1971). Athletic activity in adolescence as an etiological factor in degenerative hip disease. *Journal of Bone and Joint Surgery, 53B*, 406–419.

Neumann, D. A. (1989). Biomechanical analysis of selected principles of hip joint protection. *Arthritis Care and Research, 2*, 146–155.

Nordemar, R., Ekblom, B., Zachrisson, L., & Lundquist, K. (1981). Physical training in rheumatoid arthritis: A controlled long-term study: I. *Scandinavian Journal of Rheumatology, 10*, 17–23.

Noyes, F. R., Matthews, D. S., Mooar, P. A., & Grood, E. S. (1983). The symptomatic anterior cruciate deficient knee. *Journal of Bone and Joint Surgery, 65A*, 163–173.

Panush, R. S., & Brown, D. G. (1987). Exercise and arthritis. *Sports Medicine, 4*(1), 54–64.

Rejeski, W. J., Ettinger, Jr., W. H., Schumaker, S., James, P., Burns, R., & Elam, J. T. (1995). Assessing performance-related disability in patients with knee osteoarthritis. *Osteoarthritis and Cartilage, 3*, 157–167.

Roberts, J., & Burch, T. (1938). (USPHS Publication No. 1000, Series II, No. 15). Washington, DC: U.S. Public Health Service.

Robinson, W. D. (1985). Management of degenerative joint disease. In W. M. Kelley, E. D. Harris, S. Ruddy, & C. B. Sledge (Eds.), *Textbook of rheumatology* (2nd ed.). Philadelphia: Saunders.

Saal, J. (1990). Dynamic muscular stabilization in the nonoperative treatment of lumbar pain syndromes. *Orthopaedic Review, 19*, 691–700.

Short, C. L. (1947). Arthritis in the Mediterranean theater of operations: Incidence of joint disease. *New England Journal of Medicine, 236*, 383–395.

Simkin, P. A. (1995). Why this joint and why not that joint? *Scandinavian Journal of Rheumatology, 24* (Suppl. 101), 13–16.

Sledge, C. B., Sternberg, J. J., & Tsukamoto, S. (1981). Communication between synoviocytes and chondrocytes: Effect of hydrocortisone and other agents. *Seminars in Arthritis and Rheumatism, 11,* 136–137.

Sokoloff, L. (1969). *The biology of degenerative joint disease* (pp. 5–23). Chicago, IL: University of Chicago Press.

Sprague, R. (1983). The acute cervical joint lock. *Physical Therapy, 63,* 1439–1444.

Stankovic, A., Mitrovic, D., & Ryckewaert, A. (1980). Prevalence of degenerative lesions in articular cartilage of the human knee joint: Relationship with age. In J. G. Peyron (Ed.), *Epidemiologie de l'arthrose* (pp. 94–98). Paris: Geigy.

Suomi, R., & Lindauer, S. (1997). Effectiveness of the Arthritis Foundation Aquatic Program on strength and range of motion in women with arthritis. *Journal of Aging and Physical Activity, 5,* 341–351.

Swanson, A. B., & de Groot-Swanson, G. (1985). Osteoarthritis in the hand. *Clinics in Rheumatic Diseases, 11*(2), 393–420.

Twomey, L., & Taylor, J. (1987). The lumbar spine, low back pain and physical therapy. In L. Twomey & J. Taylor (Eds.), *Physical therapy of the low back* (pp. 303–315). New York: Churchill Livingstone.

Van de Putte, L. B. A. (1995). Why the joint? *Scandinavian Journal of Rheumatology, 24* (Suppl. 101), 7–9.

van Saase, J. L., van Romunde, L. K., Cats, A., Vandenbroucke, J. P., & Valkenburg, H. A. (1989). Epidemiology of osteoarthritis: Zoetermeer survey: Comparison of radiologic osteoarthritis in a Dutch population with that in 10 other populations. *Annals of Rheumatic Disease, 48,* 271–280.

Vincelette, P., Laurin, C., & Levesque, H. (1972). The footballer's ankle and foot. *Canadian Medical Association Journal, 107,* 873–877.

Ware, J. E., & Sherbourne, C. D. (1992). The MOS 36-item short-form health survey (SF-36): I: Conceptual framework and item selection. *Medical Care, 30,* 473–483.

Washington, E. (1978). Musculoskeletal injuries in theatrical dancers: Site, frequency and severity. *American Journal of Sports Medicine, 2,* 75–98.

Weinberger, M., Tierney, W. M., & Booher, P. (1989). Common problems experienced by adults with OA. *Arthritis Care and Research, 2*(3), 94–99.

Wood, P. H. N. (1976). Osteoarthritis in the community. *Clinics in Rheumatic Diseases, 2,* 495–507.

Zayer, M. (1980). Osteoarthritis following Blount's disease. *International Orthopaedics, 4,* 63–66.

6

FIBROMYALGIA SYNDROME

I. Jon Russell, MD, PhD, Jeanne L. Melvin, MS, OTR, FAOTA, and Mima Siegel, PT

Fibromyalgia syndrome (FMS) is a chronic, painful disorder characterized by widespread discomfort and tenderness to palpation at anatomically defined "tender points." The term *fibromyalgia* refers to pain perceived to be in the muscles and fibrous soft tissues. *Syndrome* refers to the somewhat variable spectrum of associated symptoms. (This terminology reflects a symptomatic classification, even though the perpetuating mechanism is probably a central neuroendocrine disorder.)

Population Affected

The nationwide prevalence of FMS is not known, but an epidemiological study conducted in Wichita, KS, found prevalence rates of 3.4% in women and 2% overall (Wolfe, Ross, Anderson, Russell, & Herbert, 1995b). Adult women develop FMS seven to nine times more often than men. About five million persons in the United States have FMS, and the frequency is similar in every country of the world studied to date (Wolfe, 1993). The peak age of onset is in the mid fifth decade (Wolfe, Ross, Anderson & Russell, 1995a), but persons at any age can be affected, including children and elderly persons (Buskila et al., 1993). FMS is present in about 5% to 10% of all patients in a general medicine clinic and in about 10% to 20% of patients in rheumatology clinics (Goldenberg, Simms, Geiger, & Komaroff, 1990). The annual direct cost of FMS to the U.S. economy for medical and rehabilitative care is estimated to exceed $12 billion (Wolfe et al., 1997b). Lost wages, domestic burdens, and compromised quality of life must be added to the direct cost to determine the real cost of FMS to patients and society.

Diagnosis

Until recently, a prevalent belief was that patients with FMS exhibited no objective abnormalities. As a result, the disorder was diagnosed on the basis of the subjective symptoms. Initially, the most convincing evidence that FMS is an integrated syndrome was the relative consistency of the symptoms from one patient to another.

In 1990, the American College of Rheumatology (ACR) published classification criteria for FMS (Wolfe et al., 1990) to help define and standardize patient selection for research studies. These criteria are now likewise applied as diagnostic criteria. Before these criteria became available, physicians first ruled out all other conditions that could cause widespread pain before they could make the diagnosis of FMS. Now, FMS is diagnosed when a person meets the published classification criteria, even when there are concomitant conditions. The ACR diagnostic criteria are a highly sensitive and specific means of identifying affected persons (Table 1). FMS diagnosis requires a history of widespread body pain for at least 3 months and a physical finding of pain induced by 4 kg palpation pressure/cm^2 at 11 of the 18 anatomically defined tender points (Figure 1). A wide range of systemic manifestations referred to as *associated symptoms* may accompany FMS, but they are not required for diagnosis (Table 2). Associated symptoms are not included in the diagnostic criteria because they can occur in persons without FMS and because their inclusion did not improve the sensitivity of the criteria for distinguishing persons with FMS from patients with other chronic disorders (Wolfe et al., 1990). For a given person with FMS, it is important document the nature and extent of associated symptoms and to track the person's progress during treatment.

Etiology

The pathogenesis of FMS was at first thought to reside in the skeletal muscles near the location of the pain. In fact, several uncontrolled studies reported observing microscopic abnormalities in the muscles of patients with FMS, but ultrastructural study failed to identify any specific abnormality (Yunus, Kalyan-Raman, Masi, & Aldag, 1989). When a carefully controlled study of muscle metabolism used deconditioned control subjects to match inactive patients with FMS, magnetic resonance spectroscopy failed to identify abnormalities in muscle metabolism, which indicates that muscle abnormalities detected in earlier studies may have been confounded by deconditioning (Simms, 1996). Other studies of muscle strength that appeared to distinguish patients with FMS from control subjects may have suffered, in part, from differences in voluntary effort. Therefore, soft-tissue tenderness in FMS cannot be explained by primary muscle abnormalities, either structural or functional (Simms, 1996).

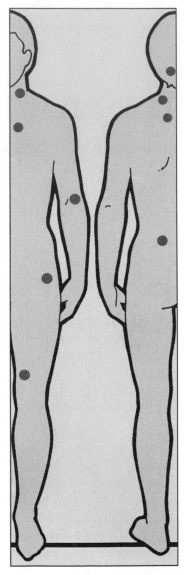

Figure 1. The dots indicate the 18 tender points evaluated to diagnose FMS. There are 9 on each side of the body. *Note.* From *Fibromyalgia: Getting Healthy*, by J. Melvin, 1996, Bethesda, MD: American Occupational Therapy Association. Copyright 1996 by the American Occupational Therapy Association. Reprinted with permission.

On the other hand, independently confirmed laboratory findings in FMS now include persistently elevated levels of cerebrospinal fluid substance P (a neuropeptide that facilitates pain

Table 1. The 1990 American College of Rheumatology Criteria For the Classification of Fibromyalgia Syndrome (Criteria developed to define patients included in research)

- **From history:** Widespread musculoskeletal pain (axial skeleton and all four extremities) for at least 3 months
- **From exam:** Reproducible tenderness (described as "painful") with 4 kg of palpation pressure or less at 11 of 18 anatomically defined tender points (See Figure 1)

Anatomical location of bilateral tender point sites
- Occiput: near the greater occipital nerve foramen
- Cervical: the anterior aspect of the intertransverse spaces at C5–C7
- Trapezius: the midpoint of the upper trapezius border
- Scapular: above the scapular spine over the origin of the supraspinatus muscle
- Second rib: the upper rib surface lateral to the sternum at the costochondral junction
- Epicondyle: the extensor fascia 2 cm distal to the lateral epicondyle
- Gluteal: the gluteus maximus muscle near the posterior ileal origin of the gluteus medius
- Trochanter: the posterior margin of the greater trochanter
- Medial knee: the soft-tissue fascia proximal to the medial femoral condyle

Note. From "The American College of Rheumatology 1990 Criteria for the Classification of Fibromyalgia," by F. Wolfe et al., 1990, *Arthritis and Rheumatism, 33*, pp. 103–112. Copyright 1990 by Lippincott Williams & Wilkins. Reprinted with permission.

Table 2. Possible Associated Symptoms in Fibromyalgia Syndrome

All of these symptoms can occur with or without FMS, but if they start after the onset of FMS, they are likely to be associated. If they occurred before the onset of FMS, they may be aggravated by FMS.

Nervous System
Paresthesias
Balance problems
Headaches
Nonrestorative sleep
Insomnia (i.e., difficulty falling asleep, staying asleep, or waking too early)
Cognitive impairment
Panic attacks
Hypersensitivity to sensory stimuli

Skin and Circulatory Systems
Hypersensitivity
Rashes
Raynaud's phenomenon
Thermal dysregulation
- Intolerance to heat or cold
- Night sweats
Swelling in circumscribed areas

Cardiopulmonary System
Dyspnea (diaphragmatic and intercostal muscle impairment)
Costochondritis
Asthma
Allergies
Sinus congestion
Heart palpitations related to anxiety

Gastrointestinal System
Dry mouth (unrelated to medications)
Indigestion
Heartburn and esophageal reflux
Functional bowel disorder (FBD)
(e.g., gas, bloating, slow motility [constipation])
Irritable bowel syndrome (IBS)

Urinary System
Urinary frequency and dysuria (irritable bladder)

Systemic Symptoms
Fatigue

Psychological and Emotional Symptoms
Depression
Anxiety
Increased compulsivity
Hypervigilance

perception) (Russell et al., 1994; Vaeroy, Helle, Forre, Kass, & Terenius, 1988; Welin, Bragee, Nyberg, & Kristiansson, 1995), lower than normal serum serotonin levels (Hrycaj, Stratz, & Muller, 1993; Russell et al., 1992; Russell, Vipraio, & Lopez, 1993), lower than normal plasma insulin-like growth factor levels (Bennett, Clark, Campbell, & Burckhardt, 1992; Russell, Vipraio, Michalek, & Lopez, 1992), and abnormal functions of the hypothalamic-pituitary-adrenal axis (Crofford et al., 1994; Griep, Boersma, & deKloet, 1993; Tilbe, Bell, & McCain, 1988). These findings clearly indicate that the central nervous system (CNS) mechanisms for regulating pain and physiological stress are disordered in FMS.

Other abnormalities awaiting confirmation by a second study include elevated spinal fluid levels of nerve growth factor (Giovengo, Russell, & Larson, in press), histological changes in skeletal muscle vessels (Lindman, Hagberg, Bengtsson, Henriksson, & Thornell, 1995), low skeletal muscle adenosine triphosphate (ATP) (Bengtsson, Henriksson, & Larsson, 1986) and low erythrocyte ATP (findings that indicate an apparent defect in energy metabolism) (Eisinger & Ayavou, 1990; Russell & Vipraio, 1993), low serum tryptophan (the substrate for serotonin metabolism) (Russell, Michalek, Vipraio, Fletcher, & Wall, 1989), impaired transport of tryptophan across the blood–brain barrier (Yunus, Dailey, Aldag, Masi, & Jobe, 1992), increased activity of kynurenine synthesis (which diverts tryptophan away from serotonin synthesis) (Russell, Vipraio, & Acworth, 1993), decreased platelet serotonin concentration (Russell & Vipraio, 1994), increased numbers of platelet membrane reuptake receptors for serotonin (Russell et al., 1992), decreased excretion of 5-hydroxy indole acetic acid (a metabolite of serotonin) (Kang, Russell, Vipraio, & Acworth, 1998), abnormal erythrocyte carbohydrate metabolism because levels of the enzyme transketolase are low (Eisinger & Ayavou, 1990), and dramatically high serum hyaluronic acid, which may prove to be the biological equivalent of prolonged morning stiffness (Yaron et al., 1997).

These abnormalities, if confirmed, suggest that FMS is a disorder of energy metabolism, tryptophan and serotonin metabolism, and pain or sensory amplification. Until two or more investigators confirm a new finding, it is difficult to know how much credence to give to it. The confirmation of such biochemical findings will signal a major departure from the previous belief that there are no objective abnormalities in FMS.

Reliable classification criteria have made diagnosing FMS possible even in the presence of other painful conditions. This disorder can occur in conjunction with a wide variety of rheumatic, infectious, myopathic, neurological, endocrine, malignant, or psychiatric disorders. There may be unknown metabolic or neurochemical connections between FMS and recognized concomitant conditions. On the other hand, many persons with severe chronic pain, sleep disorders, illness, and depression never develop FMS. The question that remains is whether everyone is potentially susceptible to develop FMS given the right set of circumstances or whether FMS only occurs in persons with a specific genetic predisposition.

Differential Diagnosis

FMS may present as an isolated painful condition, in which case it must be distinguished from various other painful conditions. FMS can accompany other painful disorders, such as systemic lupus erythematosus, in which the contribution of symptoms from each disorder can produce a composite that is clinically more troublesome than either disorder alone.

FMS Versus Localized Soft-Tissue Pain

There are more than 100 non-arthritic conditions in which a localized soft-tissue structure of the musculoskeletal system becomes painful, often after an injury or an unusually vigorous episode of exercise. It is helpful to classify these painful localized syndromes as bursitis, tendonitis, nerve compression, enthesis, or referred pain. Most of these conditions can be identified by pressure on the tender anatomical structure. FMS is distinguished from these localized conditions when widespread pain and tenderness are present.

Table 3. Tender Points Versus Trigger Points (Borg-Stein & Stein, 1996)

Tender Points	Trigger Points
Areas of tenderness	Areas that are painful
• Muscle	muscle
• Musculotendinous junction	
• Bursa	
• Fat pad	
Symmetrical, widespread	Asymmetrical, focal
Treatment is systemic	Treatment is local
No referral pain pattern	Referral pain patterns
No taut bands	Have taut bands

FMS Versus Myofascial Pain Syndrome

It is important to distinguish FMS from myofascial pain syndrome (MPS), which is a regional pain syndrome related to an active trigger point (Travell & Simons, 1992). (See Table 3 for a comparison of trigger and tender points.) Two practical problems with the evaluation of MPS and trigger points have only recently become obvious. The first is that clinicians quite skilled in the diagnosis and treatment of MPS have exhibited poor interrater agreement when asked to examine a series of healthy control subjects interspersed randomly with persons who have MPS (Gerwin, Shannon, Hong, Hubbard, & Gevirtz, 1995; Nice, Riddle, Lamb, Mayhew, & Rucker, 1992; Wolfe et al., 1992). However, interrater reliability has improved with preexamination training (Gerwin et al., 1995). Many clinicians had erroneously believed that an person with regional MPS could gradually develop satellite sites that could eventually involve the entire body to form a widespread total-body MPS. It now seems likely that patients with widespread pain actually have FMS. These issues raise concern about the accuracy of the literature that earlier characterized the features of MPS, including its pathogenesis.

FMS Versus Cardiac Disease

A patient with FMS may experience severe chest pain that resembles angina. Palpation on the second or third costochondral junctions of the upper anterior chest in such a patient will often reproduce the pain pattern. At the same time, there will be tenderness at most of the other tender points. Sometimes it is necessary to evaluate the patient for ischemic heart disease because the two conditions can coexist.

FMS Versus Nerve Entrapment

The low back, lateral thigh, and medial knee tender points are typical anatomical locations for tenderness in FMS, but together they may seem like they are continuous and may descriptively sound like sciatica. However, if the patient has FMS, the paresthesias will not follow a dermatome, and there will be widespread tenderness and positive tender points in the upper body.

Tingling or numbness in the distal upper and lower extremities associated with FMS can sometimes mimic nerve entrapment syndromes (e.g., carpal tunnel, cubital tunnel, radiculopathy, or thoracic outlet). In FMS, the paresthesias do not follow dermatome patterns, and the electromyograms of patients with FMS are usually normal. Sometimes, the paresthesias of FMS can mimic peripheral neuropathies resulting from diabetes, heavy metal intoxication, or vitamin deficiency. In these cases, positive diagnostic tests for metabolic or toxic diseases are needed to define the etiology. Having FMS does not protect a patient from developing other disorders, so health care workers must remain alert for overlapping conditions.

FMS Versus Chronic Fatigue Immune Dysfunction Syndrome

Chronic fatigue immune dysfunction syndrome (CFIDS), which is sometimes called "chronic fatigue syndrome," is an uncommon, unusually severe cause of fatigue. Milder forms of chronic fatigue are much more common and may be caused by poor sleep, inadequate exercise, depression, poor nutrition, low thyroid, hypoxia, anemia, and various other medical conditions. Patients who do not meet the diagnostic criteria for CFIDS may have chronic fatigue but not the syndrome.

Initially, CFIDS was described in small isolated epidemics, which led to the hypothesis that the cause was a transmissible agent. The initial impressions of an infectious process have since given way to neuroendocrine explanations mainly involving the hypothalamic-pituitary-adrenal axis (Demitrack et al., 1991). Patients with CFIDS who have widespread pain (about 70%) often meet the criteria for FMS and have both conditions (Komaroff & Goldenberg, 1989).

Course and Prognosis of FMS

The severity of FMS varies greatly between persons and in the same person from time to time. Several studies have documented the natural course of FMS (Bengtsson, Backman, Lindblom, & Skogh, 1994; Felson & Goldenberg, 1986; Wolfe et al., 1997a, 1997b). These studies reported that some patients describe a rather consistent pattern of their symptoms, pain, and severity over a period of 10 to 20 years. Other patients report a more episodic course with exacerbations and partial remissions. Most patients can adapt to their symptoms sufficiently to allow them to live relatively active lives (Henriksson, Gundmark, Bengtsson, & Ek, 1992). This is not true, however, for about one third of patients (Wolfe et al., 1995a) whose symptoms have been sufficiently severe to interfere with employment, compromise the person's quality of life, and reduce the person's ability to fulfill social roles.

FMS commonly develops after trauma (Buskila, Neumann, Vaisberg, Alkalay, & Wolfe, 1997), surgery, or bereavement. One explanation is that these events cause stress, depression, and anxiety and disturb sleep. These factors may alter serotonin metabolism and neuroendocrine function, thus triggering FMS. There has been a concern that research on FMS has involved only the most severe cases. Bradley and colleagues (1994) evaluated persons in the community who had not sought medical care for FMS. They had milder symptoms and less psychiatric complications than clinic patients. This may only reflect clinical practice because many patients report having mild symptoms for years but only sought care when symptoms became severe. Alternatively, patients may seek clinical care for physical symptoms as their emotional symptoms worsen.

As with most clinical disorders, the attitude of patients with FMS toward their illness, their general coping skills, and their healthy lifestyle behaviors can be an important determinant of their ability to adapt to their symptoms. A diligent approach to seeking a physician, a therapist, and a beneficial treatment program illustrates a level of self-reliance. This self-motivation toward exploring and resolving physical, psychological, and environmental problems would likely improve the overall prognosis for FMS (Gustafsson & Gaston-Johansson, 1996).

Disability

Persons with FMS exhibit limitations of physical function nearly comparable with that of persons with rheumatoid arthritis (RA), even though these patients are limited by different factors (Cathey, Wolfe, & Kleinheksel, 1988). Both groups indicate similar levels of subjective pain (Bombardier et al., 1986). Patients with FMS are not only limited by pain and fatigue but also by cognitive impairment that diminishes their ability to organize, plan, and multitask, skills that are required for many vocations and social roles. Many patients with FMS are limited by hyperreactivity to environmental stimuli such as lights, sound, and motion (Waylonis & Heck, 1992). Some of these persons have trouble processing verbal communication, and others are limited by the depression or anxiety that are part of FMS. The contribution of cognitive impairment to disability in FMS has not been determined, but it likely plays a major role.

The actual cause of physical impairment in FMS needs further clarification because neither limited joint range of motion (ROM) nor muscle weakness correlates with the compromise in physical function. About 30% to 45% of patients with FMS have opted for early retirement or have accepted a work change that resulted in decreased job status or income. This seems to clearly indicate that some persons with FMS are not able to function as effectively as they did before the onset of FMS (Liller, Mutter, & Catlett, 1995; Wolfe et al., 1995a).

Two patient surveys (*Fibromyalgia Syndrome: Current Clinical Status*, 1994; Liller et al., 1995) found that about 10% of patients with FMS received Social Security disability payments. In many such cases, however, the basis for awarding disability payments was a concomitant condition like osteoarthritis (OA), even when careful evaluation revealed that the most troublesome symptoms were actually due to FMS. It is important to note that FMS does not resolve once disability compensation is granted (McCain, Cameron, & Kennedy, 1989; Moldofsky, Wong, & Lue, 1993), so it is unlikely that patients with FMS are defrauding the system.

RA and OA are listed by the U.S. Social Security Administration as potentially disabling conditions, but FMS is not; this understandably makes receiving disability payments more difficult for persons with FMS for comparable incapacity to accomplish a given task. It is still not clear which criteria should be used in any nonterminal pain condition to establish the inability to accomplish any regular compensable work. Therapists must develop functional capacity evaluations that fairly document physical limitations in patients with FMS.

Medical Management

Clearly, the correct diagnoses must be made, and concomitant illnesses must be addressed appropriately. Education about FMS is critical for medical management and in enlisting the patient's active participation in self-management (Russell, 1996). There are various educational media available for FMS (Box 1), but there is no substitute for one-on-one education from an informed

---

Box 1
Resources

Organization Resources

The Arthritis Foundation
1330 West Peachtree Street
Atlanta, GA 30309
1-404-872-7100 or 1-800-283-7800
Internet address: www.arthritis.org

This organization provides an excellent booklet on FMS and on specific medications at no charge, aquatic and land-based exercise classes, and the Fibromyalgia Self-Help Course nationwide. Some chapters offer a free health video lending library. The organization can refer patients to rheumatologists with a special interest in FMS.

The Arthritis Society
National Office
250 Bloor Street East, Suite 901
Toronto, ON M4W 3P2
1-416-967-1414 or 1-416-967-7171 (fax)
Internet address: www.arthritis.ca

This organization offers specialized patient care programs, recreational exercise programs, resource libraries, and consumer education material.

CFIDS Association of America
P.O. Box 220398
Charlotte, NC 28222-0398
1-800-442-3437

Fibromyalgia Alliance of America
P.O. Box 21990
Columbus, OH 43221-0990
1-614-457-4222, 1-888-717-6711 (United States only), or 1-614-457-4222 (fax)

This organization provides patient education and support group resources and publishes *The Fibromyalgia Times* newsletter.

Interstitial Cystitis Association
51 Monroe Street
Suite 1402
Rockville, MD 20850
1-301-610-5300 or 1-301-610-5308 (fax)
Internet address: www.ichelp.org

National Chronic Pain Outreach
   Association, Inc.
7070 Old Georgetown Road
Suite 100
Bethesda, MD 20814-2429
1-301-652-4948 or 1-301-907-0745 (fax)

National Fibromyalgia Research Association
P.O. Box 500
Salem, OR 97302

Internet address: www.teleport.com/~nfra (may have to search this site through yahoo.com or hotbot.com). This is an activist organization to promote education on and treatment of FMS. It provides an updated list of resources for FMS.

National Sleep Foundation
729 15th Street NW, 4th Floor
Washington, DC 20005
Internet address: natsleep@erols.com

Internet Resources

Searching "Fibromyalgia" on the Internet brings up an extensive array of resources and sales pitches.

- The Mining Company Guide to Arthritis (http://arthritis.miningco.com/msub15.htm) provides an extensive number of resources, fact sheets, interactive opportunities, and links to other Internet resources

(continued)

Box 1 (continued)

on FMS and other rheumatic diseases. They provide excellent education material. (*Note.* You may have to search "arthritis and mining company" to find this site.)

- The Fibromyalgia Network (www.fmnetnews.com)

- The British Columbia Fibromyalgia Society (www.alternatives.com/bcfms) provides a current list of excellent fibromyalgia Web links.

- *The Journal of SLEEP* (www.leland.stanford.edu/dept/sleep/journal) provides scientific abstracts pertaining to sleep research.

- The Amazon Bookstore (amazon.com) lists all the books published on FMS.

- Abledata (www.abledata.com) is a national database on adaptive equipment and assistive devices.

- One Step Ahead News (www.osanews.com) is the Web's on-line news magazine for persons with disabilities and provides excellent links to other sites related to coping with disabilities, including one on the Americans With Disabilities Act (www.osanews.com/Links/ada.htm).

Professional Publications

Journal of Musculoskeletal Pain
Quarterly, $50 per year
Haworth Medical Press, 1-800-342-9678

Journal of Musculoskeletal Medicine
Cliggot Publishing Company
Box 4010
Greenwich, CT 06830

Arthritis Care and Research (the *Journal of the Association of Rheumatology Health Professionals*)

American College of Rheumatology
60 Executive Park South
#150
Atlanta, GA 30329
Internet address: www.rheumatology.org

---

health care provider to help patients achieve individual goals. Reassurance that the symptoms are real and make sense can help the patient to have confidence in the diagnosis and treatment.

Self-management training plays an especially important role for patients with FMS who are hypersensitive to medications and may experience side effects from normal doses. Medications are often started at pediatric doses or at half of a normal adult dose. Many patients with FMS simply do not want to take medications. For this reason, patients appreciate nonpharmacological approaches such as rehabilitation.

Herbal Products and Supplements

There are numerous herbs that have been historically used to increase calmness or encourage deeper sleep. There is little or no scientific documentation of these claims in relation to FMS, but these herbs do not appear to be harmful. The most common "relaxing herbs" used as teas are mint, chamomile, anise passion flower, valerian root, and hops. These herbs are considered to be antispasmodic and aid digestion by relaxing the gastrointestinal tract. Teas that contain citrus, strong spices, or rose hips are used by some persons for revitalization in the afternoon but are too stimulating for use in the evening. Valerian root can be taken in capsule form and has been found to be a mild to moderate hypnotic substance (Balderer & Borbely, 1985; Lindahl & Lindwall, 1989). There are several products in pill form that combine the above herbs and claim to improve sleep. One homeopathic product, Calms Forte (P & S Laboratories, a division of Standard Homeopathic Company, Los Angeles, CA) has been helpful for one author (J.M.) to achieve deeper sleep in patients who cannot tolerate medications. Calms Forte contains hops, oats, chamomile, calcium, magnesium, and phosphates. The dosage is from 1 to 6 tablets a day. Calms Forte does not encourage dependence. Kava kava extract is currently popular as an herbal sleep aid, but some patients stop taking it because of excessive dreaming or nightmares. There are reports of serious side effects with pure kava kava (Tinsley, 1999), and it should not be taken with medications prescribed to enhance sleep or with benzodiazepines.

Melatonin is considered to be a natural product, but it is actually a brain hormone produced during sleep. It is effective for short-term treatment of jet lag and shift-work adjustment, but there are no long-term studies regarding its side effects when used for chronic sleep disorders. It does cross the placenta and is not advisable for pregnant women. Because it is involved in the regulation of adolescent maturation, there is substantial concern about its use in children. Patients with FMS produce increased amounts of melatonin (L. J. Crofford, personal communication, 1998).

Malic acid. The use of a malic acid-magnesium combination in the treatment of patients with FMS has its origin in a research study (Russell, Michalek, Flechas, & Abraham, 1995) that found no clear benefit in the low-dose (1,200 mg malic acid/day plus 300 mg magnesium hydroxide) placebo-controlled phase but did find substantial benefit with higher dosages in an open-label, follow-up phase in which a placebo effect could not be excluded. In large doses, malic acid and magnesium hydroxide may reduce fatigue and exhaustion. This combination seems to be quite safe except for mild diarrhea caused by the magnesium in some patients. For persons with abnormal kidney function, this product could dangerously elevate magnesium levels and cause muscle weakness.

5-Hydroxy tryptophan (5-HTP). 5-HTP is a metabolic intermediate in the conversion of the amino acid tryptophan to serotonin. Administering 5-HTP orally is believed to increase serotonin production. One research study (Caruso, Sarzi Puttini, Cazzola, & Azzolini, 1990) has shown that 5-HTP is helpful in reducing the painful symptoms and insomnia of FMS. Caution is advised when combining this drug with other serotonergic drugs. Clinical experience indicates that it may take 2 to 3 months for benefits of 5-HTP to become apparent, and outcome is highly variable. Side effects are fairly minimal, but a contaminant in some preparations was blamed for inducing eosinophilia myalgia syndrome (Mayo Clinic Health Oasis, 1998). The quality of nonprescription products is difficult to determine.

S-adenosyl-l-methionine (SAMe). SAMe is a naturally occurring compound in all human tissue and organs. The body produces SAMe from methionine (an amino acid) and ATP (an energy-producing compound). SAMe is a supplement that reduces inflammation and improves depression. It has been used a prescription medication in Europe for years. In 1989, the U.S. Food and Drug Administration withdrew its support of SAMe during the evaluation process because of concerns over manufacturing methods (the substance is unstable and disintegrates if not properly processed). It became available in the United States in 1999 as an over-the-counter supplement for "joint health" and "emotional well-being." All of the studies reporting positive outcomes with SAMe involved daily injections or high daily doses. There are no studies documenting its effectiveness as a low-dose supplement.

SAMe (800 mg/day orally) has been evaluated in patients with FMS in Europe with mixed results. One study (Jacobsen, Danneskiold-Samsoe, & Andersen, 1991) showed a reduction in pain, tenderness, fatigue, morning stiffness, and mood. In another study using 600 mg of intravenous SAMe (Volkmann et al., 1997), there was improvement in subjective perception of pain and overall well-being, but there was no change in objective measures. The side effects of SAMe are minimal.

Guaifenesin. Guaifenesin is most readily available as an ingredient in cough syrup. It was theorized to aid FMS by reducing urate crystal formation, but the basis for that theory is unclear. Popularized on the Internet, guaifenesin was evaluated in a controlled, blinded trial and was shown not to be effective in reducing the symptoms of FMS (Bennett, 1996a).

Medications for Sleep

Ever since FMS was identified as involving a sleep disorder (Moldofsky, Scarisbrick, England, & Smythe, 1975) and serotonin deficiency (Russell et al., 1992), the focus of medical management has been on medications that improve sleep by increasing the availability of serotonin.

Tricyclic antidepressants. Amitriptyline (Elavil) is the most commonly used drug of its type for FMS because studies have demonstrated its effectiveness (Carette, McCain, Bell, & Fam, 1986; Wolfe et al., 1997c). However, amitriptyline has the strongest anticholinergic effect of all tricyclics, which results in symptoms like dry mouth, constipation, urinary retention, weight gain, increased appetite, blurred vision, tachycardia, hypotension in elderly persons, "drug hangover," and increasing restless leg syndrome (Ware, 1983). All of the tricyclics (clomipramine [Anafranil], desipramine, doxepin [Sinequan], impramine [Tofranil], and nortriptyline [Pamelor]) have the potential to cause these side effects. Many tricyclics have less anticholinergic activity than amitriptyline but have not been scientifically tested in FMS.

Tricyclic muscle relaxant. Cyclobenzaprine (Flexeril) has proved effective in improving sleep, which is not surprising because it is structurally similar to amitriptyline.

The use of low-dose tricyclic drugs in FMS is subject to CNS adaptation (tachyphylaxis) after 3 to 4 months of continuous use. This may result from an increase in the numbers of cell surface reuptake receptors for serotonin and norepinephrine, which can defeat the drug's effectiveness. One author's (I.J.R.) approach to tricyclic tachyphylaxis is to discontinue the tricyclic drug after 3 to 4 months of continuous use and substitute low-dose alprazolam (Xanax) for 1 month. Alprazolam is then stopped, and the tricyclic is resumed. This cycle is repeated 4 times a year. Alprazolam is a benzodiazepine and can be addictive, so it must be used with caution in patients with a history of drug addiction.

Trazodone (Desyrel). This antidepressant is believed to be beneficial in FMS and exhibits a lower frequency of side effects than amitriptyline, but it has not been as rigorously studied. Trazodone is an antidepressant in a category by itself. It is used at bedtime to improve sleep similar to the way in which tricyclics are used.

Antihistamines. Most nonprescription sleep aids contain antihistamines that cause drowsiness (e.g., Tylenol-PM contains acetaminophen and diphenhydramine [Benadryl]). These agents may be helpful for the insomnia of FMS, but they have not been properly studied in this condition. "Nondrowsy" antihistamines usually keep persons awake at night. Side effects from sedating antihistamines may include drug hangover and dry mouth.

Hypnotic drugs. Drugs such as flurazepam hydrochloride (Dalmane), triazolam (Halcion), and temazepam (Restoril) have never been options for long-term treatment of FMS or chronic sleep disorders because they have been shown to work for only short periods of time, create dependence and tolerance, and then cause a rebound insomnia when reduced or discontinued. They are primarily used for acute sleep disorders, postsurgical sleep problems, and jet lag, but they do not relieve pain (Moldofsky, Lue, Mously, Roth-Schechter, & Reynolds, 1996). Zolpidem tartrate (Ambian), a newer, nonbenzodiazepine hypnotic, has been effective in reducing the severity of the insomnia in FMS. Zolpidem tartrate may cause a form of physical dependence that is exhibited by a rebound insomnia when it is discontinued after nightly use for more than 2 weeks. One author (I.J.R.) recommends that zolpidem tartrate be used intermittently for no more than 1 to 3 consecutive nights with many nights of nonuse between periods of use.

Analgesics

Nonsteroidal anti-inflammatory drugs. For decades, nonsteroidal anti-inflammatory drugs (NSAIDs) have been inadequate in controlling the symptoms of FMS. Most patients report that they have tried several NSAIDs with some benefit, especially ibuprofen or naproxen. Patients with FMS should only use NSAIDs if the drugs are clearly beneficial because the risk of bleeding peptic ulcers from these drugs can be life-threatening. NSAIDs can additionally cause fluid retention, tinnitus, and confusion in high doses.

Tramadol (Ultram). This drug is sold by prescription as an analgesic. Although it is known to stimulate the μ–opioid receptor, tramadol has only a minimal risk of dependence because it acts like amitriptyline on serotonin and norepinephrine reuptake receptors. In a recent study, moderate doses of this drug dramatically reduced the symptoms, especially the pain, of FMS (Russell, Bennett, Katz, & Kamin, 1997). Potential side effects may include nausea, weight loss, dizziness, and itching. The frequency of these adverse symptoms may be reduced by starting therapy with half of a tablet (25 mg) at bedtime for 2 weeks and gradually increasing the dosage thereafter.

Narcotic analgesics. Examples of these drugs include meperidine (Demerol), morphine, codeine, oxycodone (Percodan), hydrocodone bitartrate (Vicodan), propoxyphene (Darvon), fentanyl (Duragesic), and pentazocine (Talwin). Their use in the treatment of FMS is very controversial, and there are no supportive clinical research studies. Patients quickly develop a tolerance to these drugs and need increasing doses to have any effect; patients then get to a point of experiencing the side effects while still experiencing pain. Patients who appear to need narcotic analgesics should be referred to a chronic pain program for training in behavioral management. Narcotic analgesics can be sedative and cause mental slowing and drowsiness; depress respiration and heart rate, which can affect exercising; and cause constipation (which increases fatigue), nausea, weight loss, dizziness, and itching.

Corticosteroid drugs. Even though abnormalities in the diurnal rhythm of cortisol production have been documented (Crofford et al., 1994), one study that specifically addressed the use of corticosteroids in the treatment of FMS failed to detect a benefit (Clark, Tindall, & Bennett, 1985).

Clinical Features and Associated Symptoms

Musculoskeletal System

There has long been speculation that the skeletal muscles of persons with FMS are abnormal, but there is a paucity of evidence for any specific histological muscle abnormality. Type II muscle atrophy has been reported (Yunus & Kalyan-Raman, 1989), but that would be expected in patients with FMS who are physically inactive. The cause is more likely related to the lack of exercise than to the primary pain process. There is evidence of decreased circulation and hypoxia (Bennett et al., 1989), thickening of the small arterioles (Lindman et al., 1995), and decreased ATP content of FMS skeletal muscles (Bengtsson et al., 1986), but the relationship of these findings to painful symptoms remains speculative.

During fitness and strength testing, persons with FMS performed worse on a second set of tests than on the first set of tests, presumably because the first set increased severity of unpleasant symptoms. However, unknown physiological changes may contribute to poor muscular endurance (Mengshoel, Saugen, Forre, & Vollestad, 1995; Verstappen, van Santen-Hoeufft, van Sloun, & Bolwijn, 1995).

The muscles in the neck, shoulders, and upper back (i.e., trapezius, posterior cervical, and rhomboids) are vulnerable to postural stress, fatigue, strain, and emotional tension that probably result in more discomfort for a patient with FMS than for an otherwise healthy person. These factors can affect healing from cervical trauma. In an Israeli study of 102 persons with cervical spine injuries, 21% developed posttrauma FMS compared with 1.7% of 59 patients with leg fractures (Buskila et al., 1997).

A unique neurophysiological relationship between the postural (trunk) muscles and the psyche may exist that does not appear to exist in the peripheral muscles. The slumped, round-shouldered posture reflective of depression is believed to result from a combination of posterior trunk inhibition and anterior trunk stimulation (Lowen, 1973). Conversely, the chest-high, shoulder-protracted stance of someone who is exuberant reflects posterior stimulation and anterior inhibition. Our language reflects this process as "shouldering burdens" and "embracing triumph."

Pain or aching is the major complaint of patients with FMS. The pain has been likened to that of being physically traumatized from head to toe. The symptoms of spontaneous widespread pain, diffuse soft-tissue tenderness, and tenderness to palpation at the tender points tend to be bilateral and symmetrical. Typically, the pain is constant, although the severity and location of pain may vary from hour to hour and day to day with different phases of the menstrual cycle, variation of sleep quality, and changes of the seasons. In one study of 554 patients with FMS, 70% reported that their symptoms were aggravated by noise, lights, stress, and weather (Waylonis & Heck, 1992). Patients typically believe that their pain worsens so consistently with changes in the weather that they can predict a fall in the barometric pressure, but recent research has failed to confirm that impression (Viitanen, Kautiainen, & Isomaki, 1995).

Morning stiffness in the muscles (not the joints) is a common complaint of patients with FMS. This stiffness tends to last for 30 min to 4 hr in the morning like the stiffness of RA. Patients often have difficulty distinguishing between stiffness and pain or aching.

Stiffness in the hands is a common complaint, and FMS may or may not be associated with some objective swelling. There may be difficulty distinguishing this pattern from OA, but the stiffness duration is usually much too long for OA. Patients may think their joints are stiff when in fact the stiffness appears to be in the muscles. Patients with mild, relatively asymptomatic OA may perceive increased pain from affected joints when their pain threshold is lowered by FMS.

A distinction must be made between tender points in FMS and trigger points associated with MPS. Persons with FMS have excessive tenderness in tender points that are predictable areas of tenderness in muscles, tendons, bursa, and fat pads. These tender points become unusually tender as the pain threshold becomes low and pain amplification develops in FMS. Despite the tenderness associated with a tender point, the tissue appears to be structurally normal (Borg-Stein & Stein, 1996). Pressure at tender points does not cause referral of pain to distant zones of reference as with trigger points, although in some cases the anatomical location of the tender point and trigger point may be similar. In other words, tender points are not pathological in and of themselves but rather reflect systemic hypersensitivity and therefore are not treated locally (Table 3) (Borg-Stein & Stein, 1996).

A few patients with FMS may additionally have one or more trigger points somewhere in their musculature, which indicates that MPS can be a concomitant problem in FMS (Granges & Littlejohn, 1995; Hong, Hsueh, & Simons, 1995), but trigger points in patients with FMS are often more resistant to traditional trigger point injection therapy than a classic MPS trigger point would be (Hong et al., 1995). Active trigger points are painful and electrically abnormal (Simons, Hong, & Simons, 1995c), and they benefit from direct treatment, either manual therapy or injection. They are believed to reside near a central end-plate zone or in a spindle fiber in a skeletal muscle "taut band" that can exhibit a "twitch response" when firmly stroked by the examiner's thumb or penetrated by a needle (Simons, Hong, & Simons, 1995a, 1995b). Palpation of the trigger point elicits referred pain in what is called a "zone of reference" (Travell & Simons, 1992). There is now growing consensus regarding the finding of spontaneous electrical activity at trigger point sites in a rabbit model that mimics the findings in humans (Hubbard & Berkoff, 1993; Simons et al., 1995a, 1995b, 1995c).

In one author's (J.M.) experience, there is another phenomenon that appears to be unique to FMS and is best described as "shortening" of all or part of the muscle in a manner that is clinically different from tightness or spasm. The patient does not report pain in the muscle, which is typical of a spasm, but rather they report a sharp pain (like a knife stab) at the tendon insertion at the end of range. This is common in the hip adductor, extensor carpi radialis and brevis, and finger interossei muscles, but it can occur anywhere. If this problem is detected, it can be resolved by carefully and gently stretching the affected muscle. It is helpful to ask patients, "Do you have sharp pain in the muscles with certain motions?" The pain location must be at an enthesis or tendon attachment to indicate this type of problem.

Subcutaneous nodules of fibro-fatty tissue (myogeloses) are symptomatic of FMS. They are benign and are not painful, although palpation of tissue over them may be tender. These nodules are found in healthy persons as well, and there is no evidence that they occur with greater frequency in persons with FMS (Yunus & Kalyan-Raman, 1989).

Tendon involvement. Patients with FMS exhibit tenderness to palpation or pain at certain ligament and tendon insertion sites. One explanation of this problem is that the *enthesis*, the portion of the tendon that attaches to the bone, endures maximum strain during activity because it is the point at which soft tissue attaches to hard tissue. As the pain threshold lowers with FMS, the brain detects pain messages from such overused or abused body structures. Clinically, this can be easily mistaken for tendonitis, but there is no visible inflammation, redness, or swelling. This problem is now referred to as a *noninflammatory enthesopathy.* It is most common in the extensor carpi ulnaris and extensor carpi radialis longus and brevis insertions, but it can occur in all entheses. Noninflammatory enthesopathy is common in the insertions of the interossei muscles, which results in pain over the volar aspect of the metacarpal heads. The location of pain distinguishes the problem from metacarpophalangeal synovitis, which is felt over the dorsum of the joints. Immobilization and cold modalities, similar to those for simple traumatic tendonitis, do not seem to be effective.

Many patients report that they have "joint pain" or "arthritis." It is critical to determine whether these patients have pain deep in the joint (typical of arthritis) or whether the pain is in the tendons and ligaments around the joint (typical of noninflammatory enthesopathy). In lower-extremity and larger joints, patients can distinguish the difference when it is explained to them, but discriminating palpation may be necessary to distinguish between FMS and arthritis in the hands.

Neurological System

Persons with FMS often report paresthesias (mostly tingling, occasionally crawling, or numbness) (Goldenberg, 1987) in their hands, arms, legs, and face. The paresthesias may be confined to the fingertips or fingers or occur in a glove pattern. They do not follow a dermatomal pattern, and this allows the clinician to distinguish FMS paresthesias from other nerve entrapment syndromes. Paresthesias are likely a manifestation of widespread hypersensitivity or sensory amplification, but this has not been proved. Many patients with FMS have been erroneously diagnosed with carpal tunnel syndrome, even though objective signs (e.g., pain in an anatomical distribution, positive Phalen's, decreased sensory perception at the fingertips, and weakness of the opponens pollicus muscle) and diminished sensation are lacking. These patients often unnecessarily undergo invasive nerve conduction studies or even surgery before being correctly diagnosed with FMS (Goldenberg, 1987). These symptoms wax and wane over time but do not progress into serious nerve injury. If the paresthesias are due to FMS, night wrist orthoses generally are not helpful because they are designed for carpal tunnel syndrome, but they may prevent positional strain on the wrist and hand. If they prove helpful in a trial, they are justified when desired by the patient.

Headaches are experienced by half or more of the patients with symptomatic FMS (Yunus, Masi, Calabro, Miller, & Feigenbaum, 1981). True migraine headaches are not much more common in FMS than in other major illnesses, although they may be slightly more common in younger patients. The more typical cause of head pain in FMS is a muscle contraction, a so-called "tension headache." It is a dull, pressure-like ache over the occipital area spread diffusely in the skull or forehead around one eye or both. These headaches are associated with tender points in the suboccipital muscle insertion areas, other muscles in the scalp, and deep cervical ligaments. This type of head pain can be associated with facial numbness and paresthesias of the scalp crown. If severe or chronic, tension headaches can interfere substantially with the patient's quality of life and make working, reading, or accomplishing daily activities even more difficult. A probable cause of headache in FMS is chronic sleep loss.

Patients who report dizziness, lightheadedness, and a feeling of weakness or fatigue when rising from a sitting position (orthostatic intolerance) may have mild autonomic neuropathy (i.e., neurally mediated syncope or hypotension). These symptoms should be reported to the patient's physician (Clauw, Radulovic, Heshmat, & Barbey, 1995). In the therapy clinic, this problem can be evaluated by taking the patient's pulse while sitting and standing. A decrease of 30 beats/min or more in addition to the above symptoms indicates the need for a medical evaluation. A tilt table test provides the objective evidence to make a diagnosis (Bou-Holaigah et al., 1997; Clauw, Radulovic, Katz, Baraniuk, & Barbey, 1995). Mild autonomic neuropathy can be helped with mineralocorticoid medications like fludrocortisone (Florinef) and with compression stockings. It is interesting that this neurological problem affects cardiac function even at night when patients are at rest (Martinez-Lavin, Hermosillo, Rosas, & Soto, 1998).

Cognitive impairment. Patients report difficulty learning and retaining information, processing information quickly, finding the right word, following a conversation while thinking of what to say next, reading concentration and retention, organizing, and planning and prioritizing goals (Fransen & Russell, 1996). Actual confusion (e.g. "I had to stop the car—I had no idea where I was or where I was going") is more common in CFIDS than in FMS. In all of these cognitive functions, the person is able to do the tasks but does them more slowly than normal, and that slowness is dysfunctional compared with their norm before the onset of FMS (Cote & Moldofsky, 1997). For example, if mental integration of the concepts in the first sentence of a paragraph is slowed, the person can become lost while attempting to process the concepts in the second sentence, and so forth. By the end of the paragraph, the patient cannot recall what he or she has read. Fatigue, pain, stress, depression, or anxiety tend to reduce concentration and focus, so there are many factors to consider in attempting to improve cognitive functioning. Cognitive problems improve as the sleep disorder is effectively managed and, in one author' (J.M.) experience, completely resolve if the patient is able to correct the sleep disorder behaviorally without medications (i.e., wake fully rested five out of seven mornings a week).

Motor planning. Problems with balance and clumsiness have emerged as a common symptom of FMS. One explanation is that motor planning slows along with other cognitive skills. For example, patients can see a doorway but cannot integrate the information quickly enough to avoid walking into it.

Muscular weakness. A small percentage of patients present with weakness as a complaint, yet they test within normal limits on a manual muscle examination. Sometimes weakness can be acute and described as "I walked to the end of the block and couldn't take another step. I had to sit down on the curb," or "I was going up stairs, and it felt like my foot was nailed to the floor. I couldn't lift it up." But after resting a bit, these patients are able to move. This problem improves as the FMS improves. Its etiology and mechanism are unknown.

Skin, Circulation, and Thermal Regulation

Skin hypersensitivity is reported as both diffuse and in circumscribed areas and is often described as "feeling like a sunburn" or like an "Indian burn" (i.e., the sensation of having the skin of the forearm twisted in opposite directions). Light touch can be painful for these patients, which illustrates the severity of pain amplification.

Swelling can be subjective or objective. Patients may report a subjective sense of swelling in the hands without objective or visible changes. This is referred to in the literature as *subjective swelling*. It is a characteristic feature of FMS and is typically bilateral. Subjective swelling appears to reflect the sensation of stiffness that patients experience, as in "my hands feel stiff as if they were swollen." Diffuse swelling of the hands, face, or total body is not part of FMS but may represent "idiopathic edema" (Deodhar, Fisher, Blacker, & Woolf, 1994; Yucha & McKay, 1992), a fluid retention imbalance resulting from an elevation of aldosterone, an adrenal hormone. Swelling is treated with a specific diuretic, spironolactone (Aldactone), and a healthy, low-salt diet. These patients should evaluate the role medications such as NSAIDs and tricyclics may play in fluid retention and weight gain.

It is not uncommon for patients to present with circumscribed areas of swelling anywhere on the extremities or trunk, such as a 2-in. area of swelling over the extensor muscles in the forearm or over the wrist. This phenomenon is frequently misdiagnosed as tendonitis or "tennis elbow" or is attributed to inflammation of the underlying structure. There is no warmth or redness, and the swelling does not respond to NSAIDs. The swelling does not appear to be inflammatory, and no treatment is indicated because the swelling is transitory.

Raynaud's phenomenon is reported in about one third of patients with FMS compared with 10% in the general population (Bennett et al., 1991; Vaeroy et al., 1988). Raynaud's phenomenon may be associated with paresthesias and pain in the fingers.

Many patients with FMS report problems with temperature dysregulation (i.e., their ability to adapt to heat or cold). These patients are often cold when others are hot or vice versa. Some patients develop a distracting intolerance to heat or cold. In other words, if a room becomes too cool for them, instead of just being uncomfortable and going on with the task at hand, they find it impossible to think or concentrate until the room is warmer. Hypersensitivity to cold may contribute to muscle stiffness.

Night sweats usually occur between 3:00 and 4:00 A.M. and can be associated with sleep disorders and thermal dysregulation (Glotzbach & Heller, 1994). In perimenopausal women, a hormonal deficiency should be ruled out. A few patients report increased daytime sweating (hyperhidrosis). This is a condition made worse by anxiety and may respond to β-blocker drugs like propranolol HCl (Inderal).

Reticular skin discoloration or vascular mottling that resembles livedo reticularis occurs in a small number of patients and is generally present in both upper extremities but is most visible in the lower extremities (Caro, Wolfe, Johnston, & Smith, 1986). This sign may lead clinicians to mistakenly diagnose reflex sympathetic dystrophy.

Cardiopulmonary System

There are no specific cardiac conditions linked to FMS. However, a rapid heart rate or palpitations may accompany anxiety or be related to the anticholinergic effect of tricyclic medications. There appears to be a definable overlapping prevalence of mitral valve prolapse concomitant with FMS, but the reason for the association is not known. The connection may be hypermobility (double-jointedness), which occurs in 40% of patients with FMS.

In one study (Lurie, Caidahl, Johansson, & Bake, 1990), patients with chronic primary FMS had impaired respiratory function. Patients demonstrated lower maximum inspiratory and expiratory pressures than healthy control subjects; however, spirometric values were normal. Patients with exertion dyspnea had lower respiratory pressures than those without. These findings were attributed to possible respiratory muscle dysfunction. In another study of 84 patients with primary FMS, 84% reported having dyspnea (Caidahl, Lurie, Bake, Johansson, & Wetterqvist, 1989). The severity of the perceived dyspnea correlated with a lower exercise capacity and heart rate on bicycle exercise tests. Weiss, Kreck, and Albert (1998) reported on two cases of severe, chronic episodic dyspnea associated with FMS. One plausible explanation for dyspnea in FMS is the chest pain that accompanies taking a deep breath when the patient has costochondritis at several levels. All patients with FMS who have dyspnea should have a medical workup because the dyspnea should not automatically be attributed to FMS.

Allergies may be considered an associated symptom if they begin or become worse after the onset of FMS. In one study, 38% of patients presenting with rhinitis at an allergy clinic met the diagnostic criteria for FMS (Cleveland, Fisher, Brestel, Esinhart, & Metzger, 1992). On the other hand, Clauw and associates (1996) found no evidence of allergies in many patients with FMS who perceived themselves to be allergic.

Gastrointestinal System

Functional bowel disorder (FBD), which includes any altered bowel function that is not related to inflammation such as constipation or slow motility (not related to diet) and excessive gas or bloating, is almost universal with FMS. Data on irritable bowel syndrome (IBS), a subtype of FBD, suggest that IBS is present in 30% to 60% of patients with primary FMS (Veale, Kavanaugh, Fielding, & Fitzgerald, 1991; Yunus, Masi, & Aldag, 1989).

IBS is characterized by periodically altered bowel habits (diarrhea or constipation) associated with excessive gas and lower abdominal cramping or distention that are usually relieved by bowel movements. There are no abnormalities on colonoscopy examination to suggest organic disease. For these reasons and others, the symptoms of IBS are probably somehow related to emotional stress, but that assertion is difficult to prove objectively. The unpredictability of the bowel symptoms can cause patients to curtail their social or community activities, which further isolates them and increases their anxiety. There is additional evidence that adults with primary IBS have a high frequency of childhood physical and sexual abuse (Scarinci, McDonald-Haile, Bradley, & Richter, 1994; Walker, Katon, Roy-Byrne, Jemelka, & Russo, 1993), but the frequency of abuse in patients with FMS is no different than the frequency of abuse in the general population (Russell, Russell, Cuevas, & Michalek, 1992).

Self-management of IBS includes elimination of substances that can increase gut motility such as fatty and spicy foods, caffeine, alcohol, nicotine, and (for some persons) raw vegetables and certain fruits. A high-fiber, low-fat diet with bulk fiber supplements is recommended for both IBS and constipation caused by slow motility.

Some clinicians recommend a fiber supplement and a benzodiazepine such as alprazolam (Xanax) to reduce the effect of catecholamines on bowel motility. If the bowel problem is associated with FMS or is aggravated by it, treatment of the FMS may improve the bowel problem, and thus drug management of the FMS is the priority. Treatment is the same whether the active problem at any point is diarrhea or constipation. Patients with slow motility often can reduce constipation by increasing water intake, eating a high-fiber diet, or using a fiber supplement such as Metamucil.

Adult-onset lactose intolerance is common in the general population and can overlap with FMS. This is evaluated by having patients eliminate all dairy products from their diets for 2 weeks; if the symptoms abate, the patient is likely to have some form of lactose intolerance. Then the patient must determine which dairy foods do not cause gastrointestinal distress. Persons who are lactose intolerant can often eat dairy products if they drink LactAid milk or take LactAid pills (Ortho-McNeil) after eating dairy products to help digest lactose.

Indigestion and gastric reflux problems (heartburn) are likewise common in FMS. Self-management includes eating in a relaxed atmosphere, self-relaxation before eating, chewing food well, and (for some patients) papaya digestive enzyme tablets help break down fiber and aid digestion. Herbal teas such as chamomile, mint, and anise aid digestion by providing fluid and perhaps relaxing the gastrointestinal tract. Medications such as H2-antagonists (Cimetidine, Zantac, Pepcid) and omeprazole (Prilosec) can help manage symptoms.

Gynecological and Urinary Systems

Premenstrual syndrome often worsens all of the symptoms of FMS (Hapidou & Rollman, 1998) and can seriously disrupt sleep in some patients. These patients may need a specific medication plan to manage sleep disruption from PMS. Concomitant endometriosis is not uncommon and is another source of pain that affects the serotonin system. Pain amplification from FMS may magnify the pain from endometriosis.

A small proportion (less than 30%) of patients with FMS exhibit hypersensitivity of their bladders, which causes urinary frequency (Wallace, 1990; Yunus, 1994). Generally, there is aching in the pelvic area but no burning sensation or fever to suggest an infection. Urinary frequency may result from high water intake to lose weight or to compensate for mouth dryness caused by tricyclic antidepressants. This problem is referred to as *interstitial cystitis* (IC), which is a bladder disorder characterized by intolerable bladder discomfort and histological changes in the bladder mucosa. The numbers of leukocytes typical of an infection will be lacking as will bacteria for cultures. There is considerable overlap of IC and FMS. There are specific dietary recommendations, self-management techniques, and new medications for IC. Patients with this problem should be referred to an urologist with expertise in treating the disorder or to the Interstitial Cystitis Association (Box 1).

Fatigue

For many patients, fatigue is more limiting than the pain of FMS and is the main factor limiting the ability to accomplish self-care, work, and community activities. Several factors contribute to fatigue, including a chronic lack of deep restorative sleep (which is probably the most important factor), chronic persistent pain that can be physically and emotionally draining, emotional distress and depression, and deconditioning from inadequate physical exercise and poor nutrition.

As mentioned earlier, ATP was low in the tender areas of muscles (Bengtsson et al., 1986). In addition, FMS erythrocytes exhibit substantially lower than normal levels of erythrocyte ATP, but the ATP deficiency did not correlate with a patient's subjective symptoms of fatigue (Eisinger, Plantamura, & Ayavou, 1994; Russell & Vipraio, 1993).

Fatigue management training is a critical aspect of comprehensive rehabilitation for FMS. For additional information on fatigue management, see chapter 8 in this volume on systemic lupus erythematosus.

Insomnia and Nonrestorative Sleep

Insomnia (i.e., difficulty falling or staying asleep) or seeming to sleep through the night but waking unrefreshed (i.e., nonrestorative sleep) are among the most prominent features of FMS contributing to fatigue. Patients may have difficulty falling asleep or prolonged latency (the time required to fall asleep), difficulty staying asleep (multiple nocturnal awakenings), or awaking too early in the morning (from 3:00 to 5:00 A.M.) and being unable to return to sleep. Even when patients appear to sleep, their sleep pattern may be deficient in the restorative slow-wave stage of sleep (delta wave, stages 3 and 4 of non–rapid eye movement [REM] sleep) (Anch, Lue, MacLean, & Moldofsky, 1991; Moldofsky, 1982, 1989). As a result, they tend to wake exhausted and feel achy and stiff, as if they had been "hit by a truck." Starting the day tired increases irritability and reduces one's tolerance of stress and pain. This creates a vicious cycle. Loss of restorative sleep can be tolerated by a healthy person for a few days, but patients with FMS face the same set of seemingly insurmountable problems with insomnia day after day and month after month.

Moldofsky and associates (1975) identified an alpha electroencephalogram non-REM sleep disorder in patients with FMS that is characterized by alpha (rapid waves associated with a more alert state) intrusions into deep slow-wave sleep, which results in disturbed deep sleep. This pattern is not unique to FMS, however, and can be found in persons who do not have FMS. Education in sleep hygiene and behavioral methods for improving sleep is critical to treatment.

Visual and Auditory Changes

The most frequent vision complaint of patients with FMS is transient blurred vision that is not helped by changing eyeglasses. This has been identified as "latency in accommodation" (i.e., initial blurring when adjusting vision to near or far). Patients frequently report aching around the eyes, which apparently results from FMS involvement of the eye muscle. One study found impaired eye mobility related to brainstem function (Rosenhall, Johansson, & Orndahl, 1987a), which could likewise represent slowed neuronal transmission.

In an informal study, Sadun (1992) evaluated the eye function of patients in a chronic fatigue syndrome support group and found that patients exhibited latency of accommodation, decreased range of duction (eye mobility), double vision, bouncing images, and primary horizontal nystagmus (23% of 44 patients).

A study on hearing indicated a slight decrease in auditory perception in a small percentage of patients with FMS who had auditory testing, which again indicates abnormal auditory brainstem response (Rosenhall, Johansson, & Orndahl, 1987b). This impairment may likewise reflect slowed neuronal transmission.

Psychological Manifestations

Depression is present in about 30% to 40% of patients with FMS, a value nearly identical to that of patients with RA (Ahles, Khan, Yunus, Spiegel, & Masi, 1991). The frequency of clinical depression in the general population is about 10%, and depression affects about 20% of persons with various medical illnesses. Depression is an important problem for some patients with FMS, but FMS is not likely to be the cause of the disorder. Depression is more likely a consequence of chronic pain, insomnia, and functional limitation, as is believed to be the case in RA.

The frequency of lifetime diagnoses of depression and anxiety disorders in patients with FMS ranges from 26% to 71% and has been associated with higher levels of pain and functional disability as well as increased use of medical services. These findings suggest that early identification and effective treatment of psychological distress may reduce health care costs and improve overall health for patients with FMS (Bradley, 1998).

Rehabilitation for FMS

Because FMS appears to result from a central neuroendocrine imbalance, rehabilitation interventions should teach patients self-regulation of the neuroendocrine system through control of thoughts, feelings, and behaviors and not focus solely on the muscle symptoms that are secondary to the central disorder. Self-management training is the model of intervention for chronic illness that allows therapists to address the full scope of symptoms through self-regulation (Boutaugh & Brady, 1998). Outcomes research on the self-help courses sponsored by the Arthritis Foundation have demonstrated that self-management training in a straight education format for persons with arthritis can result in a 15% to 30% improvement in addition to benefits from medication (Hirano, Laurent, & Lorig, 1994; Lorig & Holman, 1993). In a therapy setting in which the therapist can evaluate the patient and develop individual goals, self-management training can be even more effective than in a classroom format. Self-management training provides patients with a complex set of skills and attitudes that can help to improve health, reduce symptoms, improve functional capacity, and foster optimal involvement in daily activities (Boutaugh & Brady, 1998). For persons with FMS, self-management training includes patient education on self-management of associated symptoms and sleep disorders, stress management, relaxation and deep breathing, independent exercise, cardiovascular fitness, coping skills, fatigue management, and healthy nutrition (Bennett et al., 1996; Burckhardt, Mannerkorpi, Hedenberg, & Bjelle, 1994; Rosen, 1994). Missing from this list is cognitive retraining. This aspect of treatment for FMS is poorly understood. As therapists learn to improve cognitive skills in FMS, cognitive retraining should be incorporated into self-management training. This approach does not include hands-on manual therapy or clinic-based modalities. It is a process of teaching patients how to change their physiology through behavior. The patient must be an active participant in his or her care and establish mutually agreed-on goals that are realistic for the treatment period at the outset of treatment. Involving family members is often quite helpful.

There is a distinct benefit of shaping the neurophysiology of the condition through multiple directions versus only one. In research, the more interventions applied, the greater the outcome. Multidisciplinary treatment has proved to be more effective than sequential treatment for patients with severe FMS (Bennett, 1996b; Bennett et al., 1996). A controlled evaluation of the effectiveness of biofeedback and relaxation training, exercise, and a combination treatment group for patients with FMS demonstrated that all three interventions improved self-effectiveness for physical function, but the outcome was best maintained over a 2-year period by the group that received combination treatment (Buckelew et al., 1998).

Therapists in an outpatient rehabilitation clinic must organize a team approach with a psychotherapist and a nutritionist on a consultative or referral basis. The Arthritis Foundation sponsors the Fibromyalgia Self-Help Course and will train professional volunteers in how to conduct the course (Box 1).

As the patient responds to a comprehensive health and fitness program, the muscle pain usually lessens before the muscle tenderness, stiffness, or tightness does. The key to maintaining health with FMS is staying on a health and fitness program until the muscles are no longer tender (Melvin, 1996). In rehabilitation settings, therapists encounter three types of patients with FMS.

- Persons with primary (idiopathic) FMS who have had a chronic, long-term course with a recent decrease in function
- Persons with "reactive FMS" that began after a trauma or specific emotional event
- Persons referred for treatment of a specific disorder such as carpal tunnel syndrome, OA, RA, fracture, joint surgery, and so forth who have concomitant FMS (this is sometimes referred to as *secondary FMS*, and for these patients, treatment of FMS may not be their main priority). Although the initiating etiology may differ among FMS patient subgroups, FMS signs and symptoms are similar across subgroups.

For patients with reactive FMS, the self-management model still applies, but it must be balanced with treatment of the regional injuries or initiating event. Acute injuries naturally must be treated, and reactive FMS is usually diagnosed after the patient has been treated for the acute injury and has not responded to treatment within a normal time frame. At this point, it may be more beneficial to treat the FMS through self-management training and then, once it is under control, reevaluate and treat the regional injury.

Role of the Physical Therapist

The role of the physical therapist in a self-management training program includes conducting a musculoskeletal evaluation to determine which symptoms are part of FMS and which are concomitant problems; this includes the identification of MPS and trigger points for treatment. The physical therapist likewise provides patient education on FMS (e.g., how FMS affects the muscles, how to perform effective stretching techniques, and the value of fitness training). Early in the program, physical therapy education should include proper body mechanics, use of posture and positioning to control symptoms, and flare-up management strategies. Diaphragmatic breathing as well as relaxation techniques should be a part of physical therapy, and the physical therapist should include these techniques in the stress management training section as well. Patient education in the use of thermal modalities at home, self-myofascial release, and techniques for applying pressure to trigger points is additionally helpful. The physical therapist should provide the patient with a simple, effective home program and refer the patient to community-based exercise and education programs. Therapeutic strategies that encourage a patient to be dependent on clinic-based modalities or hands-on therapy do not empower the patient or encourage long-term self-management.

Role of the Occupational Therapist

Occupational therapists contribute to the rehabilitation team by providing musculoskeletal evaluation of upper-extremity symptoms, FMS education, fatigue management education (pacing, planning, prioritizing, time management, energy conservation), evaluation of factors interfering with sleep, and sleep hygiene education. Occupational therapists likewise evaluate postural strain during activities of daily living (ADL), ergonomic work environments, leisure activities, and sleep. They educate patients about available adaptive methods and equipment to reduce postural strain to the neck, shoulder region, and back. ADL equipment plays a limited role for patients with FMS because the goal is to improve functional capacity. Depending on the role of other team members, the occupational therapist's role may include stress management training, relaxation training, communication and assertiveness training, and value clarification (Rosenfeld, 1993; Zelik, 1984). Ideally, occupational therapists will be involved in cognitive skill evaluation and training as this area of intervention is developed.

Role of Other Health Professionals

Team members must teach stress management and relaxation training; cognitive concepts for managing stress and pain; self-regulation of thoughts, feelings, and behaviors; techniques for mood stabilization; coping skills training; and techniques for controlling cognitive distortions (Sandstrom & Keefe, 1998) and then assist the patient with psychosocial adjustment. This role could be provided by a psychologist or a licensed clinical social worker. A biofeedback therapist could provide stress management training. A registered dietitian skilled in high-level wellness and nutrition for high energy and self-management of functional bowel disorders, gastric reflux, slow motility, lactose intolerance, and allergies can be a terrific asset to an FMS treatment program. Many patients need education in basic healthy nutrition.

Exercise

Moldofsky and colleagues (1975) were the first to report that physical conditioning may mitigate the influence of disturbed stage IV sleep. They found that athletic students reported less musculoskeletal complaints than nonathletic students when their deep sleep was disturbed. Since that time, physical conditioning has been a cornerstone of FMS treatment. Studies evaluating the effectiveness of regular exercise with aerobic conditioning and flexibility components have shown an increase in aerobic fitness and reductions in tender points, myalgia scores, symptom reporting, fatigue, depression, and anxiety (Burckhardt et al., 1994; Martin et al., 1996; McCain, 1986; McCain, Bell, Mai, & Halliday, 1988; Wigers, Stiles, & Vogel, 1996). Although many patients must begin with a stretching program, a combination of aerobic conditioning, strengthening, and flexibility has been found more effective than simple flexibility exercises (McCain et al., 1988), relaxation training alone (Martin et al., 1996), or stress management training alone (Wigers et al., 1996). In one study, patients who received 6 hr of training in exercising independently showed greater improvement on the Fibromyalgia Impact Questionnaire (FIQ) on long-term follow-up than those who received a 6-week self-management education course alone (Burckhardt et al., 1994). Patients reported that exercise helps to reduce anxiety, improve endurance, facilitate relaxation, and support restful sleep.

Exercise that increases the heart rate (aerobic exercise) is beneficial in part because it improves circulation and thereby provides nutrition for tissues (e.g., tendons, joints, ligaments, and muscles). It improves the functioning and health of every cell in the body. Other benefits of exercise, such as increased self-esteem, better posture, increased energy, and improved mood, are important to persons with chronic pain (Greist et al., 1979; Johnsgard, 1989). The effect that exercise has on improving mood is attributed to increasing brain serotonin levels.

Evaluating the patient's "training index" after exercise at the beginning and the end of the treatment program can provide objective documentation of progress.

The training index = % maximum heart rate × duration (minutes per session) × frequency (number of sessions per week)

Determining an accurate training index in patients taking certain medications (e.g., narcotic analgesics, β-blockers) may not be possible. Bennett and colleagues (1996) reported a 200% increase in the training index in patients with FMS during a 6-month multidisciplinary program.

A regular aerobic exercise program is beneficial for nearly everyone with FMS. Most patients will need to "begin low and go slow." Start with an intensity and duration of exercise that the patient can readily tolerate and then gradually add rigor to the program as the patient's conditioning response allows. The goal should be to plan an exercise program that the patient can accomplish without exacerbating symptoms and that is sufficiently enjoyable for the patient to voluntarily continue on a regular basis. The patient must finish the workout feeling that he or she can do more rather than feeling exhausted. The patient must be confident that he or she can complete the routine successfully.

Some general principles apply rather specifically to exercise for patients with FMS. Initially, patients are often fearful of active exercise and fatigue easily, so it is helpful to start treatment by teaching them deep breathing, positioning, and passive stretching to decrease symptoms (e.g., lying on a towel roll between the shoulder blades). Initially, the home exercise program should be simple to avoid increasing patients' anxiety about accomplishing another activity in a daily life that is already difficult.

The issue of eccentric versus concentric contraction has been raised because eccentric movement requires more motor control and stronger muscle contraction than concentric movement does. Eccentric movement is difficult for patients with FMS who already have problems with motor control and strength. For these patients, building muscle strength through concentric exercise is better, especially at the beginning of the treatment program. This advice likewise applies to the way patients use their muscles in performing routine daily activities.

Some persons, often those who have always been exercise enthusiasts, are already involved in a good exercise program at the time of diagnosis. This observation highlights the fact that exercise alone is inadequate in treating FMS. It must be combined with restorative sleep, nutrition, and medication. The typical exercise for these active patients is swimming, running, or other aerobics. It is important to determine how patients are exercising. Is their manner of exercising (e.g., tension, vigor, and style) placing undue physical stress on their muscles, causing exhaustion, or disturbing sleep? If they are exercising appropriately, perhaps therapy could focus more on sleep quality, stress management, and relaxation in the work environment.

Patients with severe pain who report that even gentle exercise increases their pain may trigger a flare-up by doing too much work around the home. Patients not only have trouble learning how to exercise properly but also determining which daily household activities they are capable of doing and how much they should do. Often the therapist works with the patient in the clinic on a progressive fitness program, and the patient unwittingly does normal activities at home that are too strenuous. The resulting flare-up may be blamed incorrectly on the fitness routine, so it is helpful for the patient to have a plan for progressing both their fitness program and daily and avocational activities in a coordinated fashion (Melvin, 1996) (Box 2).

Exercise Classes

It is best to begin with a gentle exercise class two to three times per week that begins with a warm-up period followed by active exercise that moves the entire musculature in integrated spiral or functional patterns and ends with a cool-down period. The emphasis should be active versus resistive toning. The class should be led by an exercise instructor who understands FMS and does not push patients beyond their individual limits. The therapist must be able to give participants confidence in their bodies and teach the exercises in a way that lessens the fear of exercise. One way to do this is to include body awareness techniques before and after an exercise and to teach patients how to modify exercises accordingly. Especially in group sessions, patients should be instructed how to control the rate of program advancement. After patients are able to successfully participate in a mild, active movement, nonimpact program, they should be encouraged to gradually advance to greater cardiovascular conditioning. It is wise to limit the exercise to 20 or 30 min per session and to 3 days per week. Patients need at least 1 less active day between each session.

Box 2
How To Help Patients Exercise Successfully Without Flaring Up

---

1. *Create a fitness program goal.* Determine the ideal fitness program for the patient as if the patient did not have FMS (e.g., participating in a nonimpact aerobics class three times a week and doing a 30- to 45-min stretching program on the nonexercise days).

2. *Create a 10-step plan to progress toward the goal.* The first step is to determine the exercise level the patient is capable of doing now. The 10th step is the program goal. Some patients may only need 5 steps. Patients unable to walk around the block may need 15 steps. Why so many steps? Steps force the creation of a *gradual* progression. Most persons with FMS who have trouble exercising do too much too fast.

3. *The goal is to accomplish each step in the plan without increasing symptoms (causing a flare-up) before proceeding to the next step.*

4. *If the first step increases the patient's symptoms, it is too hard, too fast, or too much.* Break the first step into three or four smaller steps. This is where most patients have trouble. They are used to doing so much that simple, beginning exercises seem like nothing. But if the exercises make the patient flare-up, they are too difficult.

Note. From *Fibromyalgia: Getting Healthy*, by J. Melvin, 1996, Bethesda, MD: American Occupational Therapy Association. Copyright 1996 by the American Occupational Therapy Association. Reprinted with permission.

The muscles of patients with FMS need more time to repair and recover because deficiency in stage IV sleep can result in low production of growth hormone and insulin-like growth factor-1, which are involved in the repair of muscles after exercise. Many patients choose to continue to participate in a group exercise class to maintain their motivation but add individual swimming or walking to their personal regimen.

For how long must persons with FMS exercise? Studies indicate that patients must be in a full fitness program (aerobic strengthening and flexibility 3 hr a week) for at least 12 to 20 weeks before showing consistent gains (McCain, 1986; McCain et al., 1988). Bennett and colleagues (1996) recommended that patients participate in aerobic exercise three to four times a week at about 70% of maximum heart rate for 20 to 30 min. A patient may take 6 to 12 months to build up slowly to this level. (The authors find that many patients can make excellent progress without achieving this target heart rate.)

Exercise for Persons With Severe FMS

Most patients require 3 to 12 months to reach their fitness goals. Patients make progress only by completing each step successfully. If the patient has increased pain from one step to another, pushing to the next step is only going to worsen the pain. Patients who report that gentle exercise or walking increases their pain need a prefitness program.

Example of a prefitness program.

Step 1. Relaxation training (with or without biofeedback)

Step 2. Deep breathing program five times a day (to increase oxygen to muscles and mobilize the rib cage muscles)

Step 3. Guided active ROM exercises to tolerance without additional stretching (only when this can be tolerated without flaring up should the patient move on to the next step)

Step 4. Daily active ROM exercises performed independently at home for at least 1 week

Step 5. Build up to a gentle stretching program 30 to 45 min a day at home

Step 6. Gradually advance until the patient can do a full stretch of each muscle group daily (only after this can be tolerated without flaring up for 1 week should the patient progress to the next step)

Step 7. Begin a stretch-and-tone, water exercise, or nonimpact aerobic exercise class. Start with 20 min two times a week. Participate the first 20 min, rest during the middle, and participate in the relaxation cool-down, or do half of the exercises and repetitions. When this can be tolerated, increase participatory time as indicated below (this is combined with the home stretching program on nonclass days)

Step 8. Class exercises 30 min two times a week

Step 9. Class exercises 40 min two times a week

Step 10. Full exercise class two times a week

Step 11. Add a third class to the week

This entire process can take up to a year because there are often flare-ups or setbacks along the way. This is only one example of an exercise progression. There can be many variations, but establishing progressive steps and accomplishing each step before progressing are most important.

Fatigue Management and Sleep Retraining

The new model for treating fatigue in patients with rheumatic diseases is fatigue management training, which combines fitness training to improve functional capacity with education on how to reduce stress, improve efficiency, and conserve energy (Belza, 1990; Tach, 1990). Managing fatigue solely with energy conservation is appropriate only for patients with diseases that prevent improvement in functional capacity. Fatigue management is an ideal intervention for combining physical therapy to teach fitness training with occupational therapy to provide the education component. (See chapter 8 in this volume for more information on fatigue management and use of the Fatigue Wheel.) A multidisciplinary self-management training program for FMS should contain a fatigue management program that focuses on sleep retraining (Melvin, 1998).

The easiest way to evaluate the effect of fatigue on a patient's life is to ask the patient to rate on a 10-point scale (10=a great deal, 0=none) the extent that fatigue limits the ability for self-care (bathing, dressing, grooming), work (either employment or activities around the home), and community activities. It is helpful to give patients an overall rating of fatigue (10=the worst the fatigue has been). These assessments can be done quickly and provide objective outcomes.

Healthy sleep involves going to bed when one chooses to versus staying awake until one falls asleep; sleeping deeply; and waking up feeling rested, refreshed, and as if one has had enough sleep. This must be done on a consistent basis, for at least five mornings out of seven, without medications. (Brief awakenings do not necessarily interfere with restorative sleep.) Sleeping with the aid of medications is better than not sleeping at all, but it is not normal sleep—it is drug-induced sleep, which does not improve health in the same way that natural sleep does. Correcting the sleep disorder and healthy sleep are the keys to bringing the neuro-endocrine system back into balance. (*Note.* The physical symptoms of FMS may take 4 to 6 months to completely dissipate after a sleep disorder is fully corrected and the person has stopped taking medications.)

About 90% of patients with FMS complain of having trouble sleeping. The remaining 10% may not be aware of the impaired quality of their sleep. Some persons have lifelong sleep disorders and have never awakened feeling "rested." Their insomnia may consist of difficulty falling asleep, frequent awakening during the night, the inability to fall back to sleep, early awakening, or an alpha non-REM sleep pattern.

A sleep cycle consists of four stages of sleep (I–IV) followed by a variable period of REM sleep. Each cycle is approximately 90 to 110 min long, and there are about five cycles in an 8-hr sleep period. Stage IV sleep is "restorative" sleep. In this stage, the muscles do not move, and the brain turns into a chemistry factory and replenishes the supply of neurochemicals, including serotonin and growth hormone. The greatest amount of cellular repair takes place during this stage. REM sleep is critical for neurological health and stimulates the brain regions used in learning.

For an excellent review of basic sleep physiology, see the National Institute of Neurological Disorders and Stroke Web site (http://www.ninds.nih.gov/patients) for information titled "Brain Basics: Understanding Sleep."

Sleep evaluation should include whether patients sleep according to a daily schedule, their sleep pattern, their morning fatigue level on a scale of 1 to 10 (10=exhausted), medications that may increase or interfere with sleep, their activities between dinner and bedtime, what they have done to help their sleep, how much sleep they need to feel healthy, and their ideal sleep schedule.

Sleep retraining involves teaching patients about sleep physiology and the skills necessary to implement the recommendations below, which may include relaxation training, cognitive behavioral techniques, time management, and how to self-manage depression and anxiety. Patients should keep an activity sleep log to collect data on how their activities and behavioral interventions are altering their sleep. Rating morning fatigue, mood, and pain on a 10-point scale (10=the most severe or worst) is helpful for tracking improvements in quality of sleep because these factors are strongly influenced by stage IV sleep.

Basic sleep hygiene measures promoted by the National Sleep Foundation (Box 1) include the following:

- Caffeine should be eliminated (gradually for those who are addicted). As a compromise, patients may reduce intake to one cup of a caffeinated beverage in the morning, but if they cannot correct their sleep disorder, they must eliminate caffeine completely.
- Smokers should quit. (Bupropion hydrochloride [Wellbutrin] has been shown to be especially effective in helping patients stop smoking.)
- Avoid alcohol, especially late at night. Patients who have difficulty correcting their sleep disorders should try abstaining from alcohol for 2 weeks.
- A regular schedule is essential for retraining circadian rhythms. This schedule should likewise be observed during the weekends.
- All daytime napping should be discontinued because it reduces the patient's sleep debt (patients must be taught specific measures to increase energy besides napping).
- Exercise in the early morning or late afternoon. Vigorous exercise before bed usually increases alertness, not calmness.
- Develop a relaxing routine before bedtime. Take a warm bath, listen to music, and avoid the news.
- Have a comfortable room temperature.

There is one commonly recommended basic hygiene measure that one author (J.M.) finds detrimental to persons trying to correct sleep disorders: the recommendation "to get up if you cannot fall asleep after 30 min and read or watch television until you become tired." This strategy is recommended to reduce anxiety, but reading with a light on and watching television stimulate alertness chemicals, not sleep chemicals. It is far superior to be skilled in conscious relaxation and to slowly, systematically let go of muscle tension and let the body surrender to the mattress. The focus on relaxation can be done as a meditation and can foster a focus on thoughts instead of a focus on problems.

Other sleep retraining techniques that one author (J.M.) finds effective for patients with FMS include the following:

- External time cues that can alter circadian rhythms are called *zeitgebers* (German for "time givers"). The spectrum of early morning light is a zeitgeber. Having a regular nightly routine can be a zeitgeber.
- Patients should specifically take measures to make themselves fully alert within an hour of waking in the morning (or to their premorbid level), including eating breakfast, showering, reading, watching television, going outside, or exercising, rather than adapting to the sluggishness.
- Patients should relax after dinner and not engage in work activity that stimulates a "second wind."
- Herbal teas after dinner can help calm, especially chamomile, mint, and anise. Teas with citrus, spice, and, of course, caffeine should be avoided.

- If patients worry in bed about what they have to do the next day, the best solution is for them make a list of the next day's activities so that they can relax and not worry that they are going to forget to do something.

- To start, patients should create a 1-hr transition time before desired sleep time solely for calming activities. A calming activity is one that makes the patient tired, sleepy, or more relaxed. Reading is not always calming; novels are written in a page-turning formula to keep the reader's attention. Knitting may be relaxing for an expert but frustrating for a novice. Warm tub baths are not relaxing for everyone. Almost all patients need to do at least a 2-week trial of no television 1 hr before sleep to determine how the electronic stimulation of television affects their sleep.

- When you turn off the lights to go to sleep, the brain begins to produce melatonin; white light is perceived as sunlight and turns off melatonin production and disturbs sleep chemistry (Kalsbeek et al., 1999). Patients who need a light on should use a nightlight with a red bulb. The room should be dark and the television turned off.

- To reduce the irritation of noises inside or outside the room, ear plugs and white noise machines are helpful. Sometimes a small fan can create adequate white noise.

- The mattress should be firm (no sagging) but have thick cushioning on top. Regular eggcrate foam pads are thin, and for some a 2-in. foam pad (from a foam store) can make a tremendous difference in sleep comfort.

- The bed should only be used for sleep and sex and not for office work so that the brain can condition itself to associate sleep with the bed.

- Patients should make an arrangement with family members not to talk about stressful subjects for 1 hr before bedtime.

Most patients require 4 to 6 weeks to learn the skills to implement these recommendations.

Nutrition

Nutrition may offer an opportunity to change the brain chemistry. Food can be used to energize the mind and body or to calm them down. Food can alter energy level, mood, cognitive ability, and sleep. FMS tends to make a person hypersensitive to stimuli and potentially to drugs and certain foods such as sugar, sweeteners, chocolate, caffeine, red meat, wine, or alcohol. Most patients voluntarily eliminate offending foods from their diet.

For Fatigue and Cognition

A healthy diet (i.e., one low in fats, free of sugar, high in complex carbohydrates, and moderate in protein) can optimize energy, facilitate participation in physical activities, reduce stress, and improve sleep. If a person is feeling energetic, he or she is more likely to exercise during the day and then sleep better at night. Fat lowers metabolism; after eating a high-fat meal, a person does not burn calories at the same rate, which can contribute to weight gain and fatigue.

Foods that improve energy likewise tend to improve mental alertness. Studies on functional and psychological performance before and after different meal compositions found that the behaviors associated with norepinephrine and dopamine were increased the most after a high-protein, low-fat meal (complex carbohydrates were not influential in this context). This meal had more of an effect at breakfast compared with lunch and at lunch compared with dinner (Wurtman, 1984, 1987). In other words, a high-protein, low-fat meal (with or without a complex carbohydrates) especially at breakfast and lunch is the best meal to eat for high energy and mental alertness and can be an important component of a comprehensive fatigue management program. Wurtman (1984, 1987) does not specify a specific number of protein grams. The effect can be evident with 9 g of protein, such as in a cup of yogurt, but some patients may need more to have the desired effect (e.g., 12 g or more at breakfast). Other options for protein besides eggs include egg substitutes, fruit juice smoothies made with protein powder, low-fat cottage cheese and fruit, and toasted soy granules or nuggets (2 tablespoons=11 g protein) can be added to cold or hot cereals to change a low-protein meal into a high-protein one.

For Mood

Serotonin is metabolized from the amino acid tryptophan, and manipulating serotonin through diet has been explored. The same study protocol described above for tyrosine was applied to tryptophan (Wurtman, 1984). The type of meal that maximizes tryptophan uptake is a high-carbohydrate, protein-poor meal (a vegetarian meal with a starch, such as vegetables and rice, vegetarian pasta and salad). This is because a high-protein meal will supply lots of other amino acids to bind up the available tryptophan in protein synthesis. A high-carbohydrate meal provides glucose to carry the free tryptophan to the brain. Simple carbohydrates such as sucrose in cookies and candy qualify as serotonin boosters, which is why they are called "comfort foods." From this perspective, dinner had more of an effect than lunch, and lunch had more of an effect than breakfast. After eating a high-carbohydrate, protein-poor meal, test subjects reported feeling more calm or "centered" and less tense and stressed, had improved concentration and focus, and were less distractible, depressed, and anxious. Patients interested in reducing fatigue and improving alertness through nutrition should eat a high-protein, low-fat breakfast and lunch and a complex carbohydrate (vegetables and starches), protein-poor dinner. This does not have to be a rigid diet, but it is helpful to follow it enough to experience its benefits (Melvin, 1996).

For Sleep

Specific foods and substances can encourage or directly interfere with sleep. For example, highly acidic foods such as tomatoes, citrus fruits or juices, or wine consumed late at night can disrupt sleep. Vitamins, especially C and B, can disturb sleep. All supplements for improving energy should be taken in the morning. Alcohol, especially wine, can induce sleep but causes a rebound insomnia several hours later and fragmented sleep during the night. Alcohol consumption or lack of sufficient water intake can lead to dehydration, fatigue, headaches, and disturbed sleep (Zarcone, 1994).

Caffeine is a known stimulant to the CNS and remains in the system for a long time, up to 14 hr for the average person (Zarcone, 1994). Patients with FMS are even more sensitive to caffeine than the average person; for some, a cup of coffee in the morning can keep caffeine-sensitive persons awake late into the evening. Caffeine competes for receptor sites on the inhibitory adenosine neurotransmitter, which reduces overall inhibition and increases anxiety and irritability. Even patients who could drink coffee before bedtime all their lives can become sensitive to caffeine once they develop a sleep disorder. Persons addicted to caffeine may need to eliminate it for 6 to 10 weeks to have the full therapeutic benefit (Zarcone, 1994). Chocolate desserts may provide sufficient xanthene derivatives to affect some persons. (Xanthene is the stimulant in coffee, tea, and cocoa.)

Research indicates that nicotine affects the dopamine receptors but has much the same effect as caffeine on sleep, mood, and daytime performance (Zarcone, 1994). In addition, nicotine is a vasoconstrictor that can further impede circulation to tight hypoxic muscles. Patients with sleep disorders should stop smoking. If they cannot stop, they should not smoke after 7:00 P.M., especially not in the middle of the night.

Diet interventions that may improve sleep include a carbohydrate snack and no protein before bedtime to boost serotonin. Persons who like to drink milk to aid sleep may continue to do so (this most likely works because the high levels of calcium and magnesium that milk contains are muscle relaxants). Patients are encouraged to try both techniques and determine which works the best for them.

Outcome Evaluation

Bennett and colleagues (1996) used a broad range of outcome measures to evaluate their multidisciplinary program. They have found the following to be the most sensitive to change: the FIQ (Burckhardt, Clark, & Bennett, 1991), the Quality of Life Questionnaire (Burckhardt, Clark, & Bennett, 1993), the Coping Strategies Questionnaire (Rosenstiel & Keefe, 1983), and the aerobic training index described earlier. Two authors (J.M. and M.S.) have found that having patients rate their eight worst symptoms and two areas of functional disability on a 0 to 10 scale (10=the worst the symptom has been) is helpful for tracking improvement in a range of symptoms.

Conclusion

FMS is probably a result of a central neuroendocrine imbalance. Patients with FMS have a broad range of symptoms, all of which may be influenced by their pain, mood, nutrition, sleep, and level of fitness. To be effective, the rehabilitation intervention must teach patients self-regulation of the neuroendocrine system and not focus solely on the muscle symptoms that are secondary to the central disorder. The model of intervention that allows therapists to address the full scope of symptoms through self-regulation is self-management training.

References

Ahles, T. A., Khan, S. A., Yunus, M. B., Spiegel, D. A., & Masi, A. T. (1991). Psychiatric status of patients with primary fibromyalgia, patients with rheumatoid arthritis, and subjects without pain: A blind comparison of DSM-III diagnoses. *American Journal of Psychiatry, 148*, 1721–1726.

Anch, A. M., Lue, F. A., MacLean, A. W., & Moldofsky, H. (1991). Sleep physiology and psychological aspects of the fibrositis (fibromyalgia) syndrome. *Canadian Journal of Psychology, 45*, 179–184.

Balderer, G., & Borbely, A. A. (1985). Effect of valerian on human sleep. *Psychopharmacology (Berl)*, *87*(4), 406–409.

Belza, B. (1990). The impact of fatigue on exercise performance. *Arthritis Care and Research*, *7*, 176–180.

Bengtsson, A., Backman, E., Lindblom, B., & Skogh, T. (1994). Long-term follow-up of fibromyalgia patients: Clinical symptoms, muscular function, laboratory tests: An eight year comparison study. *Journal of Musculoskeletal Pain*, *2*, 67–80.

Bengtsson, A., Henriksson, K. G., & Larsson, J. (1986). Reduced high energy phosphate levels in the painful muscles of patients with primary fibromyalgia. *Arthritis and Rheumatism*, *29*, 817–821.

Bennett, R. M. (1996a). Guaifenesin as treatment for fibromyalgia: A 1 year double-bind, placebo-controlled study. *Arthritis and Rheumatism*, *39*(Suppl. 2), S27.

Bennett, R. M. (1996b). Multidisciplinary group programs to treat fibromyalgia patients. *Rheumatic Disease Clinics of North America*, *22*(2), 351–367.

Bennett, R. M., Burckhardt, C. S., Clark, S. R., O'Reilly, C. A., Wiens, A. N., & Campbell, S. M. (1996). Group treatment of fibromyalgia: A 6 month outpatient program. *Journal of Rheumatology*, *23*, 521–528.

Bennett, R. M., Clark, S. R., Campbell, S. M., & Burckhardt, C. S. (1992). Low levels of somatomedin C in patients with the fibromyalgia syndrome: A possible link between sleep and muscle pain. *Arthritis and Rheumatism*, *35*, 1113–1116.

Bennett, R. M., Clark, S. R., Campbell, S. M., Ingram, S. B., Burckhardt, C. S., Nelson, D. L., & Porter, J. M. (1991). Symptoms of Raynaud's syndrome in patients with fibromyalgia: A study utilizing the Nielsen test, digital photoplethysmography, and measurements of platelet alpha 2-adrenergic receptors. *Arthritis and Rheumatism*, *34*, 264–269.

Bennett, R. M., Clark, S. R., Goldberg, L., Nelson, D., Bonafede, R. P., Porter, J., & Specht, D. (1989). Aerobic fitness in patients with fibrositis: A controlled study of respiratory gas exchange and [133]xenon clearance from exercising muscle. *Arthritis and Rheumatism*, *32*, 454–460.

Bombardier, C. J., Ware, J. R., Russell, I. J., Larson, M., Chalmers, A., & Read, J. L. (1986). Auranofin therapy and quality of life in patients with rheumatoid arthritis: Results of a multicenter trial. *American Journal of Medicine*, *81*, 565–578.

Borg-Stein, J., & Stein, J. (1996). Trigger points and tender points: One and the same? Does injection treatment help? *Rheumatic Disease Clinics of North America*, *22*(2), 305–322.

Bou-Holaigah, I., Calkins, H., Flynn, J. A., Tunin, C., Chang, H. C., Kan, J. S., & Rowe, P. C. (1997). Provocation of hypotension and pain during upright tilt table testing in adults with fibromyalgia. *Clinical and Experimental Rheumatology*, *15*, 239–246.

Boutaugh, M. L., & Brady, T. J. (1998). Patient education for self-management. In J. Melvin & G. Jensen (Eds.), *Rheumatologic rehabilitation series: Volume 1: Assessment and management* (pp. 219–258). Bethesda, MD: American Occupational Therapy Association.

Bradley, L. A. (1998). Pain management interventions for patients with rheumatic diseases. In J. Melvin & G. Jensen (Eds.), *Rheumatologic rehabilitation series: Volume 1: Assessment and management* (pp. 259–278). Bethesda, MD: American Occupational Therapy Association.

Bradley, L. A., Alarcon, G. S., Triana, M., Aaron, L. A., Alexander, R. W., Stewart, K. E., Martin, M., & Alberts, K. (1994). Health care seeking behavior in fibromyalgia: Associations with pain thresholds, symptom severity, and psychiatric morbidity. *Journal of Musculoskeletal Pain*, *2*, 79–87.

Buckelew, S. P., Conway, R., Parker, J., Deuser, W. E., Read, J., Witty, T. E., Hewett, J. E., Minor, M., Johnson, J. C., Van Male, L., McIntosh, M. J., Nigh, M., & Kay, D. R. (1998). Biofeedback/relaxation training and exercise interventions for fibromyalgia: A prospective trial. *Arthritis Care and Research*, *11*, 196–209.

Burckhardt, C. S., Clark, S. R., & Bennett, R. M. (1991). The fibromyalgia impact questionnaire: Development and validation. *Journal of Rheumatology, 18*, 728–733.

Burckhardt, C. S., Clark, S. R., & Bennett, R. M. (1993). Fibromyalgia and quality of life: A comparative analysis. *Journal of Rheumatology, 20*,475–479.

Burckhardt, C. S., Mannerkorpi, K., Hedenberg, L., & Bjelle, A. (1994). A randomized, controlled clinical trial of education and physical training for women with fibromyalgia. *Journal of Rheumatology, 21*, 714–720.

Buskila, D., Neumann, L., Vaisberg, G., Alkalay, D., & Wolfe, F. (1997). Increased rates of fibromyalgia following cervical spine injury: A controlled study of 161 cases of traumatic injury. *Arthritis and Rheumatism, 40*, 446–452.

Buskila, D., Press, J., Gedalia, A., Klein, M., Neumann, R., Bohm, R., & Sukenij, S. (1993). Assessment of non-articular tenderness and prevalence of fibromyalgia syndrome in children. *Journal of Rheumatology, 20*, 368–370.

Caidahl, K., Lurie, M., Bake, B., Johansson, G., & Wetterqvist, H. (1989). Dyspnea in chronic primary fibromyalgia. *Journal of Internal Medicine, 226*(4), 265–270.

Carette, S., McCain, G. A., Bell, D. A., & Fam, A. G. (1986). Evaluation of amitriptyline in primary fibrositis: A double-blind, placebo-controlled study. *Arthritis and Rheumatism, 29*, 655–659.

Caro, X. J., Wolfe, F., Johnston, W. H., & Smith, A. L. (1986). A controlled and blinded study of immunoreactant deposition at the dermal-epidermal junction of patients with primary fibrositis syndrome. *Journal of Rheumatology, 13*, 1086–1092.

Caruso, I., Sarzi Puttini, P., Cazzola, M., & Azzolini, V. (1990). Double-blind study of 5-hydroxytrytophan versus placebo in the treatment of primary fibromyalgia syndrome. *Journal of International Medical Research, 18*(3), 201–209.

Cathey, M. A., Wolfe, F., & Kleinheksel, S. M. (1988). Functional ability and work status in patients with fibromyalgia. *Arthritis Care and Research, 1*, 85–98.

Clark, S., Tindall, E., & Bennett, R. M. (1985). A double blind crossover trial of prednisone versus placebo in the treatment of fibrositis. *Journal of Rheumatology, 12*, 980–983.

Clauw, D., Gaumond, E., Radulovic, D., Pandri, P., Ali, M., Foong, S., & Baraniuk, J. N. (1996). The role of true IgE-mediated allergic mechanisms in the "allergic" symptoms of fibromyalgia [Abstract]. *Arthritis and Rheumatism, 39*(Suppl.), S277.

Clauw, D. J., Radulovic, D., Heshmat, Y., & Barbey, J. T. (1995). Heart rate variability as a measure of autonomic function in patients with fibromyalgia (FM) and chronic fatigue syndrome (CFS) [Abstract]. *Journal of Musculoskeletal Pain, 3*(Suppl. 1), 78.

Clauw, D. J., Radulovic, D., Katz, P., Baraniuk, J., & Barbey, J. T. (1995). Tilt table testing as a measure of dysautonomia in fibromyalgia [Abstract]. *Journal of Musculoskeletal Pain, 3*(Suppl. 1), 10.

Cleveland, C. H., Jr., Fisher, R. H., Brestel, E. P., Esinhart, J. D., & Metzger, W. J. (1992). Chronic rhinitis: An underrecognized association with fibromyalgia. *Allergy Proceedings, 13*(5), 263–267.

Cote, K. A., & Moldofsky, H. (1997). Sleep, daytime symptoms, and cognitive performance in patients with fibromyalgia. *Journal of Rheumatology, 24*, 2014–2023.

Crofford, L. J., Pillemer, S. R., Kalogeras, K. T., Cash, J. M., Michelson, D., Kling, M. A., Sternberg, E. M., Gold, P. W., Chrousos, G. P., & Wilder, R. L. (1994). Hypothalamic-pituitary-adrenal axis perturbations in patients with fibromyalgia. *Arthritis and Rheumatism, 37*, 1583–1592.

Demitrack, M. A., Dale, J. K., Straus, S. E., Laue, L., Listwak, S. J., Kruesi, M. J., Chrousos, G. P., & Gold, P. W. (1991). Evidence for impaired activation of the hypothalamic-pituitary-adrenal axis in patients with chronic fatigue syndrome. *Journal of Clinical Endocrinology and Metabolism, 73*, 1224–1234.

Deodhar, A. A., Fisher, R. A., Blacker, C. V., & Woolf, A. D. (1994). Fluid retention syndrome and fibromyalgia. *British Journal of Rheumatology, 33*(6), 576–582.

Eisinger, J., & Ayavou, T. (1990). Transketolase stimulation in fibromyalgia. *Journal of the American College of Nutrition, 9,* 56–57.

Eisinger, J., Plantamura, A., & Ayavou, T. (1994). Glycolysis abnormalities in fibromyalgia. *Journal of the American College of Nutrition, 13,* 144–148.

Felson, D. T., & Goldenberg, D. L. (1986). The natural history of fibromyalgia. *Arthritis and Rheumatism, 29,* l522–l526.

Fibromyalgia syndrome: Current clinical status and needs assessment: Testimony before the U.S. House of Representatives Appropriations Subcommittee on Labor, Health and Human Services, (1994, 1 February) (testimony of I.J. Russell).

Fransen, J., & Russell, I. J. (1996). *The fibromyalgia helpbook.* St. Paul, MN: Smith House Press.

Gerwin, R. D., Shannon, S., Hong, C.- Z., Hubbard, D., & Gevirtz, R. (1995). Identification of myofascial trigger points: Inter-rater agreement and effect of training [Abstract]. *Journal of Musculoskeletal Pain, 3*(Suppl. 1), 55.

Giovengo, S. L., Russell, I. J., & Larson, A. A. (in press). Increased concentrations of nerve growth factor (NGF) in cerebrospinal fluid of patients with fibromyalgia. *Journal of Rheumatology.*

Glotzbach, S. F., & Heller, H. C. (1994). Temperature regulation. In M. H. Kryger, T. Roth, & W. C. Dement (Eds.), *Principles and practice of sleep medicine* (2nd ed., pp. 260–276). Philadelphia: Saunders.

Goldenberg, D. L. (1987). Fibromyalgia syndrome: An emerging but controversial condition. *Journal of the American Medical Association, 257,* 2782–2787.

Goldenberg, D. L., Simms, R. W., Geiger, A., & Komaroff, A. L. (1990). High frequency of fibromyalgia in patients with chronic fatigue seen in a primary care practice. *Arthritis and Rheumatism, 33,* 381–387.

Granges, G., & Littlejohn, G. (1995). Prevalence of myofascial pain syndrome in fibromyalgia syndrome and regional pain syndrome: A comparative study. *Journal of Musculoskeletal Pain, 1,* 19–35.

Greist, J. H., Klein, M. H., Eischens, R. R., Faris, J., Gurman, A. S., & Morgan, W. P (1979). Running as treatment for depression. *Comparative Psychiatry, 20,* 41–54.

Griep, E. N., Boersma, J. W., & deKloet, E. R. (1993). Altered reactivity of the hypothalamic-pituitary-adrenal axis in the primary fibromyalgia syndrome. *Journal of Rheumatology, 20,* 469–474.

Gustafsson, M., & Gaston-Johansson, F. (1996). Pain intensity and health locus of control: A comparison of patients with fibromyalgia syndrome and rheumatoid arthritis. *Patient Education and Counseling, 29,* 179–188.

Hapidou, E. G., & Rollman, G. B. (1998). Menstrual cycle modulation of tender points. *Pain, 77,* 151–161.

Henriksson, C., Gundmark, I., Bengtsson, A., & Ek, A. C. (1992). Living with fibromyalgia: Consequences for everyday life. *Clinical Journal of Pain, 8,* 138–144.

Hirano, P. C., Laurent, D. D., & Lorig, K. (1994). Arthritis patient education studies, 1987–1991: A review of the literature. *Patient Education Counseling, 24*(1), 9–54.

Hong, C.-Z., Hsueh, T.-C., & Simons, D. G. (1995). Difference in pain relief after trigger point injections in myofascial pain patients with and without fibromyalgia [Abstract]. *Journal of Musculoskeletal Pain, 3*(Suppl. 1), 60.

Hrycaj, P., Stratz, T., & Muller, W. (1993). Platelet 3H-imipramine uptake receptor density and serum serotonin in patients with fibromyalgia/fibrositis syndrome. *Journal of Rheumatology, 20,* 1986–1987.

Hubbard, D. R., & Berkoff, G. M. (1993). Myofascial trigger points studied by needle electromyography. *Spine, 18*(13), 1803–1807.

Jacobsen, S., Danneskiold-Samsoe, B., & Andersen, R. B. (1991). Oral S-adenosylmethionine in primary fibromyalgia: Double-blind clinical evaluation. *Scandinavian Journal of Rheumatology, 20*(4), 294–302.

Johnsgard, K. W. (1989). *The exercise prescription for depression and anxiety*. New York: Plenum Press.

Kalsbeek, A., Cutrera, R. A., Van Heerikhuize, J. J., Van Der Vliet, J., & Buijs, R. M. (1999). GABA release from suprachiasmatic nucleus terminals is necessary for the light-induced inhibition of nocturnal melatonin release in the rat. *Neuroscience, 91*(2), 453–461.

Kang, Y.- K., Russell, I. J., Vipraio, G. A., & Acworth, I. N. (1998). Low urinary 5-hydroxy indole acetic acid in fibromyalgia syndrome: Evidence in support of a serotonin-deficiency pathogenesis. *Myalgia, 1*, 14–21.

Komaroff, A. L., & Goldenberg, D. (1989). The chronic fatigue syndrome: Definition, current studies and lessons for fibromyalgia research. *Journal of Rheumatology, 19*(Suppl.), 23–27.

Liller, T. K., Mutter, J. B., & Catlett, J. L. (1995). *Fibromyalgia: A multi-dimensional profile*. Fairfax, VA: Fibromyalgia Association of Greater Washington.

Lindahl, O., & Lindwall, L. (1989). Double blind study of a valerian preparation. *Pharmacology Biochemistry, and Behavior, 32*(4), 1065–1066.

Lindman, R., Hagberg, M., Bengtsson, A., Henriksson, K. G., & Thornell, L.-E. (1995). Capillary structure and mitochondrial volume density in the trapezius muscle of chronic trapezius myalgia, fibromyalgia and healthy subjects. *Journal of Musculoskeletal Pain, 3*, 5–22.

Lorig, K., & Holman, H. (1993). Arthritis self-management studies: A twelve year review. *Health Education Quarterly, 20*, 17–28.

Lowen, A. (1973). *Depression and the body: The biological basis of faith and reality*. New York: Coward, McCain and Geohegan.

Lurie, M., Caidahl, K., Johansson, G., & Bake, B. (1990). Respiratory function in chronic primary fibromyalgia. *Scandinavian Journal of Rehabilitative Medicine, 22*(3), 151–155.

Martin, L., Nutting, A., MacIntosh, B. R., Edworthy, S. M., Butterwick, D., & Cook, J. (1996). An exercise program in the treatment of fibromyalgia. *Journal of Rheumatology, 23*, 1050–1053.

Martinez-Lavin, M., Hermosillo, A. G., Rosas, M., & Soto, M. E. (1998). Circadian studies of autonomic nervous balance in patients with fibromyalgia: A heart rate variability analysis. *Arthritis and Rheumatism, 41*, 1966–1971.

Mayo Clinic Health Oasis. (1998, August 31). *Diet supplements use caution* [On-line]. Available: www.mayohealth.org/mayo/9808/htm/diet__sb.htm

McCain, G. A. (1986). Role of physical fitness training in the fibrositis/fibromyalgia syndrome. *American Journal of Medicine, 29*(Suppl. 3A), 73–77.

McCain, G. A., Bell, D. A., Mai, F. M., & Halliday, P. D. (1988). A controlled study of the effects of a supervised cardiovascular fitness training program on the manifestations of primary fibromyalgia. *Arthritis and Rheumatism, 31*, 1135–1141.

McCain, G. A., Cameron, R., & Kennedy, J. C. (1989). The problem of long-term disability payments and litigation in primary fibromyalgia: The Canadian perspective. *Journal of Rheumatology, 19*(Suppl.), 174.

Melvin, J. L. (1998). Fibromyalgia syndrome: Comprehensive self-management training (featuring the program at Cedars-Sinai Medical Center). In *OT practice* (pp. 39–45). Bethesda, MD: American Occupational Therapy Association.

Melvin, J. L. (1996). *Fibromyalgia: Getting healthy*. Bethesda, MD: American Occupational Therapy Association.

Mengshoel, A. M., Saugen, E., Forre, O., & Vollestad, N. K. (1995). Muscle fatigue in early fibromyalgia. *Journal of Rheumatology, 22*, 143.

Moldofsky, H. (1982). Rheumatic pain modulation syndrome: The interrelationships between sleep, central nervous system, serotonin and pain. *Advances in Neurology, 33*, 51–57.

Moldofsky, H. (1989). Sleep and fibrositis syndrome. *Rheumatic Disease Clinics of North America, 15*, 91–103.

Moldofsky, H., Lue, F. A., Mously, C., Roth-Schechter, B., & Reynolds, W. J. (1996). The effect of zolpidem in patients with fibromyalgia: A dose ranging, double blind, placebo controlled, modified crossover study. *Journal of Rheumatology, 23*, 529–533.

Moldofsky, H., Scarisbrick, P., England, R., & Smythe, H. (1975). Musculoskeletal symptoms and NREM sleep disturbance in patients with "fibrositis syndrome" and healthy subjects. *Psychosomatic Medicine, 37*, 341–351.

Moldofsky, H., Wong, T. H. M., & Lue, F. A. (1993). Litigation, sleep, symptoms and disabilities in post-accident pain (fibromyalgia). *Journal of Rheumatology, 20*, 1936.

Nice, D. A., Riddle, D. L., Lamb, R. L., Mayhew, T. P., & Rucker, K. (1992). Intertester reliability of judgements of the presence of trigger points in patients with low back pain. *Archives of Physical Medicine and Rehabilitation, 73*, 893–898.

Rosen, N. B. (1994). Physical medicine and rehabilitation approaches to the management of myofascial pain and fibromyalgia syndromes. *Bailliere's Clinical Rheumatology, 8*(4), 881–916.

Rosenfeld, M. S. (1993). *Wellness and lifestyle renewal*. Bethesda, MD: American Occupational Therapy Association.

Rosenhall, U., Johansson, G., & Orndahl, G. (1987a). Eye motility dysfunction in chronic primary fibromyalgia with dysesthesia. *Scandinavian Journal of Rehabilitation Medicine, 19*(4), 139–145.

Rosenhall, U., Johansson, G., & Orndahl, G. (1987b). Neuroaudiological findings in chronic primary fibromyalgia with dysesthesia. *Scandinavian Journal of Rehabilitation Medicine, 19*(4), 147–152.

Rosenstiel, A. K., & Keefe, F. J. (1983). The use of coping strategies in chronic low back pain patients: Relationship to patient characteristics and current adjustment. *Pain, 17*(1), 33–44.

Russell, I. J. (1996). Fibromyalgia syndrome: Approaches to management. *Bulletin on the Rheumatic Diseases, 43*, 1–4.

Russell, I. J., Bennett, R. M., Katz, W. A., & Kamin, M. (1997). Efficacy of Ultram™ (tramadol HCl) in the treatment of fibromyalgia syndrome: Preliminary analysis of a randomized, placebo-controlled study. *Arthritis and Rheumatism, 40*(Suppl.), S117.

Russell, I. J., Michalek, J. E., Flechas, J. D., & Abraham, G. E. (1995). Treatment of fibromyalgia syndrome with Super Malic: a randomized, double blind, placebo controlled, crossover pilot study. *Journal of Rheumatology, 22*, 953–958.

Russell, I. J., Michalek, J. E., Vipraio, G. A., Fletcher, E. M., Javors, M. A., & Bowden, C. A. (1992). Platelet 3H-imipramine uptake receptor density and serum serotonin levels in patients with fibromyalgia/fibrositis syndrome. *Journal of Rheumatology, 19*, 104–109.

Russell, I. J., Michalek, J. E., Vipraio, G. A., Fletcher, E. M., & Wall, K. (1989). Serum amino acids in fibrositis/fibromyalgia syndrome. *Journal of Rheumatology, 19*(Suppl.), 158–163.

Russell, I. J., Orr, M. D., Littman, B., Vipraio, G. A., Alboukrek, D., Michalek, J. E., Lopez, Y., & MacKillip, F. (1994). Elevated cerebrospinal levels of substance P in patients with fibromyalgia syndrome. *Arthritis and Rheumatism, 37*, 1593–1601.

Russell, I. J., Russell, S. J., Cuevas, R. E., & Michalek, J. (1992). Early life traumas and confiding in fibromyalgia syndrome (FS). *Scandinavian Journal of Rheumatology, 94*(Suppl.), S14.

Russell, I. J., & Vipraio, G. A. (1993). Red cell nucleotide abnormalities in fibromyalgia syndrome. *Arthritis and Rheumatism, 36*(Suppl.), S223.

Russell, I. J., & Vipraio, G. A. (1994). Serotonin (5HT) in serum and platelets (PLT) from fibromyalgia patients (FS) and normal controls (NC). *Arthritis and Rheumatism, 37*(Suppl.), S214.

Russell, I. J., Vipraio, G. A., & Acworth, I. (1993). Abnormalities in the central nervous system (CNS) metabolism of tryptophan (TRY) to 3-hydroxy kynurenine (OHKY) in fibromyalgia syndrome (FS) [Abstract]. *Arthritis and Rheumatism, 36*(Suppl.), S222.

Russell, I. J., Vipraio, G. A., & Lopez, Y. M. (1993). Serum serotonin in fibromyalgia syndrome, rheumatoid arthritis, osteoarthritis, and healthy normal controls. *Arthritis and Rheumatism, 36*(Suppl.), S223.

Russell, I. J., Vipraio, G. A., Michalek, J., & Lopez, Y. G. (1992). Insulin-like growth factor (IGF1) in fibromyalgia, rheumatoid arthritis, osteoarthritis and healthy normal controls: Roles of diagnosis, age, sex and ethnic origin [Abstract]. *Arthritis and Rheumatism, 35*(Suppl.), S160.

Sadun, A. (1992). *Presentation on eye involvement in chronic fatigue syndrome.* Presentation at the Conference on Chronic Fatigue Syndrome and the Brain, Los Angeles, CA.

Sandstrom, M. J., & Keefe, F. J. (1998). Self-management of fibromyalgia: The role of formal coping skills training and physical exercise training programs. *Arthritis Care and Research, 11*, 432–447.

Scarinci, I. C., McDonald-Haile, J., Bradley, L. A., & Richter, J. E. (1994). Altered pain perception and psychosocial features among women with gastrointestinal disorders and history of abuse: A preliminary model. *American Journal of Medicine, 97*, 108–118.

Simms, R. W. (1996). Is there muscle pathology in fibromyalgia syndrome? *Rheumatic Disease Clinics of North America, 22*(2), 245–266.

Simons, D. G., Hong, C.- Z., & Simons, L. S. (1995a). Nature of myofascial trigger points, active loci [Abstract]. *Journal of Musculoskeletal Pain, 3*(Suppl. 1), 62.

Simons, D. G., Hong, C.- Z., & Simons, L. S. (1995b). Spike activity in trigger points [Abstract]. *Journal of Musculoskeletal Pain, 3*(Suppl. 1), 125.

Simons, D. G., Hong, C.- Z., & Simons, L. S. (1995c). Spontaneous electrical activity of trigger points [Abstract]. *Journal of Musculoskeletal Pain, 3*(Suppl. 1), 124.

Tach, B. (1990). Fatigue in rheumatoid arthritis: Conditions, strategies and consequences. *Arthritis Care and Research, 3*, 65–70.

Tilbe, K., Bell, D. A., & McCain, G. A. (1988). Loss of diurnal variation in serum cortisol, growth hormone and prolactin in patients with primary fibromyalgia. *Arthritis and Rheumatism, 31*(Suppl.), S99.

Tinsley, J. A. (1999). The hazards of psychotropic herbs. *Minnesota Medicine, 82*(5), 29–31.

Travell, J. G., & Simons, D. G. (1992). *Myofascial pain and dysfunction: The trigger point manual* (2nd ed.). Baltimore: Williams & Wilkins.

Vaeroy, H., Helle, R., Forre, O., Kass, E., & Terenius, L. (1988). Elevated CSF levels of substance P and high incidence of Raynaud phenomenon in patients with fibromyalgia: New features for diagnosis. *Pain, 32*, 21–26.

Veale, D., Kavanagh, G., Fielding, J. F., & Fitzgerald, O. (1991). Primary fibromyalgia and the irritable bowel syndrome: Different expressions of a common pathogenic process. *British Journal of Rheumatology, 30*, 220–222.

Viitanen, J., Kautiainen, H., & Isomaki, H. (1995). Changes in atmospheric pressure do not influence the pain of patients with primary fibromyalgia. *Journal of Musculoskeletal Pain, 3*, 77–82.

Volkmann, H., Norregaard, J., Jacobsen, S., Danneskiold-Samsoe, B., Knoke, G., & Nehrdich, D. (1997). Double-blind, placebo-controlled cross-over study of intravenous S-adenosyl-L-methionine in patients with fibromyalgia. *Scandinavian Journal of Rheumatology, 26*(3), 206–211.

Walker, E. A., Katon, W. J., Roy-Byrne, P. P., Jemelka, R. P., & Russo, J. (1993). Histories of sexual victimization in patients with irritable bowel syndrome or inflammatory bowel disease. *American Journal of Psychiatry, 150*, 1502–1506.

Wallace, D. J. (1990). Genitourinary manifestations of fibrositis: An increased association with the female urethral syndrome. *Journal of Rheumatology, 17*, 238–239.

Ware, J. C. (1983). Tricyclic antidepressants in the treatment of insomnia. *Journal of Clinical Psychiatry, 44*, 25–28.

Waylonis, G. W., & Heck, W. (1992). Fibromyalgia syndrome: New associations. *American Journal of Physical Medicine and Rehabilitation, 71*, 343–348.

Weiss, D. J., Kreck, T., & Albert, R. K. (1998). Dyspnea resulting from fibromyalgia. *Chest, 113*(1), 246–249.

Welin, M., Bragee, B., Nyberg, F., & Kristiansson, M. (1995). Elevated substance P levels are contrasted by a decrease in met-enkephalin-arg-phe levels in CSF from fibromyalgia patients [Abstract]. *Journal of Musculoskeletal Pain, 3*(Suppl. 1), 4.

Wigers, S. H., Stiles, T. C., & Vogel, P. A. (1996). Effects of aerobic exercise versus stress management treatment in fibromyalgia: A 4.5 year prospective study. *Scandinavian Journal of Rheumatology, 25*(2), 77–86.

Wolfe, F. (1993). The epidemiology of fibromyalgia. *Journal of Musculoskeletal Pain, 1*, 137–147.

Wolfe, F., Anderson, J., Harkness, D., Bennett, R. M., Caro, X., Goldenberg, D. L., Russell, I. J., & Yunus, M. B. (1997a). Health status and disease severity in fibromyalgia: Results of a six center longitudinal study. *Arthritis and Rheumatism, 40*, 1571.

Wolfe, F., Anderson, J., Harkness, D., Bennett, R. M., Caro, X., Goldenberg, D. L., Russell, I. J., & Yunus, M. B. (1997b). Work and disability status of persons with fibromyalgia. *Journal of Rheumatology, 24*, 1171.

Wolfe, F., Anderson, J., Harkness, D., Bennett, R. M., Caro, X., Goldenberg, D. L., Russell, I. J., & Yunus, M. B. (1997c). A prospective, longitudinal, multicenter study of service utilization and costs in fibromyalgia. *Arthritis and Rheumatism, 40*, 1560–1570.

Wolfe, F., Ross, K., Anderson, J., & Russell, I. J. (1995a). Aspects of fibromyalgia in the general population: Sex, pain threshold, and fibromyalgia symptoms. *Journal of Rheumatology, 21*, 151.

Wolfe, F., Ross, K., Anderson, J., Russell, I. J., & Hebert, L. (1995b). The prevalence and characteristics of fibromyalgia in the general population. *Arthritis and Rheumatism, 38*, 19–28.

Wolfe, F., Simons, D. G., Fricton, J., Bennett, R. M., Goldenberg, D. L., Gerwin, R., Hathaway, D., McCain, G. A., Russell, I. J., Sanders, H. O., & Skootsky, S. A. (1992). The fibromyalgia and myofascial pain syndromes: A preliminary study of tender points and trigger points in persons with fibromyalgia, myofascial pain syndrome and no disease. *Journal of Rheumatology, 19*, 944–951.

Wolfe, F., Smythe, H. A., Yunus, M. B., Bennett, R. M., Bombardier, C., Goldenberg, D. L., Tugwell, P., Campbell, S. M., Abeles, M., Clark, P., Fam, A. G., Farber, S. J., Fiechtner, J. J., Franklin, C. M., Gatter, R. A., Hamaty, D., Lessard, J., Lichtbroun, A. S., Masi, A. T., McCain, G. A., Reynolds, W. J., Romano, T. J., Russell, I. J., & Sheon, R. P. (1990). The American College of Rheumatology 1990 Criteria for the Classification of Fibromyalgia. *Arthritis and Rheumatism, 33*, 160–172.

Wurtman, R. J. (1984). Effects of foods and nutrients on brain neurotransmitters. *Current Concepts in Nutrition, 13*, 103–112.

Wurtman, R. J. (1987). Dietary treatments that affect brain neurotransmitters: Effect on calorie and nutrient intake. *Annals of the New York Academy of Science, 499*, 179–190.

Yaron, I., Buskila, D., Shirazi, I., Neumann, L., Elkayam, O., Paran, D., & Yaron, M. (1997). Elevated levels of hyaluronic acid in the sera of women with fibromyalgia. *Journal of Rheumatology, 24*, 2221–2224.

Yucha, C., & McKay, S. (1992). Idiopathic edema. *ANNA Journal, 19*(1), 29–32.

Yunus, M. B. (1994). Fibromyalgia syndrome: Clinical features and spectrum. *Journal of Musculoskeletal Pain, 2*, 5–21.

Yunus, M. B., Dailey, J. W., Aldag, J. C., Masi, A. T., & Jobe, P. C. (1992). Plasma tryptophan and other amino acids in primary fibromyalgia: A controlled study. *Journal of Rheumatology, 19*, 90–94.

Yunus, M. B., & Kalyan-Raman, U. P. (1989). Muscle biopsy findings in primary fibromyalgia and other forms of nonarticular rheumatism. *Rheumatic Disease Clinics of North America, 15*, 115–134.

Yunus, M. B., Kalyan-Raman, U. P., Masi, A. T., & Aldag, J. C. (1989). Electron microscopic studies of muscle biopsy in primary fibromyalgia syndrome: A controlled and blinded study. *Journal of Rheumatology, 16*, 97–101.

Yunus, M. B., Masi, A. T., & Aldag, J. C. (1989). A controlled study of primary fibromyalgia syndrome: Clinical features and association with other functional syndromes [Review]. *Journal of Rheumatology, 19*, 62–71.

Yunus, M., Masi, A. T., Calabro, J. J., Miller, K. A., & Feigenbaum, S. L. (1981). Primary fibromyalgia (fibrositis): Clinical study of 50 patients with matched normal controls. *Seminars in Arthritis and Rheumatism, 11*, 151–171.

Zarcone, V. P. (1994). Sleep hygiene. In M. H. Kryger, T. Roth, & W. C. Dement (Eds.), *Principles and practice of sleep medicine* (2nd ed., pp. 542–546). Philadelphia: Saunders.

Zelik, L. L. (1984). The use of assertiveness training with chronic pain patients. In F. S. Cromwell (Ed.), *Occupational therapy and the patient with pain* (pp. 109–118). New York: Haworth Press.

7

RHEUMATOID ARTHRITIS

Marilyn Sanford, PhD, PT, Stuart L. Silverman, MD, FACP, FACR, and Terri Wolfe, OTR/L, CHT

Rheumatoid arthritis (RA) is a chronic inflammatory disease with symmetrical polyarticular inflammation, morning stiffness, malaise, and fatigue. It is a systemic disease affecting not only synovial joints but also blood vessels, the heart, lungs, eyes, and other systems (extra-articular involvement).

Population Studies

The prevalence of definite RA is approximately 0.8% of the population in many countries. RA can affect any race. There is an increasing incidence with age that continues into the seventh decade. The incidence rate is for females is two to three times the rate for males at all ages with the greatest difference between genders in persons less than 50 years of age (Silman & Hochberg, 1993).

Diagnosis

The diagnosis of RA is made primarily on the basis of findings of a symmetrical polyarthritis, usually involving the hands, that has persisted for more than 60 days with morning stiffness and frequent systemic fatigue and malaise. Any synovial joint may be affected, but those most commonly involved are the second and third metacarpophalangeal (MCP) joints, the second and third proximal interphalangeal (PIP) joints of the hands, the metatarsophalangeal (MTP) joints, wrists, knees, elbows, and, less commonly, the shoulder, hip, and distal interphalangeal (DIP) joints (Arnett et al., 1988). In the shoulder and hip joints, pain on motion (in lieu of tenderness or swelling) suggests inflammation (Hawley & Wolfe, 1992).

Rheumatoid factor (RF) is found in about 85% of patients with RA, but it is not a specific test for RA, and it can be present in healthy persons (Singer & Plotz, 1956). The presence of RF correlates with severe and unremitting disease, nodules, and extra-articular manifestations. The level of RF correlates loosely with disease severity and is of little value in predicting the course of the disease. Some patients may be RF negative early in the disease and then become RF positive (Anderson, 1997).

Table 1. 1988 Revised American Rheumatism Association Criteria for Classification of Rheumatoid Arthritis* (Arnett, et al., 1988)

Criteria	Definition
1. Morning stiffness	Morning stiffness in and around the joints lasting at least 1 hr before maximal improvement
2. Arthritis of three or more joint areas	At least three joint areas have simultaneously had soft-tissue swelling or fluid (not bony overgrowth alone) observed by a physician; the 14 possible joint areas are (right or left) PIP, MCP, wrist, elbow, knee, ankle, and MTP joints
3. Arthritis of hand joints	At least one joint area swollen as above in wrist, MCP, or PIP joints
4. Symmetrical arthritis	Simultaneous involvement of the same joint areas as in criterion 2 on both sides of the body (bilateral involvement of PIP, MCP, or MTP joints is acceptable without absolute symmetry)
5. Rheumatoid nodules	Subcutaneous nodules over bony prominences, extensor surfaces, or in juxta-articular regions observed by a physician
6. Serum RF	Demonstration of abnormal amounts of serum RF by any method that has been positive in less than 5% of healthy control participants
7. Radiographic changes	Radiographic changes typical of RA on posterior-anterior hand and wrist X-rays, which must include erosions or unequivocal bony decalcification localized to or most marked adjacent to the involved joints (OA changes alone do not qualify)

*For classification purposes, a patient is said to have RA if he or she has satisfied at least 4 of the above 7 criteria. Criteria 1–4 must be present for at least 6 weeks. Patients with two clinical diagnoses are not excluded. Designation as classic, definite, or probable RA is not to be made.

Other helpful laboratory tests include the erythrocyte sedimentation rate (ESR), which measures the rate at which erythrocytes become sediment in serum in a test tube. A rate of more than 20 mm/hr indicates inflammation. Measurement of C-reactive protein may be used to monitor inflammation. It is possible but rare for a patient with active RA to have a normal ESR. Other laboratory abnormalities in RA include hypergammaglobulinemia, anemia, eosinophilia, thrombocytosis, and occasional hypocomplementemia (Anderson, 1997).

Classification

Criteria for RA (Table 1), described as "classification" criteria rather than "diagnostic" criteria, have been developed to promote uniformity in research studies (Arnett et al., 1988). It is now recognized that these criteria identify persons with quite different courses of disease, including at least three clinical types of presentation over time (Table 2).

Persons with type I RA have a self-limited inflammatory polyarthritis that is frequently a postviral syndrome that often resolves without a visit to a health professional. Type II RA involves patients who have persistent disease, although it does not lead to major long-term consequences and is manageable with traditional therapies. Type III RA is a progressive disease that, even with traditional therapies, has followed a natural history characterized by radiographic damage, declines in functional status, work disability, and premature mortality within 10 to 15 years in most

Table 2. Subtypes of Clinical Courses of Patients Who May Meet Classification Criteria for Rheumatoid Arthritis

	Type I	Type II	Type III
Type of polyarthritis	Self-limited process	Minimally progressive disease	Progressive disease
Predominant site of identification	Population studies, occasionally in the clinic	Clinical settings (unusual)	Clinical settings (typical)
Estimated proportion of the next 100 patients with RA to be seen by a rheumatologist (%)	5–20	5–20	60–90
RF+ (%)	<5	60–90	60–90
Odds of HLA DR-4	1:1	3–5:1	3–5:1
Meet criteria for RA 3–10 years later (%)	0 (by definition)	90–100 (a few may have a different diagnosis)	90–100 (a few may have a different diagnosis)
Response to traditional treatment approach	Long-term treatment not needed	Good, although some progression is usually seen	Disease progression continues despite treatment
Markers to distinguish from other types	RF, HLA DR-4	Course of 30–180 days, baseline clinical markers	Course of 30–180 days, baseline clinical markers

Note. From "How Many Types of Patients Meet Classification Criteria for Rheumatoid Arthritis [Editorial]?" by T. Pincus and L. F. Callahan, 1994, *Journal of Rheumatology, 21*, pp. 1385–1389.

patients. Most patients who meet the criteria for RA in the population have type I RA, although the self-limited process generally resolves within 6 months. However, more than 50% of patients seen in clinical settings (up to 80% in rehabilitation settings) have type III RA. These three types cannot be necessarily distinguished definitively by laboratory tests or other studies, although patients with types II and III are more likely to have RF and carry the human lymphocyte antigen (HLA) DR-4 (Pincus & Callahan, 1994).

Radiographic Findings

Radiographs of RA at an early stage indicate the presence of juxta-articular osteopenia and soft-tissue swelling. Further progression results in cartilage destruction evident radiographically as joint space narrowing and bony erosion. Although more than half of the patients with RA have radiographic abnormalities within the first 2 years of disease, most patients do not have malalignment on the radiograph or joint deformity on physical examination until after 5 years of disease. A normal radiograph does not exclude a diagnosis of RA. Indeed, this may indicate the optimal circumstances to initiate aggressive treatment. (See chapter 4 in this volume for a discussion and illustrations of typical radiographic findings.)

Functional Evaluation

An important development in rheumatology during the last 15 years has been the development and clinical use of functional status questionnaires. The most widely used questionnaires include the Health Assessment Questionnaire (HAQ) (Hawley & Wolfe, 1992) and its modified version (MHAQ) (Pincus et al., 1989). These questionnaires, which are completed by the patient, have been effective in monitoring clinical status in clinical trials. Other questionnaires such as the Arthritis Impact Measurement Scale (AIMS) (Meenan, Gertman, & Mason, 1980; Meenan, Mason, Anderson, Guccione, & Kazis, 1992) have been used in specialized studies.

Scores on the MHAQ are correlated with other clinical measures of patient status, including joint count, radiographs, and laboratory tests. Among all measures of RA, the MHAQ has been found to be the most representative single measure (including radiographs and laboratory tests) to describe patient status (Pincus et al., 1989). The MHAQ provides a permanent record of functional status, pain, fatigue, global status, learned helplessness, psychological distress, and medications. It is as effective as any clinical measure used to predict mortality from RA for 5 to 15 years, including radiographic and laboratory tests (Pincus, Wolfe, & Callahan, 1994).

Self-report functional status questionnaires can be an effective way to document functional disability and may be the only way to quantitatively measure pain, fatigue, and psychological distress. They may provide an optimal method to document whether care of a patient with RA (or any rheumatic disease) is effective over time. Questionnaires may help determine the relative effectiveness of different therapies from the perspective of function.

Course and Prognosis

The course of RA is unpredictable because the natural history of RA includes at least three types as noted above, and the course of disease in individual patients with type III progressive disease may vary considerably both from patient to patient and within the same patient at different periods.

Patients who have a spontaneous remission generally recover within 6 months. One condition often associated with great improvement is pregnancy. This period of excellent control is usually followed in the postpartum period by more severe disease at a time that is considerably difficult for the patient. It is important to prepare for this likelihood during the pregnancy while the patient is feeling well.

Measures of inflammatory activity (e.g., ESR, number of tender joints, and patient global status) may improve over 5 years as a result of medication. However, joint destruction and functional disability may continue to progress (Callahan et al., 1997).

Substantial radiographic progression has been found in all longitudinal studies of patients with RA. Radiographic damage in RA is often seen within the first 2 years of disease. Increases in radiographic scores are more rapid during early versus late disease (Fuchs & Pincus, 1992).

Most treated patients have shown severe declines in functional status as measured by physical tests of function (e.g., grip strength, dexterity), patient activities of daily living (ADL) status as measured by questionnaire (Pincus et al., 1989), or work disability as measured by analyses of drug therapies used in the 1970s and 1980s. These declines occur over long periods and are unexplained by age.

Work disability has been reported after 5 years in 60% to 70% of patients with RA who are younger than 65 years of age and had been working at disease onset (Pincus et al., 1984; Yelin, Meenan, Nevitt, & Epstein, 1980).

Patients with RA die at an earlier age than expected for persons of the same age and gender (Pincus & Callahan, 1989). Immediate causes of death are similar to those in the general population. Earlier death in patients with RA, whether attributed to RA or other causes, is associated with more severe disease. Predictors of earlier death include more involved joints and poorer functional status, older age, lower socioeconomic status, and cardiovascular comorbidity. Five-year survival rates are in the range of 45% to 55% in patients with the poorest functional status compared with 85% to 95% in persons with favorable values (Pincus & Callahan, 1989). More recent data since the use of methotrexate has shown improved survival rates of patients with the poorest levels of functioning. Callahan and associates (1997) showed improved 5-year survival rates of 70% in patients with the poorest levels of functioning. Furthermore, the number of patients with the poorest functional status has decreased from 80% of patients in 1978 (Pincus et al., 1989) to 25% of patients in 1990 (Callahan et al., 1997) with resulting decreases in disability.

Drug Therapy

The goal in treating RA is to obtain clinical remission; however, this is usually not achieved. By using the American College of Rheumatology (ACR) preliminary criteria for remission (5 out of 6 of the following criteria: absent morning stiffness less than 15 min and no fatigue, joint pain, joint tenderness, joint or tendon sheath swelling, or elevation of the ESR). Wolfe and Pincus (1994) found short-term remission in about 20% of patients and sustained remission in less than 8% of patients.

Four types of drugs are important in patient management: nonsteroidal anti-inflammatory drugs (NSAIDs), disease-modifying antirheumatic drugs (DMARDs) such as methotrexate, corticosteroids, and analgesic drugs.

Nonsteroidal Anti-inflammatory Drugs

The prototype NSAID is aspirin, which was traditionally regarded as the mainstay of management of RA. However, the use of aspirin is quite limited because doses in the anti-inflammatory range frequently result in a high frequency of complaints of gastrointestinal distress and bleeding. Long-term use of high doses of aspirin is not possible for most patients. Buffered or enteric-coated aspirin (Ecotrin) is more likely to be tolerated longer by patients.

Nonacetylated salicylates (Disalcid, Trilasate) have reduced gastrointestinal toxicity compared with aspirin but may not be as effective as acetylated salicylates. Various nonaspirin NSAIDs have been developed, including ibuprofen, naproxen, ketoprofen, indomethacin, diclofenac, meclofenamate, piroxicam, and sulindac.

Cyclo-oxygenase 2 (COX-2) inhibitors (Celebrex) are newly available. These decrease the gastrointestinal toxicity of NSAIDs by selective inhibition of prostaglandins that mediate inflammation in the joint and not the prostaglandins that protect the gut and kidneys.

Disease-Modifying Antirheumatic Drugs

Once called "second-line drugs" because they were used only after milder drugs such as NSAIDs failed, DMARDs are now used initially in the treatment of RA because they may retard disease progression. Specific drugs in this category include methotrexate, antimalarials, injectable and oral gold agents, sulfasalazine, penicillamine, azathioprine, cyclosporin, and cyclophosphamide. These drugs were formerly called *remission-inducing drugs*, but we now recognize that many patients do not achieve an adequate response or do not maintain a response due to toxicity or lack of effectiveness (Cash & Klippel, 1994).

Methotrexate is used more than all of the other DMARDs combined, primarily because it is more effective and tolerated longer than other second-line drugs in most patients (Pincus, Marcum, & Callahan, 1992). Methotrexate reduces radiological progression. The toxicity of low-dose methotrexate appears to be less than that of many NSAIDs. Methotrexate is associated with hematological and hepatic side effects. Low-dose folic acid or leucovorin calcium may reduce toxicity.

Leflunomide (Arava) was the first DMARD created specifically for RA. It reduces activation of the immune system in patients with RA by disrupting pyrimidine synthesis and hence DNA. It may be used alone as a substitute for methotrexate. Arava was generally well tolerated in clinical studies, with the most common side effects being reversible diarrhea, rash, alopecia (transient hair loss), and elevated liver function tests (Rozman for the Leflunomide Investigators' Group, 1998).

The antimalarial drugs chloroquine and hydroxychloroquine (Plaquenil) are effective for some patients with RA but are not as effective as methotrexate. This class of drugs has been associated with retinal injury that results initially in loss of color vision. This side effect is rare, but patients should have periodic eye examinations while taking these drugs.

Injectable gold salts in the form of gold sodium thiomalate (Myochrysine or Aurolate), aurothioglucose (Solganal), or oral gold (auranofin) have been a traditional mainstay in treating RA but are now used less often than methotrexate. Primary toxicities include hematological and renal problems and involve diarrhea with the oral preparation.

Sulfasalazine is the most widely used second-line drug in Europe in the late 20th century. The dosage is generally 1,000 to 2,000 mg twice a day. Toxicities include rash and gastrointestinal symptoms.

Azathioprine is an immunosuppressive drug with hematological and gastrointestinal toxicity.

Cyclophosphamide is used primarily for rheumatoid vasculitis in doses of 50 to 200 mg/day. It is not used in most patients because of the risks of leukemia and hemorrhagic cystitis that leads to cancer of the bladder endothelium.

Cyclosporin is a newer agent for patients with aggressive disease in whom methotrexate has not been effective. Cyclosporin reduces radiological progression. It can have renal toxicity.

Biological Modifiers

Anticytokine therapy. Cytokines are chemical messengers of the immune system that play an important role in the development, persistence, and destructiveness of joint inflammation. The cytokines that appear to be the most important in RA are interleukin-1, tissue necrosis factor alpha (TNF-α), interleukin-6, and granulocyte-macrophage colony stimulating factor, which are products of activated macrophages rather than T-cells. (Firestein & Zvaifler, 1997).

Etanercept (Enbrel). TNF-α is a proinflammatory cytokine that leads to synovitis and joint destruction. Etanercept binds to TNF and prevents it from binding to target cells. Etanercept is the first of a new class of drugs known as *biological modifiers* (sometimes called "biologics"). It is administered twice weekly by injection. It appears to be safe, well tolerated, and able to produce rapid, notable decreases in disease activity for at least 6 months, even in patients with longstanding RA. A sustained effect requires continued administration. Unlike DMARDs, etanercept requires no laboratory evaluation or monitoring. Its major limitation is its cost, which is about $13,000 a year (Moreland et al., 1999).

Analgesic Drugs

Analgesic medications such as acetaminophen with small amounts of codeine (Vicodin, Tylenol with codeine, etc.) are often used in addition to NSAIDs and DMARDs to provide added pain relief for the damaged joint in which anti-inflammatory therapy is not effective. The use of strong narcotic analgesics should be discouraged, but these drugs are occasionally appropriate to care for a patient with end-stage RA to improve quality of life.

Corticosteroids

Corticosteroids have a long history in the treatment of RA. Corticosteroids suppress inflammation but do not prevent disease progression. Although long-term use in high doses of more than 20 mg of prednisone a day inevitably leads to considerable toxicity in terms of osteoporosis, diabetes, obesity, hypertension, or infection, low doses of 7.5 mg or less have become widespread in most clinical settings in the United States. Patients taking low-dose corticosteroids do not have cushingoid features (e.g., moon facies, a fat pad on the dorsum of the neck, purpura, striae) but may still develop bone loss. High-dose corticosteroids are often used for vasculitis. Low-dose corticosteroids are often used in the period between onset of therapy with second-line drugs and onset of effect (Williams, 1993).

Corticosteroids may be given periodically as an intramuscular (parenteral) injection of 40 to 80 mg of a long-acting preparation or as intra-articular injections into a particularly painful joint. Many authorities recommend immobilization of the injected joint for 48 hr, but others believe that mobility is not contraindicated after injection. For example, injection of the carpometacarpal (CMC) joint plus splinting often achieves better results than injection alone (E. Nalebuff, personal communication). (See chapter 3 in this volume for more details on specific drugs.)

Overview of Clinical Drug Use

A few principles concerning the clinical use of drugs for RA are presented to provide an overview of their administration.

- Recognition of severe long-term outcomes in RA and limited long-term effectiveness of current therapies suggest that an optimal treatment strategy in RA is to control inflammation as aggressively as possible early in the disease. It is appropriate to use as much medication (including NSAIDs, DMARDs, prednisone, anticytokine therapy, and combinations of several drugs) as needed (McCarthy, Harman, Grassanovich, & Qian, 1995; Wilske, 1993; Wolfe & Pincus, 1994). All data indicate that poor clinical status is associated with poor outcomes and that drug therapy is effective but not remission inducing. Early consultation with a rheumatologist is essential.

- Drug treatment of RA is not curative; however, control of the consequences of RA is a realistic goal that requires ongoing medication on an indefinite basis.

- Inflammatory activity is reversible, whereas damage to the joint resulting from inflammation is irreversible. Therefore, the traditional advice that use of second-line drugs should be reserved until there is evidence of damage such as radiographic erosions is no longer followed. A patient is a candidate for second-line drugs once the diagnosis of RA is established and at a relatively early stage (Semble, 1995).

- Individual patients respond differently to various second-line drugs. No single drug is optimal for all patients. Some patients may require combination therapy.

- The doses required for methotrexate, azathioprine, or prednisone to be effective for RA are considerably lower than doses used in the treatment of cancer or to suppress rejection in transplant patients. Therefore, the benefit-to-toxicity ratio is considerably better for patients with RA treated with cytotoxic or immunosuppressive drugs than for other types of patients treated with these drugs.

- At least 20 years are required for definitive evidence that new approaches to therapy for RA have improved outcomes. However, reports from many centers suggest that functional outcomes are improving greatly, particularly with the widespread use of early methotrexate.

The therapist may play an important role in patient decision making about medication. Patients may be hesitant to start aggressive medical treatment. Unfortunately, by the time it is obvious to the patient that aggressive treatment is needed, some irreversible damage has likely already occurred, and it is probably too late to gain the most optimal benefits of treatment. The therapist must reinforce the benefits of early aggressive treatment. Patients must continue treatment even when in a state of apparent remission or when there is "no evidence of disease" to maintain their status. Therapists can help patients by reinforcing these concepts.

Although these drugs have been documented as effective in clinical trials, the only drugs in clinical use that are continued by more than 50% of patients for longer than 2 years and by more than 20% of patients for longer than 5 years are methotrexate and corticosteroids (Pincus et al., 1992).

Therefore, each drug other than methotrexate and the corticosteroids is effective for about 1 in 5 persons and is not effective for long periods in 4 out of 5 patients.

Rehabilitation: A Self-Management Model

The foundation of therapy for RA should be patient education that emphasizes self-management. The chronic nature of RA necessitates patient and family member education to promote informed decision making. In the 1970s and 1980s, patient education focused on teaching patients about the disease, medications, joint protection, exercises, and pain-relieving physical agents. The goal was to have patients comply with instructions.

In the 1990s, patient education evolved into teaching self-management within a wellness context. Self-management, defined by Lorig (1993) as "learning and practicing the skills necessary to carry on an active and emotionally satisfying life in the face of chronic illness", involves helping patients acquire a complex set of skills and attitudes to help maintain or improve health, slow disease progression, minimize dysfunction, and promote optimum participation in normal activities. This includes teaching patients how to use activity, exercise, nutrition, sleep, and rest not only to control symptoms but also to maximize their health.

Patient concerns may differ from that of health care providers. Patients most often visit a health care provider because of pain, functional limitations, fatigue, psychological distress, or other symptoms. Physicians may be concerned about disease activity measures such as ESRs, joint counts, and joint swelling or deformity. Health care providers must have common goals with the patient: prevention of disability, functional loss, and deterioration of quality of life.

Patients with RA, with the knowledge and support of family members, should be given resources to select activities designed to preserve or restore functional movement and locomotion (including relief of pain) to maintain and improve overall quality of life. A positive attitude toward the patient's ability to be an active self-manager is one of the most important concepts health professionals can provide for the person with RA.

Research has shown that self-management training in a group format for 2 hr a week for 7 weeks can reduce symptoms 15% to 30% in addition to the benefits attained from medication (Hirano, Laurent, & Lorig, 1994). These percentages could be even higher with individual training. Comprehensive self-management behaviors resulting from knowledge are associated with stronger feelings of self-effectiveness (i.e., the ability to control what is happening to oneself) (Taal et al., 1993). Research has substantiated the strong benefits of patient education in improving function in the RA population (Superio-Cabuslay, Ward, & Lorig, 1996).

Several studies have demonstrated that greater amounts of formal education correlate with better disease outcomes (Leigh & Fries, 1991). Providers should consider the educational background of the patient and family members and convey information in an appropriate form. Providers should be aware of cultural and personal health beliefs and identify effective methods for educating members of minority groups and those for whom the common language is not their native language (Semble, 1995). Boutaugh and Brady (1998) have written a comprehensive review on how to teach patient education for self-management of arthritis.

Multidisciplinary Approach

Optimally, effective treatment for a person with a chronic disease is provided through a multidisciplinary approach. A multidisciplinary approach may include a physician, a physical therapist, an occupational therapist, a nurse, a social worker, a psychologist, a dietitian, a pedorthist, and a vocational rehabilitation specialist. This team can effectively meet the needs of the patient who, as a result of chronic disease, has pain, fatigue, functional limitations, psychological distress, work-related disability, and financial problems. Health care providers must become aware of professionals from other disciplines in their community or institution who have expertise in helping persons with arthritis.

Ideally, a team provides this multidisciplinary approach; unfortunately, insurers may not pay for a formal team approach. When possible, occupational and physical therapy practitioners must work together to maximize patient care. Under managed care, physical therapy and occupational therapy may be limited to 6 to 12 sessions per year or per diagnosis. To avoid overlap and to facilitate care, physical and occupational therapy practitioners must coordinate care so that the needs of patients with complex polyarticular diseases can be met within limited coverage plans.

Occupational and Physical Therapy Referral

Referral to therapy is indicated early in the course of disease to maintain or increase function and especially to prevent or reduce the loss of function. Just as DMARDs should be instituted before joint damage is apparent, therapy should be instituted before joints are damaged so that the patient may learn appropriate self-management techniques.

> The key to effective management of the person with arthritis is early identification of pathodynamics that can cause secondary limitations and the prevention of those limitations. It is not possible to prevent the primary disease, but the consequences of the disease can often be controlled or reduced. (Melvin, 1989)

Referral to occupational therapy. Referral to occupational therapy is indicated for the following reasons:

- Evaluation of functional ability and upper-extremity pathology and function
- Fabrication or fitting of hand and elbow splints, braces, and orthotic devices
- Instruction in joint protection techniques, adaptive methods, and use of assistive equipment
- Instruction in fatigue and pain management
- Instruction in activities or exercises to maintain or improve hand function, joint mobility, and muscular strength
- Before and after upper-extremity surgical evaluation and treatment

Because hand involvement occurs early in the disease course, the occupational therapist may be the first or only therapist the patient visits. In these cases, the occupational therapist is responsible for determining if there is a need for a physical therapy referral. Likewise, physical therapists should screen patients for the need for occupational therapy services.

Referral to physical therapy. Referral to physical therapy is indicated for the following reasons:

- Evaluation of joint mobility, strength, endurance, gait, posture, and function
- Exercise prescription and instruction in fatigue management
- Pain management
- Gait and posture training
- Instruction in functional mobility, including the use of an assistive device
- Fabrication and fitting of lower-extremity orthoses
- Before and after surgical evaluation and treatment

Social Service Referral

Social service referral is indicated for patients with chronic diseases who have financial problems. These financial problems may result in changes in residence, the inability to afford prescription medication, lack of adherence to medical instructions, inadequate medical follow-up visits, and the inability to visit a therapist.

Psychology Referral

Patients with chronic diseases often experience psychological distress related to their functional loss (disability) and subsequent loss of their role in society (handicap). They may lose self-esteem and develop a sense of "learned helplessness." Functional outcomes may depend on their coping skills. Depression and anxiety can impair sleep, increase fatigue, and reduce functional capacity.

Vocational Rehabilitation Referral

Patients with chronic diseases often have problems maintaining a full-time job. Because of the unpredictable nature of their illness, pain, fatigue, and functional limitations may interfere with work attendance and productivity. Patients are more likely to require modifications of their workplace or help in retraining for less demanding jobs.

Evaluation

The history of the disease course, the patient's response to medications and previous rehabilitation, and an overview of functional status should be ascertained before instituting therapy. The interview offers the therapist insight into the patient's psychosocial status, including the patient's beliefs regarding the disease and what he or she views as reasonable functional goals.

Evaluation of Physical Status

Because RA is a complex, systemic illness, evaluations should be comprehensive. It is therefore important to be aware of the following factors and focus on those that are applicable to a specific patient.

- Diagnosis and onset
- Previous medical and rehabilitative management

- Joint count, distribution, inflammation, and limitations
- Morning stiffness
- Medications and complications or side effects
- Systemic manifestations (e.g., fatigue, fever, malaise, anorexia)
- Functional evaluation (e.g., ADL, gait, and endurance)
- Sleep pattern, quantity and restorative quality of sleep, and side effects of sleep medications
- Psychosocial status, depression, anxiety, family situation, and support systems
- Stress factors (emotional and physical)
- Physical demands on the patient
- Living environment
- Work, community, and avocational or recreational activities

Physical evaluation should include a careful examination of the musculoskeletal system, including joint mobility and integrity, muscle strength, tendon function, and inflammation. The examination should include evaluation of extra-articular involvement such as neurological and cardiopulmonary status and skin integrity. The presence of nodules, their size, and whether they are tender or aggravated by pressure should be noted.

The physical evaluation must indicate how proximal stability and instability will affect distal joint function, especially for the hands and feet. Joint excursion and muscle length may be evaluated by obtaining active and passive range of motion (ROM) measurements. Comparison of the two measures can help predict functional limitations. Crepitus, synovitis, muscle atrophy, and joint deformity should be noted. The time of day, morning stiffness, medication, and pain all affect the results of the evaluation, so the time of the evaluation should be documented. (Evaluation techniques for specific joints will be covered in the sections for each joint in this chapter.)

Evaluation of Function

Functional evaluation may be comprehensive or limited depending on the extent of involvement. Traditional ADL evaluations include a self-administered questionnaire or checklist to evaluate self-care skills (Backman, 1998; Melvin, 1989). For most persons with RA, an interview and questionnaire are sufficient. ADL problems can sometimes be identified with equal or greater specificity in self-administrated questionnaires than in a personal interview (Spiegel, Hirshfield, & Speigel, 1985). Thus, the self-administered ADL questionnaire becomes a useful starting point for a focused interview. The ACR functional classification for RA (Table 3) was designed to identify the functional level of patients in research studies, but it is also useful for a quick overall description of the patient.

Asking a patient to demonstrate many ADL tasks is impractical because these tasks are fatiguing and time consuming. However, for persons with severe functional limitations, observation of task performance is often the only way to obtain an accurate evaluation.

Table 3. American College of Rheumatology Revised Criteria for Classification of Functional Status in Rheumatoid Arthritis

Class	Description
I	Completely able to perform usual ADL (self-care,* vocational, and avocational)
II	Able to perform usual self-care and vocational activities but limited in avocational activities
III	Able to perform usual self-care activities but limited in vocational and avocational activities
IV	Limited ability to perform usual self-care, vocational, and avocational activities

*Usual self-care activities include dressing, feeding, bathing, grooming, and toileting. Avocational (recreational or leisure) and vocational (work, school, homemaking) activities are patient desired and age and gender specific.

Note. From "The American College of Rheumatology 1991 Revised Criteria for the Classification of Global Functional Status in Rheumatoid Arthritis," by M. C. Hochberg, R. W. Chang, I. Dwosh, S. Lindsey, T. Pincus, and F. Wolfe, 1992, *Arthritis and Rheumatism, 35,* pp. 498–502.

Evaluation of Functional Endurance and Fatigue

The patient's functional endurance and limiting symptoms should be evaluated by an interview, especially regarding the performance of everyday tasks. Patients may be interviewed about endurance when walking, stair climbing, sitting, standing, and performing instrumental ADL tasks such as grocery shopping and driving. Observational measures, such as a 5-min walk, are reasonably well tolerated by patients but are usually impractical in a short evaluation session (Oatis, 1998). (Evaluation and treatment of fatigue is discussed in chapter 8 in this volume.)

Evaluation of Pain

Pain in RA is usually multifactorial, and careful evaluation is necessary to identify probable causes. Musculoskeletal pain in RA may be caused by joint inflammation, muscle tension, strain or spasm, tendon or ligament pathology, or nerve entrapment. Muscle weakness and ligamentous laxity will predispose joints to a greater than normal amount of strain associated with daily activities. Extra-articular RA involvement such as vasculitis, pleurisy, or pericarditis can cause pain.

Therapists must perform a differential evaluation to determine whether patients have pain caused by disorders other than RA (Hayes & Petersen, 1998). Patients may experience symptoms caused by diseases of other systems such as chronic obstructive pulmonary disease, coronary artery disease, or diabetes. Osteoarthritis (OA) is a common comorbid condition in persons with RA and may exacerbate the inflammation of RA by producing bone spurs or further alterating joint biomechanics.

Widespread soft-tissue tenderness or pain above and below the waist suggests fibromyalgia syndrome (FMS) and is confirmed by the presence of at least 11 out of 18 tender points when using the ACR criteria. (See chapter 6 in this volume.) FMS is seen in many patients with RA. FMS can be triggered by any condition that disturbs sleep and is common in persons with chronic pain and fitful sleep. FMS may flare up independently of RA. An FMS flare-up may mimic a RA flare-up because, in both cases, the patient complains of widespread pain.

Pain can be evaluated by either the patient or the health care provider. The time frame is usually pain during the past two to three days. Evaluation can be completed with a visual analog scale by using a 100-mm horizontal scale with end markers that are terminal descriptors. The scale is anchored to "no pain" at the left end and "extreme pain" at the right end. Evaluation can likewise be completed with a Likert scale by using the following descriptors: none, mild, moderate, severe, and extreme. Pain can be evaluated at rest or during motion.

Treatment

Therapy Goals for Treating Joint Inflammation

Rehabilitation goals for treating joint inflammation can be related to the stages of inflammation: acute, chronic-active, and chronic-inactive. This applies to all three types of RA described earlier.

Acute stage. Therapy goals are to control inflammation through rest, splinting, and cold modalities and to maintain mobility through gentle active or active assisted exercise within the pain-free range two to three times a day.

Chronic-active stage. Patients are more mobile in this stage, so joint protection, fatigue, and pain management become more important. Exercise and activity should be increased appropriately to regain strength, mobility, and function that may have been lost during the acute stage.

Chronic-inactive stage. Persons with well-controlled RA are in a position to use self-management methods such as cardiovascular conditioning to the fullest and improve their overall health. Adaptive equipment, gait training, and instruction in fatigue management may be indicated (Table 4).

Physical Modalities

Three categories of physical agents are traditionally used in the treatment of arthritis: thermal, electrical, and aquatic or hydrotherapy. The current emphasis on self-management requires that therapists use methods that can be used in the home or on the job. Clinic-based modalities such as hot air, dry heat, whirlpools, and many electrical modalities only encourage dependence on the clinic and make home-based methods seem inferior. There is no evidence that equipment-based treatment only available in the clinic is more effective than home-based self-management methods. Cost is likewise a factor in advising against these agents (Minor & Sanford, 1993).

Cold applications decrease acute joint and tenosynovial swelling and inflammation and reduce muscle spasm and pain. Cold, not heat, is advised during an acute flare-up of arthritis. More inflamed joints may be more responsive to cold. Cold is almost always the treatment of choice for tenosynovitis, whether warmth is present or not, because swelling is the basis for impaired tendon gliding. Patients differ in their tolerance for cold versus heat both individually and with time of day. Cold applications are contraindicated for persons with cryoglobulinemia or Raynaud's phenomenon (Gerber, 1989). Commercial ice bags that remain pliable when cold are essential to contour to the joint and provide good skin contact. A thin wet cloth over the skin will protect it while allowing conduction of the cold. Dry or thick cloths can insulate the cold pack and prevent effective cooling of the body. For diffuse hand and wrist involvement, a 1-min dip in refrigerated water can be effective and easy to manage for some patients (Melvin & Michlovitz, in press).

Heat applications are effective for decreasing stiffness, muscle spasm, and pain and are appropriate for some patients once joint inflammation and swelling are under control. Heat may increase acute inflammation. Simple measures such as a warm bath, shower, or electric blanket help reduce generalized morning stiffness and facilitate exercise and activity. If the primary problem is joint swelling, heat is not recommended, although some patients nevertheless find heat somewhat comforting (Dellhag, Wollersjo, & Bjelle, 1992). Warmth is associated with comfort and probably has a psychological component in terms of pain relief.

The recent introduction of microwave-heated packs makes it easy to apply heat quickly to individual joints and body parts. Usually these packs require only 1 to 3 min in the microwave and retain the heat for 20 to 30 min, the recommended length of time for heat applications. Electrical heating pads and glove- or muff-shaped tubes are popular. Paraffin baths for inflamed RA hands generally are not recommended for most patients but are helpful for patients with OA. In chronic-inactive RA, paraffin has been shown to reduce pain but without exercise had no effect on function (Dellhag et al., 1992). An inexpensive method that has a similar effect is applying mineral oil to the hands, putting on large thin rubber gloves, and immersing the hands in hot tap water for up to 10 min (Stokes, 1996). Patients should be given written instructions that include precautions as well as guidelines for heat applications.

Deep heat, such as ultrasound and diathermy, is generally contraindicated for joint or tendon inflammation in RA because the negative effects of inflammation on joint

Table 4. Rehabilitation for Phases of Joint Inflammation

Acute Phase
Control of Inflammation
Rest, splinting, and cold modalities
Preserve joint mobility
Gentle ROM through available range and proper
    positioning
Pain management
Education, deep breathing, relaxation training, imagery,
    and stress management
Maximize health
Restorative sleep and healthy nutrition

Chronic-Active Phase
Control of Inflammation
Rest, splinting, cold modalities, joint protection tech-
    niques, foot orthoses, and assistive technology

Preserve Joint Mobility
Gentle ROM (avoid stretching the capsule)
Preserve joint stability
Joint protection and assistive technology
Preserve muscle strength
Therapeutic exercise and fitness exercise
Pain management
Education, relaxation training, thermal modalities,
    imagery, and stress management
Fatigue management
Energy conservation, education, and fitness exercise
Maximize health
Restorative sleep, healthy nutrition, fitness exercise, and
    stress management
Improve function
Assistive technology

Chronic-Inactive Phase
Reduce Stiffness
Heat modalities

Preserve Joint Mobility and Strength
Exercise for ROM and strengthening
Fatigue management
Energy conservation, education, and fitness exercise
Maximize health
Restorative sleep, healthy nutrition, fitness exercise, and
    stress management
Improve function
Assistive technology and splinting to stabilize joints

structures may be increased. Ultrasound may play a role in deep soft-tissue contractures in carefully selected cases (Schuerman, 1998). Electrical stimulation has comparatively few applications in RA. Transcutaneous electrical nerve stimulation (TENS) has received mixed reviews (Griffin & McClure, 1981) but is a method of pain management for home use in selected cases with a single damaged joint that causes a disproportionate amount of pain. TENS is not recommended for the typical pain of polyarticular arthritis (Sotosky & Lindsay, 1991).

Topical analgesics. For decades, over-the-counter topical agents with so-called counterirritant effects used to reduce or block the sensation of pain have been available (e.g., menthol, camphor, methylsalicylate). A topical pain relief agent incorporating capsaicin (an alkaloid derived from hot peppers) has been shown to be effective in reducing pain reportedly by depleting substance P from peripheral neurons (Deal, Schnitzer, & Lipstein, 1991). This agent has the drawback of needing to be applied four times a day and can burn sensitive tissue and eyes. NSAID creams (e.g., salicylic acid, diethylamine salicylate, indomethacin, naproxen, diclofenac, and piroxicam) for transdermal drug delivery are now available by prescription. Although primarily used for local soft-tissue inflammation, topical NSAIDs may play a role in the management of isolated exacerbation of a RA joint.

Manual therapies. Manual therapy techniques (e.g., passive joint mobilization or manipulation, massage, and myofascial release) can be beneficial in specific therapeutic situations, but they should not be used in lieu of self-management training. Passive manual therapies may provide pain relief in some patients, but the relief may be due in part to a psychological component from the comfort of hands-on therapy.

Passive joint mobilization during the acute phase is not advised. Other than mild manual traction used to unload joint surfaces during passive ROM exercise, mobilizing techniques are generally not indicated in RA because joint capsules and ligaments are already lax and tend toward instability. This is particularly true when there is major cartilage loss and bony erosion. Joint mobilization may be undertaken cautiously in the chronic-active and chronic-inactive stages of RA in specific and selected instances. The use of passive oscillatory techniques for pain relief in RA does not support a self-management model of care.

Depression, nonrestorative sleep, stress, and poor nutrition can all amplify pain. Teaching the patient self-management skills to reduce these factors can result in overall pain reduction (Bradley, 1998). Relaxation training, stress management, and guided imagery can be used as components of a self-management program and are powerful methods for changing one's physiology and reducing pain. Videotapes and audiotapes are available for these purposes.

Teaching patients how to manage a flare-up can increase self-effectiveness in their ability to manage and reduce pain. Writing out the plan for the patient validates the plan and enhances coping skills. The goal is to remain calm, become less fearful of each flare-up, and become progressively more skilled in bringing the exacerbation under control with rest, modalities, relaxation, positioning, and medications. Fear can amplify the inflammatory response and pain. Patients believe that they have followed the regimen of their health care provider in terms of medication and are frustrated that they have done their best. They may believe they are at fault for having a flare-up. The ability to handle a flare-up with confidence and without fear improves recovery from the exacerbation (J. L. Melvin, personal communication, 1998).

Therapeutic Exercise and Staging

Questions about exercise are the second most common type of questions asked by patients with RA after questions concerning diet. A body of evidence exists that exercise is of value in RA, even in patients with active synovitis. If muscles can be exercised and tone and bulk maintained, joints may be protected and function improved. Few patients realize the value of exercise in the treatment of their arthritis. The therapist must convey the importance of exercise and emphasize the role of muscle in stabilizing the joint. (This is true for all joints except the digit joints, in which strong muscles can increase joint deformity [Melvin, in press].) At the same time, the added benefits of exercise on the heart, lungs, and general fitness can be discussed. Exercises, especially specific exercises for individual joints, should be taught by the therapist and reviewed at a later time. If the patient is in an early active stage of disease or is frail, exercise may need to be started in a hydrotherapy pool. The warmth of the water and its buoyancy may enable the muscle to begin the strengthening process.

A comprehensive exercise prescription must consider the severity and stage of joint inflammation, joint integrity, patient preferences, and comorbid medical conditions. The therapist should consider three types of exercise: daily ROM exercises in the morning to overcome morning stiffness and start the day, specific exercises to strengthen muscles to protect a specific joint or group of joints in patients with local disease, and general fitness exercise. The patient should be instructed not only in specific exercises but also in how and when to adapt the exercise as conditions change. Exercise staging requires an exercise program that adapts the type, frequency, and amount of exercise to the stage of disease activity as well as functional activities planned for the day.

Acute stage. During the acute stage, while the joint is swollen and painful, gentle active exercise once or twice a day is advised. Melvin (1989) emphasized that, in this phase, intra-articular swelling has distended the joint capsule, and ligaments are already maximally stretched; thus, additional stretching could cause further damage. Consequently, passive ROM should be gentle and not forced. Active assisted or passive exercises may be indicated if active muscle contraction greatly increases pain either during and after movement or when active motion lags behind passive ROM. (Table 4 outlines rehabilitation for phases of joint inflammation.)

Chronic-active stage. In this phase, active exercise to maintain or increase ROM, isometric exercise (particularly with an isometric hold in different parts of the range), and short-arc isotonic exercise (possibly with light resistance) to maintain or increase strength may be instituted. Patients should exercise at least two or three times a day and increase repetitions as the inflammation subsides.

Chronic-inactive stage. In this phase, patients should continue to perform active ROM exercise, isometric strengthening exercises, and include short- to full-arc isotonic exercise with light to moderate resistance. Gentle passive stretching can be added as needed. Repetitions and exercise periods per day may be increased, and a greater intensity of functional activity may result. Low-impact exercises and activities that challenge the cardiopulmonary system should be included.

Fitness exercise. In both the chronic-active and chronic-inactive stages, regular aerobic exercise either individually or through group or community exercise programs is advisable. (See the section "Aerobic Exercise for Fitness" in this chapter.)

ROM exercise. Morning stiffness, soft-tissue swelling, muscle spasm, and soft-tissue contracture can limit joint mobility in patients with RA. Therefore, a daily individualized ROM program is essential. Patients should attempt to take each joint through its full active ROM at least once a day and preferably more often. Patients must learn how to gauge full ROM. Several repetitions may be required to reach full ROM. Active assisted ROM or gentle passive ROM is needed when pain or muscle weakness prevent active ROM. The number of repetitions and frequency of exercise should increase as inflammation subsides. Byer (1985) found notable reductions in morning stiffness by combining aquatic aerobic exercise three times a week with ROM exercise daily in the evenings.

Muscle strengthening exercise. As with ROM, muscle strengthening exercises must be adapted to the stage and severity of the disease. Strengthening exercises should be limited or eliminated when there is a disease flare-up or an acute episode of any systemic illness (Melvin, 1989). Isometric exercise is less likely to produce pain in joints than isotonic exercise and is used to maintain strength until more vigorous exercise can be resumed. Isotonic and resistive exercises are appropriate in self-management of chronic disease and should be instituted when there is minimum pain and stiffness. Warm-up and cool-down periods are an integral part of the strengthening program. Strength training is frequently prescribed on alternate days with aerobic exercise, whereas flexibility exercise (e.g., ROM, stretching) should be performed daily. Dynamic strengthening exercise is essential for healthy weight-bearing joints. Mild to moderately involved joints in persons with RA respond to low-repetition, high-resistance exercise of the knee with increased strength. High-intensity, progressive resistive exercise has been shown to improve functional performance, even in older persons taking low doses of corticosteroids (Lyngberg, Harreby, Bentzen, Frost, & Danneskiold-Samsoe, 1994).

Aerobic exercise for fitness. During the past 20 years, there has been a change in the attitude toward fitness training for patients with RA. Some of this change in attitude may relate to the increased functional level of patients with RA with more aggressive treatment. Studies have demonstrated not only the comparative safety of aerobic exercise but also improvements in self-effectiveness, aerobic capacity, and physical performance (Stenstrom, 1994). Some studies have shown the additional benefit of reduced pain. Research has demonstrated the safety and effectiveness of aerobic exercise through biking (Harkcom, Lampman, Banwell, & Castor, 1985; Ekblom, Lovgren, Aldering, Fridstrom, & Satterstrom, 1975), walking and swimming (Minor, Hewett, Webel, Anderson, & Kay, 1989), and dance (Perlman et al., 1990).

A 5-year study of persons with moderate RA who engaged in physical training revealed much slower progression of radiographic erosions of joints compared with a control group (Nordemar, Eckblom, Zachrisson, & Lundquist, 1981). Persons with RA who engaged in vigorous forms of exercise either did not change or experienced a decrease in the number of painful or swollen joints. They demonstrated improvements in pain and fatigue and notable increases in strength and walking time (Minor, 1990). There is evidence that helping patients focus on exercise goals rather than pain fosters self-effectiveness with the exercise program and improves the likelihood of achieving the benefits of exercise (Stenstrom, 1994).

The type of the fitness exercise selected is important. A stamina-building exercise that involves pacing is important. Exercises of choice include aquatics, low-impact aerobics, tai chi, dancing, and other forms of general conditioning exercise that are available in most communities. The Arthritis Foundation sponsors both aquatic and land-based exercise programs taught by instructors with spe-

---

Box 1
Resources

Equipment Resources

Silver Ring Splint™ Company
P.O. Box 2856
Charlottesville, VA 22902-2856
804-971-4052 or 804-971-8828 (fax)

Organization Resources

The Arthritis Foundation
1330 West Peachtree Street
Atlanta, GA 30309
404-872-7100 or 1-800-283-7800
Internet address: www.arthritis.org

This organization provides an excellent booklet on OA, self-management techniques, and specific medications at no charge; aquatic and land-based exercise classes; the Arthritis Self-Management Course nationwide; and a free health video lending library in some chapters. The Arthritis Foundation can refer patients to rheumatologists.

The Arthritis Society
National Office
250 Bloor Street East
Suite 901
Toronto, ON M4W 3P2 Canada
416-967-1414 or 416-967-7171(fax)
Internet address: www.arthritis.ca

This organization offers specialized patient care programs, recreational exercise pro-

grams, resource libraries, and consumer education materials.

Internet Resources

Searching "rheumatoid arthritis" on the Internet brings up an extensive array of resources and sales pitches, unproven remedies, and misinformation (11,262 listings). Hot Bot is one of the best search directories for information on diseases.

- The Arthritis Foundation and The Arthritis Society both have Web sites (see addresses above).
- The Amazon Bookstore (www.amazon.com) is the easiest online bookseller to search. There are more than five self-help books on OA.
- Abledata (www.abledata.com) is a national database for adaptive equipment and assistive devices.
- One Step Ahead News (www.osanews.com) is the Web's online news magazine for persons with disabilities and provides excellent links to other sites related to coping with disabilities, including one on the Americans With Disabilities Act (www.osanews.com/Links/ada.htm).
- Minnesota Mining Company's guide to arthritis (http://arthritis.miningco.com/msub7.htm) has excellent resources and information.

---

cial training in adapted exercise for persons with arthritis (Box 1). The Self-Help Course includes extensive exercise instruction and has been demonstrated to reduce pain and increase function (Lorig, 1993). Audiotapes, videotapes, and printed materials are available. Many communities have exercise programs appropriate for persons with arthritis, and therapists should be aware of appropriate community resources (Haralson-Ferrell, 1998). (For a comprehensive review of this topic, see Minor [1998].)

Joint Protection Techniques

Joint protection is an approach that analyzes the patient's ADL and devises strategies to ensure that forces applied to joints can be tolerated without increasing inflammation or pain (Cordery & Rocchi, 1998). Preservation of joint structures, reduction of internal and external stresses to a joint, decreased swelling, and relief of pain have obvious benefits in the treatment of RA. On the basis of biomechanical principles that build on anatomy, the pathology of RA, and the inflammatory process, joint protection can be a powerful method for achieving these goals. The principles of joint protection for RA are listed in Table 5.

Respect for pain and maintenance of muscle strength and joint ROM are important self-management techniques for persons with RA. It is important that patients carry out activities and exercises only to the point of discomfort, not pain. Patients must be aware of their pain thresholds so that they stop activities or do not get into situations where they have to drop an object because of pain.

Joint protection incorporates a balance of rest and activity. For persons with active RA, rest and sleep should be encouraged. Balancing rest and activity can apply to repetitive hand activities. Muscles tire quickly in static holding positions. Frequent position changes and rest help reduce the effect of the activity on joint structures.

Splints and Orthoses

Splinting is an effective intervention that can be used to reduce inflammation, reduce or alleviate pain, improve function, prevent positional contractures, prevent stress injuries, and provide the postsurgical management of soft tissue (Phillips, 1989 and 1995). The therapist must understand the goal and purpose of the splint (resting, functional, or corrective), the type of splint, and whether fabricated versus prefabricated splints should be used. Correlating the goals of the patient with the goals to be achieved from the splint can increase adherence to treatment recommenda-

Table 5. Principles of Joint Protection for Rheumatoid Arthritis and Inflammatory Joint Disease (Cordery, 1998)

1. Respect pain.
2. Maintain muscle strength and joint ROM.
3. Use each joint in its most stable, anatomical, or functional plane.
4. Avoid positions of deformity and forces in their direction.
5. Use strongest joints available for the job.
6. Use correct patterns of movement.
7. Avoid staying in one position for long periods.
8. Avoid starting an activity that cannot be stopped immediately.
9. Balance rest and activity.
10. Reduce the force.

tions. The patient's ability to apply, remove, and care for the splint must be determined in advance. When patients understand the purpose of the splint and the limitations the splint may impose, they have realistic expectations that encourage adherence and greater patient satisfaction. The weight of the hand splint is a critical consideration and can reduce adherence. Heavy splints can aggravate fragile shoulders and elbows and increase upper-extremity fatigue. Heavy hand-based splints can aggravate or increase fatigue in the wrist. Another precaution is awareness that splinting one joint may increase stress on other joints (e.g., immobilization of the wrist can exacerbate inflammation of the MCP joints) (Melvin, 1989). Establishing treatment priorities is a critical aspect in the care of the patient (e.g., is it worth damaging the MCP joint to help the wrist?). The answer is probably not because better surgeries exist for the wrist than for the MCP joints. (Table 6 lists the types of RA hand involvement that can be treated with splinting. See Colditz and Melvin [in press] for a complete review of splinting for arthritis.)

Specific Joint Involvement and Treatment

Wrists

Wrist involvement is common (75% to 95% of patients) and includes synovitis of the radiocarpal joint, radioulnar joint, and intercarpal joints and tenosynovitis of the flexor tendons in the carpal tunnel and of the extensor tendon compartments (Flatt, 1983; Wilson, 1986). There is no joint between the ulna and the carpus, although there is a triangular fibrocartilage disc and space for synovitis to expand so that swelling over the ulnar styloid is often the first site of hand syn-

Table 6. Rheumatoid Arthritis Hand Involvement That Can Be Effectively Treated With Splinting (Marx, 1992)

Wrist
Synovitis
Instability and subluxation (to prevent rupture of the long digit extensor muscles)
Carpal tunnel syndrome
Tenosynovitis (volar and dorsal)

Thumb
CMC synovitis
MCP or IP synovitis or instability

MCP Joint
Synovitis
Ulnar deviation (to improve function)
Intrinsic muscle tightness (to stretch intrinsic muscles)

Fingers
Swan-neck deformity (to prevent hyperextension)
Lateral instability to stabilize during function
Boutonnière deformity in the early stage to stabilize in extension to allow antideformity exercise if reducible to stabilize during function.
Mutilans deformity to stabilize and improve function for nonsurgical candidates

ovitis. Synovitis in the radiocarpal joint can limit all wrist motions. Swelling in the distal radio-ulnar joint limits supination and pronation, and instability results in a prominent ulnar styloid (ulnar head syndrome) (Flatt, 1983; Swanson, 1995). Tenosynovitis may be either painful or painless. Flexor tenosynovitis may impede the gliding of the long finger flexors through the carpal tunnel, which prevents full active finger flexion or extension. The presence of tenosynovitis is determined by testing tendon excursion both proximally and distally. Extensor tenosynovitis generally does not impair tendon gliding; it is determined by the visual evaluation of swelling in the dorsal compartments. With severe chronic RA, cartilage loss over multiple joints in the wrist and digits can increase the ratio of long tendon length to bone length, which reduces the effectiveness of the long finger tendons. Synovitis can cause entrapment of the median nerve in the carpal tunnel and of the ulnar nerve in Guyon's canal. The synovium hypertrophies over time, which results in ligamentous laxity and subluxation that allows the carpus to slide volarly and ulnarly off the end of the radius. In most cases, the carpus rotates during this process, and the wrist becomes radially deviated on the forearm. This is referred to as the *classic RA hand pattern*. It creates a strong ulnar force on the lax and unstable MCP joints as the digits align with the forearm during functional activities, which is referred to as a *zig-zag deformity* (Flatt, 1983). If the carpus does not rotate radially but simply subluxes ulnarly, the MCP joints are not likely to develop ulnar drift.

The goal of therapy should focus on controlling inflammation and preserving function. Cold is the most effective modality for swelling of both joint synovitis and tenosynovitis. If only the wrist is involved, a rigid custom-molded splint for use during both day and night is the most effective method for controlling inflammation. If the MCP joints are inflamed and nighttime splinting is indicated, a full hand-resting splint is recommended to take all pressure off the MCP joints. A flexible wrist splint is indicated during the day to reduce compensatory stress to the MCP joints (Colditz & Melvin, in press; Melvin, 1989). Whenever possible, splints should be custom-made so that the wrist can be positioned in 10° to 20° ulnar deviation. Maintaining ulnar deviation is critical to reducing the ziz-zag deformity on the MCP joint (Flatt, 1983). In the chronic-active or chronic-inactive stages, isometric exercises provide a safe means to improve wrist and finger extensor strength to counteract the strong flexor forces. When performed in proper alignment, isometric exercises cause less pain and less joint stress. Self-management of wrist symptoms is best done through use of joint protection techniques, use of assistive devices or adaptive methods (Noaker, 1996), splints, cold modalities for inflammation, and warming techniques for stiffness. Proper evaluation is needed for the complex wrist joint with an understanding of the biomechanics of how the wrist affects the function of the hand. The wrist is the stable support for hand function (or the "pillar" of the hand) and must be well supported by either a splint, joint protection positioning, or use of assistive devices. A volar or dorsal wrist support splint can be used for wrist synovitis or tenosynovitis inflammation. (Postoperative therapy for the wrist is examined in volume 4 of this series.)

Fingers

All digit joints can be affected by RA. Occasionally, only the wrist and a few MCP and PIP joints are involved. The MCP and PIP joints tend to have more erosive disease. The classic recognizable deformity at the MCP joints, ulnar drift (Figure 1), begins with subluxation and radial deviation of the wrist as described above. Synovitis of the MCP joint distends the capsule and leads to a protective spasm of the intrinsic muscles that creates an additional volar subluxing force on the joints (Flatt, 1983). If the wrist becomes ulnarly deviated when this occurs, MCP joint alignment remains neutral or can go into mild radial drift. Treatment of the MCP joints must consider the position of the wrist (Melvin, 1989). An inability to actively extend an MCP joint (within available ROM) could be the result of the exten-

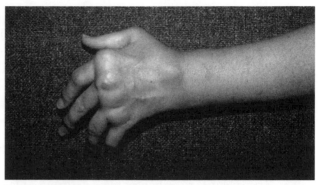

Figure 1. The hand of a 26-year-old woman with classic, severe, RA deformity pattern: radial deviation of the wrist and mcp volar dislocation and ulnar drift. Photo courtesy of Jeanne Melvin.

sor tendon migrating into the MCP ulnar valley, a rupture of the extensor tendons at the wrist level where they typically are "sawed apart" over rough carpal bones, or, in rare cases, posterior interosseous nerve entrapment.

The most common deformities at the PIP joints are flexion contractures, the boutonnière deformity, and the swan-neck deformity. The boutonnière deformity results solely from synovitis of the PIP joint that displaces the lateral bands, which creates excessive hyperextension force on the DIP joint and secondary MCP joint hyperextension. Although there are splints that maintain the PIP joint in extension, correction is generally not possible because the damage to the lateral bands that caused the deformity is severe (Flatt, 1983). Swan-neck deformity involves a pattern of MCP joint flexion, PIP joint hyperextension, and DIP joint flexion. In the RA hand, swan-neck deformity most frequently results from a combination of PIP joint (volar plate) laxity, MCP joint synovitis, and tight intrinsic muscles. In this case, progression of the deformity can be reduced by elimination of the intrinsic muscle tightness through stretching exercises and splinting (Colditz & Melvin, in press). The swan-neck deformity can begin with a mallet deformity at the DIP joint or PIP synovitis rupturing the volar plate (Nalebuff & Millender, 1975; Rizio & Belsky, 1996). Synovitis at the PIP joint can lead to lateral instability that limits precision pinch. As hand disease progresses, the first pinch that is lost is precision tip pinch, then pad-to-pad pinch. Lateral pinch is the last to be lost and is the most important to maintain because it is the power pinch (Melvin, 1989).

RA synovitis in the DIP joint is generally less severe and erosive than in the PIP or MCP joints, but synovitis can rupture the distal attachment of the extensor digitorum communis tendon and result in a mallet finger deformity. Flexor tenosynovitis of the wrist can impair proximal tendon gliding of the digitorum profundus tendon and prevent full active DIP flexion that results in limited DIP motion (Melvin, 1989). Generally, a mallet finger caused by RA is not treated the same as a mallet finger caused by trauma because the tendon is compromised by RA. The most common treatment is surgical fusion in 5° of flexion performed in conjunction with other hand surgery. When flexor tenosynovitis limits tendon gliding, cold modalities and passive ROM are necessary to prevent joint contractures and tendon shortening.

Acute MCP joint synovitis should be splinted to provide local rest to the joints to decrease inflammation and pain. Position the joint in 45° of flexion to maintain the length of the collateral ligaments. Position the wrist in 10° to 20° of ulnar deviation if possible to reduce ulnar force on the MCP joints and in 15° of extension to maximize the carpal tunnel space (when the radiocarpal joint is in neutral, the second metacarpal is in 15° of extension) (Colditz & Melvin, in press). Splinting during sleep and at rest is essential to prevent deforming positional contractures. Splinting during the daytime is determined by the degree of inflammation in the PIP joints because immobilization of the MCP joints can cause compensatory stress on the PIP joints and make them worse (Colditz & Melvin, in press; Melvin, 1989).

Splinting to immobilize the PIP joint increases the risk of stiffness because, no matter what position the joint is in, one of the collateral ligaments is slack and at risk for contracture (Flatt, 1983). Treatment for the boutonnière deformity includes passive and active ROM exercises to maintain PIP extension and DIP flexion exercises with the PIP joint as straight as possible to stretch the oblique retinacular ligament and soft tissue in an antideformity pattern. Splinting may be helpful to maintain the joint length and position after exercise. A boutonnière splint holds the PIP joint in maximal extension while allowing for DIP flexion and stretching of the oblique retinacular ligament. The splint can be fabricated from low-temperature plastic (figure-8 design) or silver (Silver Ring Splint™ Company, Charlottesville, VA). For selected cases, serial casting in conjunction with DIP flexion exercises may help reduce a mild boutonnière deformity.

For swan-neck deformities, treatment should focus on maintaining PIP flexion both actively and passively, encouraging MCP joint extension and DIP joint extension, and reducing tight intrinsic muscles. Use of functional tripoint splints that block the last 10° to 15° of extension can prevent the joint from "catching" in extension and greatly improve function (Colditz & Melvin, in press; Harrell, 1996). A removable thermoplastic splint can be fabricated by using the figure-8 design, or a Silver Ring Splint™ can be fitted. If the patient has tight intrinsic muscles, joint protection includes an analysis of hand activities that requires an intrinsic-plus position and patient instruction in alternative methods. (For an in-depth review of swan-neck deformities, see Nalebuff and Millender [1975].)

Assistive devices that enlarge grip and increase lever force can reduce stress on vulnerable digit joints. Adaptive handles that allow the wrist and MCP joints to be used in neutral alignment instead of ulnar deviation are likewise helpful (Noaker, 1996). Using the palms of the hands instead of a grip eliminates flexor forces on the MCP joints. Joint protection training and activity adaptation are major interventions for hand management.

Thumbs

Approximately 68% to 80% of the persons with RA will have thumb involvement (Flatt, 1983). Nalebuff (1984) identified five common patterns of thumb deformity.

1. *Type I.* MCP joint flexion resulting in interphalangeal (IP) joint hyperextension and CMC joint abduction (the most common type).

2. *Type II.* CMC adduction resulting in MCP hyperextension and IP flexion (similar to the OA thumb).

3. *Type III.* MCP joint synovitis resulting in ulnar ligament damage and lateral deviation of the joint and CMC joint adduction.

4. *Type IV.* MCP synovitis that results in hyperextension and IP joint flexion with no CMC limitation but with adduction posturing.

5. *Type V.* Mutilans deformity of the IP or MCP joints with osteolysis of the phalanges and shortening and instability of the thumb joints (Nalebuff & Garrett, 1976).

In addition to these deformities, there can be rupture of the IP and MCP collateral ligaments or severe erosions that cause frank instability. The extensor pollicis longus can rupture as it passes Lister's tubercle.

Ulnar nerve entrapment at the elbow or wrist can cause weakness of the adductor pollicis muscle. Median nerve entrapment in the carpal tunnel can cause weakness and atrophy of the abductor pollicis and the flexor pollicis brevis as well as sensory loss in the thumb and median-innervated fingers. Numbness or tingling in only the thumb is indicative of C6 compression.

Treatment of the thumb focuses on functional immobilization splints to control inflammation, joint protection, assistive devices to reduce deforming stress, and, in the late stages, stabilization splints to allow effective pinch and prehension skills.

In RA, the wrist is almost always involved. Splinting for CMC synovitis usually must be done in conjunction with splinting the wrist. Patients with MCP or IP joint instability do extremely well with joint fusions that provide them with pain-free, stable, and lateral pinch. Patients who are not surgical candidates can benefit greatly from MCP or IP stabilization splints made from 1/16-in. thermoplastic (Colditz & Melvin, in press).

The Nalebuff classification illustrates the dynamics of the thumb joints as a kinetic chain. In the early stages, when the joint is passively correctable, splinting can be used to alter or eliminate the deforming forces identified in the classification. For example, the initiating event in the type IV deformity is MCP synovitis and hyperextension; splinting only the MCP joint in slight flexion reduces inflammation and eliminates the deforming dynamics on the adjacent joints.

Hand-based splints can be fabricated to support the thumb in palmar abduction and allow IP flexion of the thumb with involvement of the CMC joint or with basal joint arthritis. If the MCP joint of the thumb is involved, a simple figure-8 splint can restrict movement at the MCP joint while allowing CMC joint motion and IP joint motion. Having a stable, pain-free thumb for pinch activities can greatly improve the function of a person with RA. A simple hand-based splint can make the difference in independence, self-esteem, and vocation for someone with RA and thumb involvement.

Elbows

Approximately 20% to 50% of patients with RA will have elbow involvement (Inglis, 1985). The synovial lining is common to both the elbow (humeroradioulnar) joint and the proximal radioulnar joint. Painful synovitis prompts the patient to keep the arm in flexion and pronation with consequent contractures that limit functional extension and supination. Distention and inflammatory destruction of the capsule result in a weak, unstable articulation. Flexion contractures up to 30° usually do not interfere with functional ability (Morrey, Askew, An, & Chao, 1981). A loss of 30° to 60° of extension interferes with the ability to reach and perform certain activities (e.g., donning socks). A loss of 40° to 90° of extension restricts push-off leverage for chair transfers and interferes with the mobility required for dressing. A loss of more than 90° of extension is rare, but when it occurs, it seriously restricts reach and limits dressing, perineal care, and transfers (Melvin, 1989). Extension contractures (or diminished flexion) are less frequent. They can severely limit one's ability to eat, groom, and perform personal hygiene. For example, a person who can flex the elbows to only 90° generally will not be able to eat with regular utensils.

Forearm rotation can be limited by synovitis in either the proximal or distal radioulnar joints. The restricting joint can be determined by which radioulnar joint is painful at the end of forearm rotation range. Synovitis can directly affect the ligaments supporting the elbow, which results in destruction of the annular ligaments surrounding the radial neck and makes the radial head unstable. The unopposed biceps and brachioradialis muscles then displace the radial head anteriorly toward the antecubital fossa where it can limit flexion, extension, and rotation (Morrey et al., 1981).

Ulnar entrapment neuropathy may result from a "double crush syndrome" where cervical entrapment makes the ulnar nerve more susceptible to compression at the elbow, or neuropathy may result from primary compression by synovitis in the cubital tunnel. Flexion makes the cubital tunnel more shallow and increases the vulnerability of the ulnar nerve to external pressure, which results in pain over the tunnel (sometimes termed *ulnar neuritis*).

RA may involve inflammation of the olecranon bursa that causes marked swelling over the dorsum of the elbow and interferes with desk work. This can be infectious and require antibiotic intervention. Noninfectious bursitis often responds to a corticosteroid injection. Any aggravating activities must be evaluated and eliminated; elbow sleeves can improve comfort. Chronic bursitis unresponsive to medication or conservative treatment can be successfully treated with surgery (Stewart, Manzanares, & Morrey, 1997).

Patients who are RF positive may develop rheumatoid nodules on the extensor surface of the ulna and the ulnar border of the forearm. The nodules may form over pressure areas, in which case reduction of the pressure source can reduce the size of the nodule. However, nodules may be unrelated to pressure. They tend to be painful when pressure is applied, and they can become infected.

The treatment of choice is prevention of elbow contractures with effective control of swelling, maintenance of ROM, and strengthening of the elbow extensors. An effective method for applying cold to the elbow is an ice water dip (1 to 4 min) in a wide food storage container three to four times a day (refrigerating the water keeps it cold enough). If the contracture is recent, a volar night splint may provide sufficient, sustained stretch to lengthen the soft tissues. Adaptive ADL methods and use of assistive technology can improve function. Extended handles can help compensate for lost flexion or extension. Joint protection techniques to reduce pain include reducing the lever force on the elbow joint by using the upper extremity with the elbow near the trunk rather than in an extended position and carrying items on the forearm close to the elbow. The patient should avoid heavy lifting and use lightweight equipment. Attention must be paid to protecting the skin over the olecranon and nodules if present.

For ulnar nerve irritation or neuropathy, volar splinting at night in –20° of extension (or as close to that as possible) and use of padded elbow sleeves during the day can reduce symptoms. (*Note.* The middle dorsal strap must not create pressure over the cubital tunnel.)

For rheumatoid nodules, it is important to determine whether pressure from functional activities such as leaning against a table to stand or moving around in bed are aggravating the nodule. Elimination of the pressure will reduce or eliminate the nodule. Pressure over the nodule can be reduced by applying a pad around the nodule to redistribute pressure that avoids the offending activity or the use of gel pads. Slip-on padded sleeves (e.g., Heelbos™, North Coast Medical, Morgan Hill, CA) are preferred because elbow flexion is not required to keep them in place. Lambswool cuffs should not be used because the elbow flexion required to keep them in position encourages flexion contractures.

Shoulders

The shoulder girdle is a complex structure that depends on the coordinated movement of the glenohumeral, acromioclavicular, and sternoclavicular joints and the thoracoscapular articulation. RA in the shoulder usually presents with stiffness and pain in the early stages of the disease. Synovitis of the glenohumeral joint is associated with extensive cartilage loss, capsular damage, and severe limitation of motion but comparatively little bony erosion. Severe shoulder limitation may develop because shoulder joint involvement often is not recognized until late in the disease process. Patients and caregivers may be occupied with distal joints and not be aware of major shoulder limitations until function is seriously compromised. Because only 90° of shoulder flexion and abduction and 30° of external rotation are necessary for most functional activities, a person can lose up to 50% of shoulder mobility before this interferes with ADL (Melvin, 1989).

In addition to glenohumeral synovitis, bursitis, capsular fibrosis, FMS, and referred pain from the neck are frequent sources of shoulder pain in persons with RA. Adhesive capsulitis or "frozen shoulder" is not uncommon. The rotator cuff tendons that form the superior capsule are lined with synovium and may become inflamed or torn; this is a common site of injury and pain secondary to acromiohumeral impingement in otherwise healthy persons. In RA, this area is particularly vulnerable. Similarly, the subacromial bursa and the tendon of the long head of the biceps are frequent sites of inflammation. Inflammation of the acromioclavicular joint is common in RA and may be a prime source of shoulder pain (Gordon & Hastings, 1994). The sternoclavicular joint is frequently involved in RA as well.

Shoulder pain, through reflex inhibition, produces supraspinatus muscle weakness. The muscular force couple at the glenohumeral joint is dependent on the supraspinatus muscle; weakness leads to an upward-riding humerus and accentuates the potential for impingement. Synovitis of the acromioclavicular joint narrows the suprahumeral space and adds to impingement. This cycle of events causes further damage to the rotator cuff, particularly the supraspinatus tendon, and may lead to rupture of the long head of the biceps (Mills, 1988).

Poor posture is a frequent component of shoulder pain. Rounded shoulders and a "forward" head are components of the "posture of pain." These components, plus chronic tension or weakness of the supraspinatus muscle, increase the likelihood of rotator cuff impingement and can accelerate the deterioration of the shoulder joints.

The overall objective for treatment of the shoulder is for patients to learn how to self-manage inflammation, maintain functional ROM in all planes, reduce abnormal forces and strain on the shoulder, stretch the anterior chest muscles, and maintain good posture (Feinberg & Trombly, 1989). Posture training and reminders such as checking posture in a mirror or practicing wall alignment should be learned so that the shoulders can function in an optimal position. Strengthening of the scapular muscles is usually necessary to position the scapula on the thorax to improve posture and reduce problems associated with acromiohumeral impingement.

Therapists should refer to radiographs of the shoulders for evidence of bony changes. If the humeral head is elevated or joint surfaces are irregular, vigorous attempts to increase ROM or have the patient use the shoulder in a wider arc are likely to result in increased pain and further loss of function (Gibson, 1986).

Therapy for the person with shoulder involvement should address the following areas.

- Evaluation of pathology and function, including quality of use (e.g., how the shoulders and upper extremities and trunk are positioned for activities)
- Instruction in joint protection techniques, adaptive methods, and use of adaptive equipment to reduce pain and stress, maintain joint integrity, and improve function
- Instruction in stress management and relaxation techniques to reduce postural tension in the shoulders, neck, and upper extremities
- Techniques for self-management of pain include thermal modalities, biofeedback, stress management, and relaxation therapy to control inflammation and pain, enhance mobility, and facilitate exercise
- Instruction in a home program that consists of activities or exercises to maintain or improve upper-extremity joint mobility, muscle strength, and posture of the upper body
- Instruction in simple methods for monitoring shoulder flexion, such as using a mark (or self-adhesive note) as a benchmark of maximal ROM to be touched once a day or as needed.

Temporomandibular Joint (Axial Skeleton)

The temporomandibular joints (TMJs) are frequently involved in RA. The surfaces of the joints are lined by fibrous connective tissue. A fibrous intracapsular meniscus divides the joint into upper and lower compartments. Synovitis damages these structures and causes pain. Loss of motion may limit food intake and compromise nutrition, dental care, and the administration of general anesthesia. These joints may not receive the same attention that the more peripheral joints command, and severe restriction of motion may develop.

Educate patients early about the need to maintain a functional opening between the upper and lower sets of teeth wide enough to admit two vertically held knuckles as well as gentle side-to-side motion and jaw protraction. Superficial cold applications are recommended to reduce inflammation and swelling. Chronic stiffness can be relieved by holding hot washcloths over the joints and gently stretching the muscles. This can be incorporated into morning and evening hygiene routines. Relaxation techniques are beneficial to reduce unconscious clenching and muscle spasm.

A diet of soft foods, liquid supplementation, and eating small bites of food help to maintain nutrition during disease flare-ups.

Cervical Spine (Axial Skeleton)

Cervical pain and stiffness is common early in the course of RA. Radiological evidence of cervical subluxation may be present without symptoms. OA and myofascial pain are as common in persons with RA as in the general population. Patients may complain of stiffness and pain in the neck and shoulders. Discomfort associated with muscle tension responds rather rapidly to relaxation techniques and ROM, whereas pain originating in the joints produces muscle spasm and limited mobility that will persist despite local treatment.

Chronic synovitis attacks the capsules, ligaments, and joint surfaces of the cervical vertebrae, including the atlas, the axis with the odontoid process, the atlanto-occipital joint, and the zygapophyseal (facet) and lateral interbody (Luschka) joints. The upper first to fourth cervical levels are the most common sites of inflammation, but the entire cervical spine can be involved.

The atlantoaxial joint is particularly subject to subluxation associated with stretching or rupture of the transverse ligament of the axis. Symptoms include occipital headaches from pressure on the greater occipital nerves, pain radiating to the forehead and eyes, or a positive Lhermitte's sign with an electrical shock-like sensation down the back and often into the legs or arms on neck flexion or extension. The patient may feel a "clunk" sensation as the head slips forward or may complain that the head feels as if it will "fall off." Signs of myelopathy as a result of cord compression include weakness and paresthesias in the extremities, a feeling of heaviness in the legs, new onset of impaired fine motor skills, stumbling or difficulties with gait, and bowel and bladder dysfunction (Cracchiolo, Gall, & Janisse, 1999). Instability of C1 or C2 associated with rupture of the transverse ligament may cause vertebral artery compression with dizziness, nausea, dysarthria, and nystagmus. These symptoms may be more pronounced with rotation and lateral flexion. Such symptoms must be reported to the patient's physician.

In the most severe cases, the dens may project upward through the foramen magnum and compress the brain stem. Bulbar disturbance can be sudden and fatal, or it may present with abnormal swallowing or phonation. Unilateral collapse of bony structures can produce a mechanical torticollis that is difficult to reduce and manage conservatively (Moncur & Williams, 1988).

Subluxation of the lower cervical spine is more likely to produce symptoms of nerve root irritation with symptoms of arm pain extending distal to the shoulder with or without neck pain. Nerve root compression is associated with numbness and tingling or motor weakness or may be painless and not discovered until the patient presents with cubital or carpal tunnel syndrome and a double crush syndrome becomes apparent. All patients with RA should have a neurological screening to detect cervical nerve root compression.

Passive mobilization and manipulation of the cervical spine are contraindicated in persons with RA because of ligamentous instability. Similarly, mechanical cervical traction is not recommended. Posture training, functional ROM, and isometric exercises for the neck are of value as are thermal agents for pain. When proximal and distal nerve compression is present, treatment of distal entrapment is usually unsuccessful until the proximal entrapment is treated.

Surgery in the high cervical spine appears to have a better outcome when performed earlier rather than later (Chevalier & Larget-Piet, 1994). This may relate to the length of time that even low doses of corticosteroids have been administered. Physical measures should not be attempted as a method of delaying or substituting for surgery unless the patient is not a surgical candidate.

Soft collars may provide warmth and comfort for sleeping and activity, but they do not stabilize the spine. Patients who must have the cervical spine stabilized postoperatively are adequately immobilized only with a halo device or a cervicothoracic brace. Other hard braces and soft collars do not provide immobilization (Moncur & Williams, 1988).

Proper cervical lordotic support is critical to allow muscles to relax at night, maintain optimal spinal ROM, and reduce pressure on nerve roots. Pillows can be soft and accommodative or firmer with the potential for restoring the lordotic curve.

Thoracic and Lumbar Spine, Rib Cage, and Chest (Axial Skeleton)

The synovial joints of the thoracic and lumbar spine are usually not clinically involved in RA. However, patients with RA may experience the same kind of low back pain that affects other persons. Low back protection protocols must be modified for patients with RA because many standard recommendations such as squatting to lift and standing with one foot on a low cupboard edge would increase strain on involved lower-extremity joints. Patients with RA are less at risk for back injury because they are usually less able to do heavy lifting or strenuous work.

The risk of compression fractures of the thoracic spine in postmenopausal women is greater with RA. Long-term corticosteroid use can cause osteoporosis and spinal fractures in either gender. New medications for osteoporosis can be effective in reversing demineralization. Nutritional guidelines for calcium intake for women at risk for osteoporosis is 1,500 mg/day in food or supplements. Antigravity exercises along with posture training can help mitigate the sequela of osteoporosis.

Chest pain requires a medical examination to rule out pericarditis, pleurisy, vasculitis, and coronary or pulmonary disease. The costochrondral joints can be painful (chondrodynia or costochrondritis) or can become inflamed with tender, firm, fusiform swelling (Tietze's syndrome). Costochrondral joints may respond to thermal agents for pain management. An injection of 1% xylocaine and corticosteroid can be beneficial and diagnostic (Fortin & Shadick, 1994). Deep breathing and diagonal arm movement may be added when pain permits and are useful in maintaining chest, upper trunk, and shoulder mobility and posture.

Lower Extremities

Abnormalities of alignment anywhere in the lower extremity will produce unusual stress on adjacent joints, and a cycle of increasing pain and deformity of the foot, knee, or hip may be perpetuated. Persons with progressive RA develop a typical antalgic gait, with reduced velocity and stride length, loss of the usual heel–toe pattern, and increased double limb support (Platto, O'Connell, Hicks, & Gerber, 1991). The gait produced by foot pain and deformity transmits abnormal forces to the knee where knee flexion contractures and bilateral genu valgum may develop. The abnormal knee position is associated with flexion and adduction contractures at the hip.

During active disease or after a surgical procedure involving the lower extremities, crutches or a walker may be needed to relieve pressure on one or both lower extremities. Upper-extremity involvement may preclude the use of standard hand grips on crutches or walkers, although ergonomically designed grips may be a sufficient adaptation. Platform crutches or roller walkers with forearm troughs may be required to eliminate weight bearing through the hands, wrists, or elbows. A temporary hand splint adaptation that will support the wrist and fingers while an assistive device is used has been described (Someya, Miaki, Asai, Tachino, & Nara, 1988). A single standard cane is usually contraindicated for RA because of the abnormal stress placed on the hand and wrist.

Feet and Ankles

Most patients with RA have foot symptoms early in the course of the disease, and sometimes the feet are the initial areas of complaint. Dealing effectively with foot pain in RA is a frequent rehabilitation challenge (Moncur, 1995) (Tables 7–9). The earliest RA changes in the lower extremity usually occur in the MTP joints of the toes when synovitis distends and weakens the joint capsules and ligaments. Destruction of cartilage and bone erosions further destabilize the joints. The first MTP joint often develops a characteristic hallux valgus or bunion (Figure 2), whereas the fifth MTP joint develops a "bunionette." The natural product of the gait cycle is a dorsal displacement of the lateral four toes, which are referred to as "cock-up toes" when the proximal phalanges come to rest on the necks of the metatarsals (Figure 2). The toes may eventually angle medially or laterally. Hammertoes or claw toes may likewise develop (Dimonte & Light, 1982).

The loss of toe alignment allows toe flexor and extensor tendons to displace between the metatarsal heads and "bowstring." This abnormal muscle pull, which is compounded by muscle spasm in both the intrinsic and extrinsic muscles of the foot, enhances the toe deformities. The fat pad that normally cushions the metatarsal heads migrates anteriorly, which allows the metatarsal heads to bear unrelieved weight at push-off and causes patients to feel as if they are "walking on marbles." Plantar callosities are prone to develop under the forefoot. Ulcers may develop under the metatarsal heads (Dimonte & Light, 1982; Moncur & Shields, 1983).

Metatarsalgia of the forefoot is accentuated by changes in the hindfoot. Just as angulation at the wrist contributes to abnormal forces at the MCP joints of the hand, abnormal position of the subtalar joints of the feet contributes to forefoot abnormalities. Synovitis of the subtalar and talocalcaneonavicular joints destabilizes the mechanism that normally allows the foot to be flexible enough to accommodate the weight-bearing surface during the stance phase and rigid enough to be a lever during push-off in gait. The talus rotates and slides forward on the calcaneus, and the calcaneus assumes a valgus position (Figure 3). The talonavicular joint, no longer well supported by a healthy spring ligament, becomes

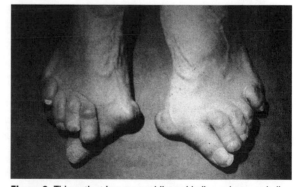

Figure 2. This patient has severe bilateral hallux valgus, and all of the MTP joints are subluxed left to right, which creates cock-up deformities. The patient has bilateral hindfoot valgus (not visible) and loss of both longitudinal and transverse arches with splaying of the forefoot. This patient is likely to need custom foot orthoses and heat-moldable shoes to accommodate the left toes overlying the large toe. (Photo courtesy of Judy Peck, MS, PT)

prominent medially and comes to rest on the supporting surface and accompanies the collapse of the longitudinal arch of the foot (Locke, Perry, Campbell, & Thomas, 1984). This pronation of the foot contributes to a spread of the metatarsals and flattening of the distal transverse arch at the forefoot, which produces a "splayed forefoot" (Platto et al., 1991).

The posterior tibialis tendon may be stretched, develop tenosynovitis, or rupture, which reduces or eliminates its function in maintaining the longitudinal arch. Pronation stretches the plantar fascia and contributes to plantar fasciitis (Moncur, 1995). Bony spurs of OA can be compounded by the bony erosions of RA, whereas malposition of the calcaneus allows shortening of the tendocalcaneus and increases the likelihood of calcaneal bursitis (Dimonte & Light, 1982). Rheumatoid nodules may form anywhere in the foot.

Footwear and orthoses. Shoes must provide ample toe room that allows the phalanges to lie straight and flat. Narrow shoes with pointed toes must be avoided because of the tendency to develop hallux valgus and overlapping toes. External supports, appropriately selected, may help retain a more normal configuration of the foot. Shoes with built-in arch supports or custom orthoses help shape the contours of the surface on which the foot moves during gait. In patients with forefoot pain but without deformity, a good-quality running shoe with a solid heel counter and arch support will often be sufficient to protect the patient's foot; if an orthosis is needed, the regular insole can be removed and replaced with an individualized orthosis (Moncur, 1995). Persons with recalcitrant metatarsalgia or who are prone to foot ulcers may benefit from evaluation of the pressure on the plantar surface so that pressure relief can be specifically built into orthoses (Mueller, 1995).

Table 7. Characteristics of Rheumatoid Arthritis in the Forefoot

Site	Problem	Characteristics
Hallux	Hallux valgus	Great toe drifts toward the fibular side of the foot; ligaments of joint and joint capsule may be destroyed by RA.
	Bunion	Synovitis, pannus, and callus formation at first MTP joint; hard or soft corns; rheumatoid nodules.
	Subluxation/ dislocation	Capsule, ligament, and tendon destruction; fibular drift complicates the ability to roll off the hallux during terminal stance.
Toes II/V	Metarsalgia	Synovitis, rheumatoid nodules, pannus formation, and the loss of fat pads under metatarsal heads causes pain and the feeling of "walking on rocks."
	Callosities	Chronic synovitis subluxation and rheumatoid nodules stimulate calluses on the plantar surface of the MTP joints and dorsum of the toes.
	Overlapping toes	MTP joint subluxation may result in toes overlapping each other.
	Hammer toes	Dorsal subluxation of the MTP joint results in MTP joint hyperextension, PIP joint flexion and DIP joint extension.
	Claw toes	Dorsal subluxation of the MTP joint results in MTP joint hyperextension, PIP and DIP flexion.

Note. Adapted from "Rheumatic Conditions and Aging," by C. Moncur, in *Physical Therapy of the Foot and Ankle* (2nd ed., pp. 121–122), edited by G. C. Hunt and T. G. McPoil, 1995, New York: Churchill Livingstone. Copyright 1995 by Churchill Livingstone. Reprinted with permission.

More attention to the management of hindfoot disease in RA is indicated (Hunt, Fromherz, & Gerber, 1987). Ankle–foot orthoses or leg–hindfoot orthoses to control the subtalar joints during gait help prevent the "cascading" effects of pronation, including the loss of the longitudinal arches of the midfoot and forefoot abduction (Moncur, 1995).

Early referral and patient education should include information about the destructive changes that can occur in RA of the foot and the importance of preventing deformity in the first place. Appropriate shoes and orthoses are essential preventive measures. (See the Appendix of at the end of this volume for guidelines on selecting shoes.)

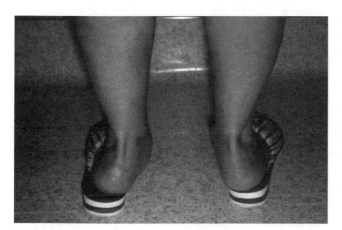

Figure 3. Hindfoot valgus is evaluated by a posterior view of the angle of the calcaneus to the tibia on weight bearing. The talus has rotated and slid forward on the calcaneus (right to left). The talonavicular joint, no longer supported by the spring ligament, has become pronated and contributes to the splayed forefoot. Patients who wear slippers to the clinic because shoes are uncomfortable need custom orthoses or adapted shoes that provide proper support and minimize pain. (Photo courtesy of Judy Peck, MS, PT)

Table 8. Characteristics of Rheumatoid Arthritis in the Midfoot

Site	Problem	Characteristics
Transverse tarsal joints	Talonavicular joint disruption	Head of talus and tuberosity of the navicular bone rotate downward and medialward, creating a pronated midfoot.
		Rupture of the posterior tibialis tendon and the ligamentous support on the medial arch facilitate the plantar motion of the talus and navicular bones.
	Calcaneocuboid joint disruption	Disruption of the soft tissues of the calcaneocuboid articulation allows the lateral arch to drop and contributes to the abnormal pes planovalgus deformity.
Intertarsal joints	Cuneonavicular joint disruption	Soft-tissue failure of the cuneonavicular articulation contributes to plantar migration of the first cuneiform and navicular bone, accentuating the pes planovalgus deformity.
	Intercuneiform joint disruption	Not usually an isolated site for RA to occur. Soft-tissue failure in these joints occurs concurrent with the other midtarsal joints in pes planovalgus. Cuneometatarsal and cubometatarsal articulation disruptions contribute to changes in the relationship between the midfoot and forefoot, including forefoot abduction (fibular drift).

Note. Adapted from "Rheumatic Conditions and Aging," by C. Moncur, in *Physical Therapy of the Foot and Ankle* (2nd ed., pp. 121–122), edited by G. C. Hunt and T. G. McPoil, 1995, New York: Churchill Livingstone. Copyright 1995 by Churchill Livingstone. Reprinted with permission.

Exercises for the feet. ROM and strengthening exercises for the intrinsic and extrinsic muscles of the foot help maintain foot function. Active and passive ROM of the toes and foot prevent contractures secondary to muscle spasm and abnormal gait. Flexion of the MTP joints, extension of the toes, abduction of the great toe, and supination of the foot are particularly important. Performed during a bath or when drying the feet after a shower, these exercises can be incorporated into daily activities (Melvin, 1989). Swimming in a warm pool is useful for patients with foot pain because swimming provides ROM and aerobic exercise (Moncur, 1995).

Particular attention should be paid to the cocontraction of toe flexors and extensors and the posterior tibialis muscles because they are key to maintaining normal position and because they produce abnormal forces once cock-up toes develop. Careful stretching of the gastrocnemius-soleus muscles helps reduce forces contributing to Achilles tendonitis or bursitis and pronation of the foot (Moncur, 1995).

Knees

As the largest synovial joint in the body, the knee is particularly susceptible to the effects of synovitis, with joint effusion, erosion of cartilage and bone, and capsular and ligamentous laxity leading to knee joint instability. Knee flexion contractures develop because flexion is the position of greatest comfort. Relatively small amounts of synovial effusion produce reflex inhibition of the quadriceps and spasm of the hamstring muscles. Quadriceps muscle weakness, whether the result of disuse, primary muscle involvement, reflex inactivity secondary to swelling and pain, or other factors, is key to reducing lower-extremity function (Stenstrom, 1994).

Patients must learn the importance of maintaining full ROM in the knee and strength in the quadriceps muscles. Frequent breaks to stand up while sitting for prolonged periods as well as

Table 9. Characteristics of Rheumatoid Arthritis in the Hindfoot

Site	Problem	Characteristics
Subtalar joint	Pain in hindfoot	Synovitis and pannus formation in the subtalar joint causes pain. Swelling may be present distal to malleoli. Pain may be elicited on palpation of sinus tarsi, on motion, or when weight bearing. Subtalar pain must be differentiated from talocrural joint pain.
	Subcalcaneal bursitis	Pain occurs beneath the Achilles tendon due to synovitis, rheumatoid nodule, or bursitis.
	Plantar fasciitis	Pain occurs at the attachment of the plantar aponeurosis to the tuberosity of the calcaneus.
	Subtalar joint disruption	Synovitis, pannus formation, destruction of the ligaments, and the attachment of the posterior tibialis to the sustentaculum tail of the calcaneus allow the head of the talus to migrate downward and medialward, creating a valgus deformity in the hindfoot; this phenomenon contributes to the formation of a planovalgus deformity in the midfoot and forefoot.

Note. From "Rheumatic Conditions and Aging," by C. Moncur, in *Physical Therapy of the Foot and Ankle* (2nd ed., pp. 121–122), edited by G. C. Hunt and T. G. McPoil, 1995, New York: Churchill Livingstone. Copyright 1995 by Churchill Livingstone. Reprinted with permission.

exercise to maintain muscle strength and ROM are essential to preserve functional knee mobility. Patients who have difficulty standing may find doing one or two quadriceps sets with each leg easier before they attempt to stand; this activity can be part of a daily exercise plan. Proper positioning with the knees in full extension while in bed is essential. Prone lying is an effective method of applying a prolonged stretch to the knees and the hips, where flexion contractures develop concomitantly with those at the knee.

Modalities for the control of pain and inflammation, particularly cold modalities, are advisable. A knee splint or brace can be used to stabilize the unstable knee during function, rest the joint, or provide a prolonged stretch. Raised chairs, toilet seats, and beds make sitting and standing less painful. Difficulty getting in and out of an automobile can be reduced if the patient sits down on the car seat and then rotates the legs in or out of the vehicle. Total knee arthroplasty is indicated if pain and functional loss are great.

Hips

The hip joints are usually not a source of complaints early in the course of RA. However, more than half of patients with RA will develop hip changes that are apparent radiographically and on clinical examination. Hip synovitis produces pain in the groin; pain may be referred to the medial aspect of the knee. The position of comfort, hip flexion, adduction, and external rotation can progress rapidly to fibrous contracture of the joint. In patients with severe disease, demineralization of pelvic bone stock may allow acetabular protrusio, in which the head of the femur deepens the acetabulum and pushes it into the pelvic cavity.

Gait is greatly altered by hip disease; pain and contracture combine to produce functional limitations. To reduce pressure in the hip joints, a bilateral gluteus medius (Trendelenberg) gait frequently develops in which the trunk shifts abruptly from side to side. Flexion contractures of the hip necessitate knee flexion and excessive extension of the lumbar spine to permit an upright posture, which increases energy costs markedly. The external rotation alters the weight-bearing line through the knee and foot, which promotes calcaneal valgus, increases weight on the medial longitudinal arch, and increases hallux valgus at push-off during ambulation. Limitation of hip motion interferes with stair climbing, comfortable sitting, sexual intercourse, perineal hygiene, foot care, and other functional activities.

Instructions in positioning for rest and ROM that will help maintain functional movement include daily prone lying and precautions about the use of pillows under the knees. Sitting with the legs crossed promotes flexion, external rotation, and adduction and should be avoided. Exercises should be directed toward hip extension and abduction ROM and strength. Assistive devices for gait, dressing, and other functional activities similar to those used for knee contracture are helpful. Total hip joint arthroplasty has been successful in relieving pain and restoring function.

Systemic and Extra-Articular Involvement

RA is commonly accompanied by systemic manifestations such as fatigue, malaise, anorexia, and weakness. Nutritional health may be complicated by both loss of appetite and pain with chewing due to painful TMJs. Decreased motivation and depression reflect the psychological burden of chronic disease and the neurobiology of pain and disturbed sleep. The rehabilitation team may offer suggestions and direct management of fatigue and sleep by providing information about fatigue management, sleep hygiene, time management, relaxation techniques, adapted equipment, therapeutic exercise, and posture training. Helping patients engage in avocational and productive activities can help reduce depression and mitigate against the losses encountered with chronic arthritis.

Extra-articular manifestations include subcutaneous nodules, cyst formation, pleurisy and other pulmonary manifestations, pericarditis, nerve entrapments, peripheral neuropathy, Felty's syndrome, Sjögren's syndrome, anemia of chronic disease, and vasculitis.

About 15% of patients with RA develop sicca syndrome, a condition of dry eyes and mouth, as a manifestation of associated Sjögren's syndrome. These complaints are treated with artificial tears, lozenges, frequent liquids, and by humidifying the environment. The Sjögren's Association has extensive educational material on ways to cope with symptoms. The Arthritis Foundation likewise has information (Box 1).

Ocular manifestations include episcleritis and scleritis.

Synovial cysts such as popliteal cysts may enlarge and rupture. They are treated by aspiration, local corticosteroid injection, and rarely with excision.

Subcutaneous nodules occur at some point in 25% to 50% of patients. When located at pressure points such as the elbow, these nodules may require protection by padding. When traumatized, nodules may require excisional surgery, but they often recur. Skin vasculitic lesions are frequent in patients with RA with the appearance of nailfold infarcts or palpable purpura. These lesions do not imply systemic vasculitis. Drugs used to treat RA can cause skin abnormalities such as ecchymoses and petechiae.

RA may involve the lung or heart. Inflammation of the pleura or pericardium is commonly seen at autopsy, as is histological evidence of interstitial lung disease. Usually manifestations are mild and asymptomatic; however, if a patient develops pleuropericardial effusions associated with shortness of breath, systemic corticosteroids may be helpful. If the pericardial effusion results in compromise, pericardiocentesis may be needed.

Neurological manifestations include myelopathies related to cervical spine instability, entrapment neuropathies, and ischemic neuropathies related to vasculitis such as mononeuritis multiplex.

Anemia of chronic disease is seen in almost all patients with active disease. However, the anemia of blood loss due to gastrointestinal bleeding is of concern in the differential because many patients with RA take NSAIDs or aspirin.

Surgical Management

More aggressive pharmaceutical management, patient education, and, ultimately, a cure for the disease may eventually prevent the need for most operative procedures in RA. Currently, however, surgery for RA continues to plays major role in management. Pain is the single most important indication for surgery in more than 90% of cases. However, surgical intervention is occasionally needed for the patient with malformed, malaligned, or ankylosed joints that may not be very painful. Both the patient and surgeon must understand what is and what is not attainable with the surgical intervention. The need for intervention should be determined preoperatively by determining the duration of disease, the extent of involvement, the previous medical treatment, the pattern of disease (is the patient improving or stable?), the effect on daily living, and the involvement of adjacent joints requiring multiple procedures.

Total joint arthroplasty is the most common operative procedure performed in RA. Primarily performed because of unremitting pain, limited motion, or severely impaired function, arthroplasty for the hip, knee, wrist, elbow, shoulder, MCP, first MTP, and TMJ joints are considered successful and are commonly performed. Improved ROM can be expected after surgery, although muscle weakness may compromise functional use. Total ankle arthroplasty has been attempted, but a satisfactory replacement has not been developed. Preoperative and postoperative programs for persons with RA who receive total joint arthroplasty must be comprehensive and incorporate clear delineation of goals, patient education, and exercise and activity prescriptions (Sledge, 1993).

Arthrodesis of unstable joints often increases function and reduces or eliminates joint pain. Joints that have extensive destruction of cartilage and bone leading to instability are candidates for arthrodesis. Common sites for arthrodesis are the spine, toes, wrist, foot, and ankle. Hindfoot procedures include triple arthrodesis in patients who have a stable tibiotalar joint. Fusion of the cervical spine is indicated for vertebral subluxations that cause neurological compromise. Arthrodesis is performed as a salvage procedure after rare complications or failures of total joint arthroplasty.

Surgery of the RA foot most commonly involves the forefoot. Metatarsal head resection and arthrodesis of the first MTP joint help reduce pain, allow toes to assume better alignment within footwear, and improve gait.

Synovectomy is a viable treatment option for the wrist, elbow, ankle, and knee if the articular surface has not been destroyed and if the patient has continued pain after at least 6 months of medical management. Synovectomy is usually done arthroscopically.

The release of tendon sheaths lined with diseased synovium may free entrapped tendons and reduce the likelihood of tendon rupture. The wrist and hand are the most common sites for synovial resection. Synovectomy and tenosynovectomy are best done in conjunction with other surgeries, particularly at the shoulder. Given the success of total joint arthroplasty, these procedures are not performed at the knee as often as they were in the past (Anderson, 1997). (A more complete review of surgery for arthritis and postoperative rehabilitation can be found in volume 5 of this series.)

Employment Issues

RA has a negative effect on the ability of patients to work in the workplace. Patients with RA may need time away from work for appointments with health care providers or for rest during a flare-up. Patients with RA may require modification of their job responsibilities or acceptance of a less demanding job or reduced hours. Patients with RA who are self-employed or who have control over the pace of their work are more likely to continue gainful employment. The Americans with Disabilities Act (Public Law 101-336) requires employers to make reasonable accommodations in work schedules and job tasks to make it possible for employees with disabilities to perform the essential functions of their job. Job visits with the approval of the employer may be helpful for some patients.

When evaluating the work environment, it is important consider the employee's total functioning and not only how hand function affects the job. Modifications must be carefully planned with the employee, who is an active member of the decision-making team, and costs to the employer or to the employee must be determined. Some examples of adaptations or changes in the workplace can include large-grip pens, writing aids, computers with voice activation or proper mouse or track ball designs, headset or speaker telephones, and book or document holders.

Home Evaluation and Therapy

Home treatment can make the difference between dependence and independence in self-care for patients who are unable to travel to a clinic. Helewa and colleagues (1991) conducted a controlled trial ($N=53$) of a 6-week comprehensive home occupational therapy program for patients with RA. Patients in the treated group had notable improvements in self-care, household management, heavy cleaning, and mobility. There was a major reduction in pain. A comprehensive evaluation was conducted on disease activity and functional ability, physical examination of joint disease activity and damage, grip strength, and morning stiffness. A specific itemized ADL assessment was used to plan treatment goals. Treatment included hand therapy, assistive device training, home adaptations, joint protection training, energy conservation education, foot management and shoe insoles and adaptations, recommendations for foot orthoses, and wheelchair prescriptions. If appropriate, patients received vocational evaluations, adaptations to work settings, methods to enhance leisure activities, psychosocial counseling , stress management education, and education on how to use community resources.

A typical home evaluation includes the therapist's understanding of the current disease activity of that patient as well as location and type of pain, level of functioning, level of fatigue, and the duration and severity of stiffness. A home visit includes determining the patient's accessibility needs. The therapist evaluates the entrance and exit to the home, steps and stairs, the doorways and halls, and bedroom, kitchen, and bathroom access. The patient's daily routine is reviewed with the therapist, and household tasks are identified. Modifications or recommendations can be made to improve energy conservation as well as accessibility with recognition of the patient's individual goals and needs. Recommendations may include the use of railings on stairs, doors with lever knobs rather than the ball knobs for opening, light switches at either end of a hallway, raised toilet seats to assist with limitations in ROM at the hip and knee, and walk-in showers or built-in bathtub seats and grab bars. In the kitchen, new modified convenience items (e.g., built-up handles) are available for persons with weakness in grip and pinch. Organization equipment such as book holders, lap desks, lazy susans, pull-out shelves, movable stools or chairs for preparing food, and power controls versus light switches may be recommended. When possible, patients should have the opportunity to try out adaptive equipment before purchasing it (Box 1).

Sexual Counseling

Health care providers are often hesitant to discuss the sexual problems of their patients. Patients with chronic diseases have the same difficulties as healthy persons with impotence, decreased libido, premature ejaculation, and orgasm dysfunction. Patients with RA may have problems with positioning, arthralgias, stiffness, muscle weakness, and fatigue. The therapist may play an important role by encouraging patients to communicate their concerns to their health care providers and to their partners. There is a wealth of information in the Arthritis Foundation's pamphlet *Living and Loving* (Box 1).

Conclusion

RA continues to be a disease that challenges patients and therapists. RA is a systemic disease with rapid progression in the first few years. The consequences of the disease are greater than the side effects of the medications. Patients are treated earlier and more aggressively with new drugs and combinations of drugs with improved patient survival and improved functional outcomes. Research has demonstrated that, in addition to taking medications, patients can further control symptoms and improve quality of life by applying self-management skills such as stress management, fatigue management, relaxation training, improved sleep, and cardiovascular exercise. The challenge for rehabilitation therapists in the new millennium is to develop effective protocols for self-management training and fatigue management that demonstrate positive outcomes for improving and sustaining functional capacity.

References

Anderson, R. J. (1997). Rheumatoid arthritis: Clinical features and laboratory. In *Primer on the rheumatic diseases* (11th ed., pp. 161–167). Atlanta, GA: The Arthritis Foundation.

Arnett, F. C., Edworthy, S. M., Bloch, D. A., McShane, D. J., Fries, J. F., Cooper, N. S., Healey, L. A., Kaplan, S. R., Liang, M. H., Luthra, H. S., Medsger, T. A., Mitchell, D. M., Neustadt, D. H., Pinals, R. S., Schaller, J. G., Sharp, J. T., Wilder, R. L., & Hunder, G. G. (1988). The American Rheumatism Association 1987 revised criteria for the classification of rheumatoid arthritis. *Arthritis and Rheumatism, 31,* 315–324.

Backman, C. (1998). Functional assessment. In J. L. Melvin & G. Jensen (Eds.), *Rheumatologic rehabilitation series: Volume 1: Assessment and management* (pp. 157–194). Bethesda, MD: American Occupational Therapy Association.

Boutaugh, M. L., & Brady, T. J. (1998). Patient education for self-management. In J. L. Melvin & G. Jensen (Eds.), *Rheumatologic rehabilitation series: Volume 1: Assessment and management* (pp. 219–258). Bethesda, MD: American Occupational Therapy Association.

Bradley, L. A. (1998). Pain management interventions for patients with rheumatic diseases. In J. L. Melvin & G. Jensen (Eds.), *Rheumatologic rehabilitation series: Volume 1: Assessment and management* (pp. 259–278). Bethesda, MD: American Occupational Therapy Association.

Byer, P. H. (1985). Effect of exercise on morning stiffness and mobility in patients with RA. *Research in Nurse Health, 8,* 275–281.

Callahan, L. F., Pincus, T., Huston, J. W., Brooks, R. H., Nance, E. P., & Kaye, J. J. (1997). *Measures of activity and damage in RA: Depiction of changes and prediction of mortality over 5 years.* Arthritis Care and Research, 10, *381–394.*

Cash, J. M., & Klippel, J. H. (1994). Second line drug therapy for rheumatoid arthritis. *New England Journal of Medicine, 330,* 1368–1375.

Chevalier, X., & Larget-Piet, B. (1994). General diseases of the spine in rheumatoid arthritis. *Current Opinion in Rheumatology, 6,* 311–318.

Colditz, J., & Melvin, J. L. (in press). Orthotic treatment for arthritis of the hand. In J. L. Melvin & E. A. Nalebuff (Eds.), *Rheumatologic rehabilitation series: Volume 4: The hand: Evaluation, therapy, and surgery.* Bethesda, MD: American Occupational Therapy Association.

Cordery, J., & Rocchi, M. (1998). Joint protection and fatigue management. In J. L. Melvin & G. Jensen (Eds.), *Rheumatologic rehabilitation series: Volume 1: Assessment and management* (pp. 279–322). Bethesda, MD: American Occupational Therapy Association.

Cracchiolo, A., III, Gall, V., & Janisse, D. (1999). Rheumatoid arthritis in the foot and ankle: Surgery and rehabilitation. In J. L. Melvin & V. Gall (Eds.), *Rheumatologic rehabilitation series: Volume 5: Surgical rehabilitation* (pp. 165–194). Bethesda, MD: American Occupational Therapy Association.

Deal, C. L., Schnitzer, T. J., & Lipstein, E. L. (1991). Treatment of arthritis with topical capsaicin: A double blind trial. *Clinical Therapeutics, 13,* 383–395.

Dellhag, B., Wollersjo, I., & Bjelle, A. (1992). Effect of active hand exercise and wax bath treatment in rheumatoid arthritis patients. *Arthritis Care and Research, 5,* 87–92.

Dimonte, P., & Light, H. (1982). Mechanics, gait deviations and treatment of the rheumatoid foot. *Physical Therapy, 12*(8), 1148–1156.

Ekblom, B., Lovgren, O., Alderin, M., Fridstrom, M., & Satterstrom, G. (1975). Effect of short-term physical training on patients with rheumatoid arthritis: A six-month follow-up study. *Scandinavian Journal of Rheumatology, 4,* 87–91.

Feinberg, J. R., & Trombly, C. A. (1989). Arthritis. In *Occupational therapy for physical dysfunction* (pp. 815–830). Baltimore: Williams & Wilkins.

Firestein, G. S., & Zvaifler, N. J. (1997). Anticytokine therapy in rheumatoid arthritis. *New England Journal of Medicine, 337,* 195–197.

Flatt, A. (1983). *Care of the rheumatoid hand* (4th ed.). St. Louis: Mosby.

Fortin, P. R., & Shadick, N. A. (1994). Arthritis and chest pain, dyspnea, and cough. In J. H. Klippel & P. A. Dieppe (Eds.), *Rheumatology* St. Louis: Mosby.

Fuchs, H. A., & Pincus, T. (1992). Radiographic damage in rheumatoid arthritis: Description by nonlinear models [Editorial]. *Journal of Rheumatology, 19,* 1655–1658.

Gerber, L. H. (1989). Rehabilitation of patients with rheumatic diseases. In W. N. Kelley, E. D. Harris, Jr., S. Ruddy, & C. B. Sledge (Eds.), *Textbook of rheumatology* (3rd ed., pp. 1728–1744). Philadelphia: Saunders.

Gibson, K. R. (1986). Rheumatoid arthritis of the shoulder. *Physical Therapy, 66*(12), 1920–1929.

Gordon, D. A., & Hastings, D. E. (1994). Rheumatoid arthritis: Clinical features: Early, progressive and late disease. In J. H. Klippel & P. A. Dieppe (Eds.), *Rheumatology* (pp. 5:3.1–5:3.14). St. Louis: Mosby.

Griffin, J. W., & McClure, M. (1981). Adverse responses to transcutaneous electrical nerve stimulation in a patient with rheumatoid arthritis. *Physical Therapy, 61*(3), 354–355.

Haralson-Ferrell, K. (1998). Community resources in comprehensive rehabilitation. In J. L. Melvin & G. Jensen (Eds.), *Rheumatologic rehabilitation series: Volume 1: Assessment and management* (pp. 393–408). Bethesda, MD: American Occupational Therapy Association.

Harkcom, T. A., Lampman, R. M., Banwell, B. F., & Castor, C. W. (1985). Therapeutic value of graded aerobic exercise training in rheumatoid arthritis. *Arthritis and Rheumatism, 28,* 32–39.

Harrell, P. (1996). Splinting of the hand. In S. T. Wegener (Ed.), *Clinical care in rheumatic disease* (pp. 83–89). Atlanta, GA: American College of Rheumatology.

Hawley, D. J., & Wolfe, F. (1992). Sensitivity to change of the Health Assessment Questionnaire (HAQ) and other clinical and health status measures in rheumatoid arthritis: Results of short term clinical trials and observational studies versus long term observational studies. *Arthritis Care and Research, 5,* 130–136.

Hayes, K. W., & Petersen, C. M. (1998). Joint and soft tissue pain. In J. L. Melvin & G. Jensen (Eds.), *Rheumatologic rehabilitation series: Volume 1: Assessment and management* (pp. 125–156). Bethesda, MD: American Occupational Therapy Association.

Helewa, A., Goldsmith, C. H., Lee, P., Bombardier, C., Hanes, B., Smythe, H. A., & Tugwell, P. (1991). Effects of occupational therapy home service on patients with rheumatoid arthritis. *Lancet, 337,* 1453–1456.

Hirano, P. C., Laurent, D. D., & Lorig, K. (1994). Arthritis patient education studies, 1987–1991: A review of the literature. *Patient Education and Counseling, 24*(1), 9–54.

Hochberg, M. C., Chang, R. W., Dwosh, I., Lindsey, S., Pincus, T., & Wolfe, F. (1992). The American College of Rheumatology 1991 revised criteria for the classification of global functional status in rheumatoid arthritis. *Arthritis and Rheumatism, 35,* 498–502.

Hunt, G. C., Fromherz, W. A., & Gerber, L. H. (1987). Hindfoot pain treated by a leg–hindfoot orthosis. *Physical Therapy, 67*(9), 1384–1388.

Inglis, A. (1985). Rheumatoid arthritis. In B. Morrey (Ed.), *The elbow and its disorders* (pp. 1984–2000). Philadelphia: Saunders.

Leigh, J. P., & Fries, J. F. (1991). Education level and rheumatoid arthritis: Evidence from five data centers. *Journal of Rheumatology, 18*(1), 24–34.

Locke, M., Perry, J., Campbell, J., & Thomas, L. (1984). Ankle and subtalar motion during gait in arthritic patients. *Physical Therapy, 64*(4), 504–509.

Lorig,, K. (1993). Self -management of chronic illness: A model for the future. *Generations,* 11–14.

Lyngberg, K. K., Harreby, M., Bentzen, H., Frost, B., & Danneskiold-Samsoe, B. (1994). Elderly rheumatoid arthritis patients on steroid treatment tolerate physical training without an increase in disease activity. *Archives of Physical Medicine and Rehabilitation, 75,* 1189–1195.

Marx, H. (1992). Rheumatoid arthritis. In B. Stanley (Ed.), *Concepts in hand rehabilitation* (pp. 395–418). Philadelphia: F. A. Davis.

McCarthy, D. J., Harman, J. G., Grassanovich, J. L., & Qian, C. (1995). Treatment of rheumatoid joint inflammation with intrasynovial triamcinolone hexacetonide. *Journal of Rheumatology, 22*(9), 1631–1635.

Meenan, R. F., Gertman, P. M., & Mason, J. H. (1980). Measuring health status in arthritis: The Arthritis Impact Measurement Scales. *Arthritis and Rheumatism, 23,* 146–157.

Meenan, R. F., Mason, J. H., Anderson, J. J., Guccione, A. A., & Kazis, L. E. (1992). AIMS2: The content and properties of a revised and expanded Arthritis Impact Measurement Scales health status questionnaire. *Arthritis and Rheumatism, 35,* 1–10.

Melvin, J. L. (1989). *Rheumatic disease in the adult and child: Occupational therapy and rehabilitation* (3rd ed.). Philadelphia: F. A. Davis.

Melvin, J. L., (in press). Therapeutic exercise and thermal modalities in the management of arthritis of the hand. In J. L. Melvin & E. A. Nalebuff (Eds.), *Rheumatologic rehabilitation series: Volume 4: The hand: Evaluation, therapy, and surgery.* Bethesda, MD: American Occupational Therapy Association.

Mills, J. A. (1988). Arthritis of the shoulder. In C. R. Rowe (Ed.), *The shoulder*. New York: Churchill Livingstone.

Minor, M. A. (1990). Physical activity and management of arthritis. *Annals of Behavioral Medicine, 13*, 117–124.

Minor, M. (1998). Exercise for health and physical fitness. In J. L. Melvin & G. Jensen (Eds.), *Rheumatologic rehabilitation series: Volume 1: Assessment and management* (pp. 351–368). Bethesda, MD: American Occupational Therapy Association.

Minor, M. A., Hewett, J. E., Webel, R. R., Anderson, S. K., & Kay, D. R. (1989). Efficacy of physical conditioning exercise in patients with rheumatoid arthritis or osteoarthritis. *Arthritis and Rheumatism, 32*, 1396–1405.

Minor, M. A., & Sanford, M. K. (1993). Physical interventions in the management of pain in arthritis: An overview for research and practice. *Arthritis Care and Research, 6*(4), 197–206.

Moncur, C. (1995). Rheumatic conditions and aging. In G. C. Hunt & T. G. McPoil (Eds.), *Physical therapy of the foot and ankle* (2nd ed.). New York: Churchill Livingstone.

Moncur, C., & Shields, M. (1983). Clinical management of metatarsalgia in the patient with arthritis. *Clinical Management, 3*(4), 7–13.

Moncur, C., & Williams, H. J. (1988). Cervical spine management in patients with rheumatoid arthritis: Review of the literature. *Physical Therapy, 68*(4), 509–515.

Moreland, L. W., Schiff, M. H., Baumgartner, S. W., Tindall, E. A., Fleischmann, R. M., Bulpitt, K. J., Weaver, A. L., Keystone, E. C., Furst, D. E., Mease, P. J., Ruderman, E. M., Horwitz, D. A., Arkfeld, D. G., Garrison, L., Burge, D. J., Blosch, C. M., Lange, M. L., McDonnell, N. D., & Weinblatt, M. E. (1999). Entanercept therapy in rheumatoid arthritis: A randomized controlled trial. *Annals of Internal Medicine, 130*, 478–486.

Morrey, B. E., Askew, L. J., An, K. N., & Chao, E. Y. (1981). A biomechanical study of normal functional elbow motion. *Journal of Bone and Joint Surgery, 63A*, 87–89.

Mueller, M. J. (1995). Use of an in-shoe pressure measurement system in the management of patients with neuropathic ulcers or metatarsalgia. *Journal of Orthopaedic and Sports Physical Therapy, 21*(6), 328–336.

Nalebuff, E. A. (1984). The rheumatoid thumb. *Clinics of Rheumatic Disease, 10*, 589–608.

Nalebuff, E. A., & Garrett, J. (1976). Opera-glass hand in rheumatoid arthritis. *Journal of Hand Surgery, 1*(3), 210.

Nalebuff, E. A., & Millender, L. H. (1975). Surgical treatment of swan-neck deformities in rheumatoid arthritis. *Orthopedic Clinics of North America, 6*(3), 733.

Noaker, J . (1996). Enhancing functional ability alternative techniques, assistive devices and environmental modification. In S. Wegener (Ed.), *Clinical care in rheumatic disease* (pp. 89–93). Atlanta, GA: American College of Rheumatology.

Nordemar, R., Eckblom, B., Zachrisson, L., & Lundquist, K. (1981). Physical training in rheumatoid arthritis: A controlled long-term study. *Scandinavian Journal of Rheumatology, 10*, 25–30.

Oatis, C. A. (1998). Locomotor dysfunction: Evaluation and treatment. In J. L. Melvin & G. Jensen (Eds.), *Rheumatologic rehabilitation series: Volume 1: Assessment and management* (pp. 195–218). Bethesda, MD: American Occupational Therapy Association.

Perlman, S. G., Connell, K. J., Clark, A., Robinson, M. S., Conlon, P., Gecht, M., Caldron, P., & Sinacore, J. M. (1990). Dance-based aerobic exercise for rheumatoid arthritis. *Arthritis Care and Research, 3*, 29–35.

Phillips, C. (1989). Management of the patient with rheumatoid arthritis. *Hand Clinics, 5*(2), 291–309.

Phillips, C. (1995). Therapist's management of patients with rheumatoid arthritis. In J. M. Hunter, E. J.

Mackin, & A. D. Callahan (Eds.), *Rehabilitation of the hand: Surgery and therapy* (4th ed., pp. 1345–1350). St. Louis: Mosby.

Pincus, T., & Callahan, L. F. (1989). Reassessment of twelve traditional paradigms concerning the diagnosis, prevalence, morbidity and mortality of rheumatoid arthritis. *Scandinavian Journal of Rheumatology, 18*(Suppl. 79), 67–96.

Pincus, T., & Callahan, L. F. (1994). How many types of patients meet classification criteria for RA [Editorial]? *Journal of Rheumatology, 21,* 1385–1389.

Pincus, T., Callahan, L. F., Brooks, R. H., Fuchs, H. A., Olsen, N. J., & Kaye, J. J. (1989). Self-report questionnaire scores in rheumatoid arthritis compared with traditional physical, radiographic, and laboratory measures. *Annals of Internal Medicine, 110,* 259–266.

Pincus, T., Marcum, S. B., & Callahan, L. F. (1992). Long-term drug therapy for rheumatoid arthritis in seven rheumatology private practices: II. Second-line drugs and prednisone. *Journal of Rheumatology, 19,* 1885–1894.

Pincus, T., Wolfe, F., & Callahan, L. F. (1994). Updating a reassessment of traditional paradigms concerning rheumatoid arthritis. In F. Wolfe & T. Pincus (Eds.), *Rheumatoid arthritis: Pathogenesis, assessment, outcome, and treatment* (pp. 1–74). New York: Marcel Dekker.

Platto, M. J., O'Connell, P. G., Hicks, J. E., & Gerber, L. H. (1991). The relationship of pain and deformity of the rheumatoid foot to gait and an index of functional ambulation. *Journal of Rheumatology, 18*(1), 38–43.

Rizio, L. & Belsky, M. R. (1996). Finger deformities in rheumatoid arthritis. *Hand Clinics, 12*(3), 531–540.

Rozman, B., for the Leflunomide Investigators' Group. (1998). Clinical experience with leflunomide in rheumatoid arthritis. *Journal of Rheumatology, 25*(Suppl. 53), 27–32.

Schuerman, S. (1998). Thermal agents for inflammatory arthritis. In J.L. Melvin & G. Jensen (Eds.), *Rheumatologic Rehabilitation series: Volume 1: Assessment and Management.* Bethesda, MD: American Occupational Therapy Association.

Semble, E. L. (1995). Rheumatoid arthritis: New approaches for its evaluation and management. *Archives of Physical Medicine and Rehabilitation, 76,* 190–201.

Silman, A. J., & Hochberg, M. C. (1993). Rheumatoid arthritis. In *Epidemiology of the rheumatic diseases.* Oxford, England: Oxford University Press.

Singer, J. M., & Plotz, C. M. (1956). The latex fixation test: Application to the serological diagnosis of rheumatoid arthritis. *American Journal of Medicine, 21,* 188.

Sledge, C. B. (1993). Reconstructive surgery in rheumatic diseases: Introduction to surgical management. In W. N. Kelley, E. D. Harris, Jr., S. Ruddy, & C. B. Sledge (Eds.), *Textbook of rheumatology* (3rd ed., pp. 108–109). Philadelphia: Saunders.

Someya, F., Miaki, H., Asai, H., Tachino, K., & Nara, I. (1988). Hand splint for rheumatoid arthritis patients during gait training after joint replacement in lower extremity. *Archives of Physical Medicine and Rehabilitation, 69,* 644.

Sotosky, J. R., & Lindsay, S. M. (1991). Use of TENS in arthritis management. *Bulletin on the Rheumatic Diseases, 40*(5), 3–5.

Speigel, J. S., Hirshfield, M. S., & Spiegel, T. M. (1985). Evaluation self care activities: Comparison of the self-reported questionnaire with an occupational therapist interview. *British Journal of Rheumatology, 24,* 357–361.

Stenstrom, C. H. (1994). Therapeutic exercise in rheumatoid arthritis. *Arthritis Care and Research, 7,* 190–197.

Stewart, N. J., Manzanares, J. B., & Morrey, B. F. (1997). Surgical treatment of aseptic olecranon bursitis. *Journal of Shoulder and Elbow Surgery, 6*(1), 49–54.

Stokes, B. (1996). Community-based physical therapy management of arthritis. In J. M. Walker & A. Helewa (Eds.), *Physical therapy in arthritis* (p. 308). Philadelphia: Saunders.

Superio-Cabuslay, E., Ward, M., & Lorig, K. (1996). Patient education interventions in osteoarthritis and rheumatoid arthritis: A meta-analytic comparison with nonsteroid anti-inflammatory drug treatment. *Arthritis Care and Research, 9,* 292–295.

Swanson, A. B. (1995). Pathogenesis of arthritic lesions. In J. M. Hunter, E. J. Mackin, & A. D. Callahan (Eds.), *Rehabilitation of the hand: Surgery and therapy* (4th ed., pp. 805–903). St. Louis: Mosby.

Taal, E., Riemsma, R. D., Brus, H. L. M., Seydel, E. R., Rasker, J. J., & Wiegmann, O. (1993). Group education for patients with RA. *Patient Education and Counseling, 20*(2/3), 177–187.

Williams, H. J. (1993). Rheumatoid arthritis: Treatment. In *Primer on the rheumatic diseases* (10th ed., pp. 93–96). Atlanta, GA: The Arthritis Foundation.

Wilske, K. R. (1993). Inverting the therapeutic pyramid: Observations and recommendations on new directions in rheumatoid arthritis based on the authors experience. *Seminars in Arthritis and Rheumatism, 23*(Suppl. 1), 11–18.

Wilson, R. L. (1986). Rheumatoid arthritis of the hand. *Orthopedic Clinics of North America, 17,* 315.

Wolfe, F., & Pincus, T. (Eds.). (1994). *Rheumatoid arthritis: Pathogenesis, assessment, outcome, and treatment.* New York: Marcel Dekker.

Yelin, E., Meenan, R., Nevitt, M., & Epstein, W. (1980). Work disability in rheumatoid arthritis: Effects of disease, social, and work factors. *Annals of Internal Medicine, 93,* 551–556.

SYSTEMIC LUPUS ERYTHEMATOSUS

Sara E. Walker, MD, MACP, Judy R. Sotosky, MEd, PT, and Jeanne L. Melvin, MS, OTR, FAOTA

Systemic lupus erythematosus (SLE) is a complex chronic inflammatory disease caused by regulatory abnormalities of the immune system. It can affect multiple organ systems including the skin, renal, cardiovascular, pulmonary, neuropsychiatric, and musculoskeletal systems (Alarcon-Segovia, 1988; Schur, 1993). Persons with SLE experience an unpredictable pattern of exacerbations ("flare-ups") and remissions of their disease in which different systems may be affected at different times. Clinical presentation commonly includes fatigue, arthralgias, arthritis, rash, and Raynaud's phenomenon (Schur, 1993). Box 1 discusses historical aspects of SLE.

Causative Factors: SLE as an Autoimmune Disease

Autoimmunity develops when antibody responses are directed against antigens that are part of the body ("self-antigens"); these antibodies are known as *autoantibodies*. It is possible for autoantibodies to form in a person who does not have an autoimmune disease. For example, some women and men have positive fluorescent antinuclear antibody tests (commonly called the *ANA test*), but they do not have SLE. ANAs are found in diseases other than SLE such as rheumatoid arthritis (RA) and scleroderma (Illei & Klippel, 1999).

Autoimmune diseases occur when autoantibodies or autoreactive cells result in damage to body organs. SLE is the prototype of an autoimmune disease. Like other autoimmune illnesses, SLE tends to cluster in family members. First-degree relatives of patients with SLE may have autoantibodies with positive ANA tests, and there is an increased probability that both twins in a monozygotic pair will be affected. SLE is often associated with defects in the immune system. Serum levels of immunoglobulin (Ig) A, specific complement proteins, lymphocyte function, erythrocyte receptors for immune complexes, and phagocytosis may be deficient or defective. SLE incidence is higher in women and may exacerbate during pregnancy or in the postpartum period. Estrogen and prolactin have the potential to stimulate disease activity, and testosterone appears to be protective. Environmental factors such as infections, drugs, ultraviolet light, and nutrition have been implicated as factors that can incite SLE (Shoenfeld, 1992).

Population Affected

SLE characteristically involves women of childbearing age and affects 8 to 10 women for every man affected. The usual age at onset is between 15 and 40 years, and SLE is rare before puberty. Although reports vary, SLE affects 1 in 2,000 persons in a general outpatient population. Prevalence of SLE in

---

Box 1
Historical Aspects of SLE

The term *lupus* (which is Latin for "wolf") was first applied to cutaneous disease in medieval times. In 1833, Biett's description of round red patches on the faces of young women was published by his pupil, Cazenave; this is considered to be the first description of SLE. Von Hebra of Vienna, Austria, used the term *butterfly* to describe the malar rash of SLE in 1845 (as cited in Smith & Cyr, 1988). In 1902, Sequeira and Balean of the London Hospital published a detailed account of woman 18 years of age whose clinical findings would be clearly recognizable today as SLE (Figure 1A) (Sequeira & Balean, 1902). She was hospitalized with a malar rash, malaise, headache, abdominal pain, edema, and hematuria. Blood and granular casts appeared in her urine, and glomerulonephritis was found at autopsy. Two years later, Osler (as cited in Smith & Cyr, 1988) described two women who probably had SLE: both developed facial erythema and renal failure.

Hargraves, Richmond, and Morton (1948) described the lupus erythematosus (LE) cell, an in vitro phenomenon that demonstrated the ability of antinuclear antibodies to damage nuclear material. This landmark discovery provided practitioners with the first relatively specific test for SLE and allowed the diagnosis to be made in a living patient. Although many pathologists now consider the LE cell test to be outmoded, it is the only diagnostic

test for SLE that can be performed in two hours in a simply equipped laboratory. Our modern concept of SLE as a multisystem disease results from the classic description published in 1954 (Harvey, Shulmar, Tumulty, Conley, & Schoenrich, 1954) and the seminal contributions of Dubois (1966), who organized a clinic for patients with SLE and authored the first major textbook on the subject. In 1957, Friou (1957) used the indirect immunofluorescence technique to demonstrate antibodies directed against nuclear targets. The ANA test is still used as a screening test for SLE. In the same year, antibodies to anti-dsDNA were reported; this antibody system is now recognized as useful in confirming the diagnosis of SLE (Buskila & Schoenfeld, 1992). Soon thereafter, it was shown that antibodies to DNA as well as a DNA-like antigen could be eluted from the kidneys of patients with SLE (Koffler, Schur, & Kunkel, 1967). This important discovery introduced the key concept that lupus nephritis is mediated by immune complexes deposited in renal glomeruli.

SLE remains a key topic for investigations in many clinics and laboratories. Important new discoveries include the finding that genetic features predispose persons to SLE (Arnett, 1993), the influences of hormones on SLE (Lahita, 1992), and the potential value of aggressive treatment for patients with severe SLE renal disease (Fox & McCune, 1994).

the United States is estimated to be as high as 50.8/100,000. In the United States, African-American and Hispanic persons have an increased incidence of the disease (Hochberg, 1992; Pisetsky, 1997).

Clinical Features and Diagnosis

The diagnosis of SLE involves identification of a systemic illness that commonly involves more than one organ system. Criteria for classifying SLE have been developed but do not necessarily apply to every person with SLE (Tan et al., 1982). These criteria are useful for distinguishing SLE from other autoimmune illnesses and for confirming the diagnosis of SLE in patients who are included in population studies and clinical trials (Tan et al., 1982).

The major clinical features of SLE include a facial rash that covers the cheeks and bridge of the nose (malar rash or "butterfly rash"), photosensitivity, and ulcers in the nose and mouth. Discoid skin lesions may appear that are red, raised patches with keratotic scaling, follicular plugging, and scarring. Discoid lupus is of interest because it may occur as an isolated skin condition or may be associated with the systemic illness of SLE. Arthralgias and nonerosive arthritis are common in SLE. Pleurisy, pericarditis, glomerulonephritis, central nervous system (CNS) complications, and hematological abnormalities (e.g., hemolytic anemia, low white blood cell count, low platelet count) may be present in patients with SLE.

Active Versus Inactive Disease

In evaluating individual patients with SLE, it is important to appreciate whether the disease is active or inactive. The patient with active disease typically "feels sick" and has manifestations of

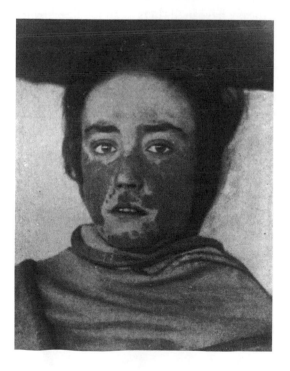

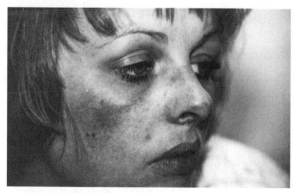

Figure 1. (A) This woman (18 years of age) was one of the first reported cases in whom the malar rash of SLE was associated with severe renal disease. *Note.* From "Lupus erythematosus: A clinical study of seventy-one cases," by J. H. Sequiera and H. Balean, 1902, *The British Journal of Dermatology, 14,* pp. 367–379. Copyright 1902 by Blackwell Science Ltd. Reprinted with permission. (B) Malar rash in a young woman with SLE. The eruption involves the bridge of the nose, the malar surfaces, and the area between the nose and the upper lip. It has telangiectatic character (small red vascular spots) and is red.

active inflammation that may include increased fatigue, fever, myalgias, skin rashes, joint pain and swelling, and pleurisy. Other symptoms during a flare-up include headaches, memory problems, and possibly other symptoms of CNS involvement and edema or findings of SLE renal disease. Tests for antibodies to double-stranded DNA (anti-dsDNA) are often positive when the disease is active, and serum levels of the third and fourth components of complement (C3 and C4) may be low. SLE is typically active when the diagnosis is first made, and disease may reactivate later after a period of drug treatment. Reactivation of SLE is referred to as a "lupus flare."

SLE usually becomes inactive after appropriate treatment is instituted. Spontaneous improvement can occur. The patient with inactive disease may feel perfectly well or may continue to have problems with fatigue or fibromyalgia syndrome (FMS). In the late stages of SLE, the disease may be suppressed adequately, but attention should be paid to the development of premature atherosclerosis, renal insufficiency, and complications of long-term treatment with corticosteroid drugs such as prednisone (Liang, Stern, & Esdaile, 1988).

Other Diseases That Resemble SLE

Undifferentiated, Overlap, and Mixed Connective Tissue Diseases

The term *undifferentiated connective tissue disease* is often used when a patient does not have enough symptoms to meet the diagnostic criteria for a specific rheumatic disease. If a patient has symptoms that are characteristic of two or more rheumatic diseases, the diagnosis may be called an *overlap syndrome* by some physicians or *undifferentiated connective tissue disease* by others. Many but not all of these cases will evolve into SLE or scleroderma over a period of years (Mukerji & Hardin, 1993). Patients with overlapping features of several connective tissue diseases may be diagnosed as having *mixed connective tissue disease*. These persons characteristically have high titers of antibodies directed against ribonuclear protein antigen and U1 small ribonucleoprotein (Kallenberg, 1993).

Sjögren's Syndrome

Sjögren's syndrome is a disorder in which the salivary and lacrimal glands are infiltrated with inflammatory cells. This leads to diminished function of the glands, which results in "sicca" symptoms (i.e., dryness of the eyes and mouth). Swelling of the parotid glands may be present. Sjögren's syndrome may occur alone as a primary disease. Secondary Sjögren's syndrome occurs when the sicca abnormalities are present in a patient with a connective tissue disease. RA is the connective tissue disease that is most commonly associated with secondary Sjögren's syndrome (Fox, 1997). However, 8% of patients with SLE have secondary Sjögren's syndrome (Andonopoulos, Skopouli, Dimou, Drosis, & Moutsoupoulos, 1990). Patients with Sjögren's syndrome should be referred to the National Sjögren's Association for the latest information on self-management of dry eyes, mouth, and skin and other symptoms (Box 2).

Autoantibodies in SLE

When diagnosing SLE, it is assumed that the patient has a positive indirect ANA test. This test is useful as a screening test because it is positive in almost all patients with SLE. On the other hand, a positive ANA test is not highly specific for SLE. Many well persons (especially elderly persons), patients taking drugs such as procainamide, and patients with other inflammatory connective tissue diseases such as RA may have a positive ANA test.

Box 2
Resources

Organization Resources
The Arthritis Foundation
1330 West Peachtree Street
Atlanta, GA 30309
1-404-872-7100 or 1-800-283-7800
Internet address: www.arthritis.org

This organization offers excellent free booklets about SLE, pain management, medications, fatigue, stress management, and exercise. Local chapters are in most states. The Arthritis Foundation provides community self-help programs in SLE management (*Systemic Lupus Erythematosus Self-Help Course* [1994]), exercise, aquatic programs, and support groups.

National Sjögren's Syndrome Association
5815 North Black Canyon Highway
Suite 103
Phoenix, AZ 85015-2200
602-433-9844 or 1-800-395-6772
Internet address:www.sjogrens.org or nssa@aol.com.

This organization offers books, videotapes, cassettes, and support.

The ROM Institute
3601 Memorial Drive
Madison, WI 53704

This company sells cassette tapes containing the *ROM Dance*. This video leads patients through a series of ROM activities with imagery and soft music to encourage relaxation. Titles include *ROM Dance in*

Sunlight, ROM Dance in Moonlight, and a seated version of the *ROM Dance*.

Lupus Foundation of America, Inc.
1300 Piccard Drive
Suite 200
Rockville, MD 20850-4303
301-670-9292 or 800-558-0121
Internet address:
http://internet-plaza.net/lupus/

This organization offers lay and professional information materials on SLE and pain, depression, kidney involvement, medications, and pregnancy. Local chapters throughout the United States provide education seminars and support groups.

Stanford Arthritis Center
Health Education Research
1000 Welch Road
#204
Palo Alto, CA 94304

This center is a source of different types of relaxation tapes specifically adapted for persons with rheumatic diseases and joint pain.

SLE Foundation
149 Madison Avenue
Suite 205
New York, NY 10016
1-212-685-4118
Internet address: www.lupuny.org

This organization provides a wide range of services for patients.

(continued)

Box 2 (continued)

Internet Resources

- A search for "systemic lupus erythematosus" on www.hotbot.com or the Alta Vista search directory will link you to all Web sites related to this topic.

- The Amazon Bookstore (www.amazon.com) lists all the books published on SLE.

- Abledata (www.abledata.com) is a national database on adaptive equipment and assistive devices.

- The Mining Company has excellent patient education material on all rheumatic diseases (http://lupus.miningco.com/msub1.htm).

Print Resources

Lupus: A Patient Care Guide for Nurses and Other Health Professionals (1997)

Available at no charge from the National Arthritis and Musculoskeletal and Skin Diseases (NAIMS) Information Clearinghouse

National Institutes of Health
1 AMS Circle
Bethesda, MD 20892-3675
1-301-718-6366
Internet address: www.nih.gov/niams

This is an excellent resource with topical patient education sheets for photocopying.

(See also volume 1, chapter 17, of this series.)

Two autoantibody systems are specific for SLE and may be used to confirm the diagnosis. A test for anti-dsDNA is positive in two thirds of patients, and about 30% of patients with SLE have positive tests for antibodies to the Sm antigen (anti-Sm).

Other autoantibodies include antibodies to Ro (anti-Ro, also known as anti-SSA) in about 40% of patients with SLE and antibodies to La (anti-La, also known as anti-SSB). Anti-Ro/SSA and anti-La/SSB occur in patients with Sjögren's syndrome. Anti-Ro/SSA is associated with subacute cutaneous lupus erythematosus (a form of lupus that is largely restricted to the skin). Antibodies against phospholipids may result in a false-positive test for syphilis and are associated with an increased tendency to develop arterial or venous blood clots (Gladman & Urowitz, 1997).

Reproduction and SLE

Family Planning

SLE primarily affects women during their childbearing years, and concerns about reproduction are common. Oral contraceptives have been implicated in causing lupus flares, but many physicians believe that contraceptives with low estrogen content are acceptable for patients with SLE (Arden, Lloyd, Spector, & Hughes, 1994). Using a diaphragm with a spermicidal jelly or having a tubal ligation are the methods least likely to exacerbate disease activity. Pregnancy should be planned only when the disease is in remission and when there is no elevation of anti-dsDNA antibody levels.

Effects of SLE Treatment on the Fetus

Prednisone is inactivated by the placenta, and doses of 60 mg/day or less do not reach the fetus. Therefore, this corticosteroid is used widely to treat pregnant women with SLE. Azathioprine and hydroxychloroquine have the potential to reach the fetus, but healthy infants have been delivered to women taking these drugs. Caution must be exercised with the use of nonsteroidal anti-inflammatory drugs (NSAIDs) during a SLE pregnancy. These drugs cross the placenta and may lead to premature constriction of the ductus arteriosus in the fetus. In addition, they affect platelet aggregation and may predispose premature infants to intracranial hemorrhage. Women should avoid pregnancy if they are taking cyclophosphamide or methotrexate.

Effects of Pregnancy on SLE

The woman with SLE who is planning to become pregnant must accept the fact that hers will be a high-risk pregnancy. The risk of a flare-up is increased during pregnancy. This topic is debated by many clinicians. There is evidence, however, that the risk of an exacerbation of SLE is increased if the disease is active at the time of conception (Mintz, Niz, Gutierrez, Garcia-Alonso, & Karchmer, 1986).

Effects of SLE on the Fetus

Fetal wastage and prematurity are increased in women with SLE. Growth and development of surviving children are believed to be normal. The neonatal SLE syndrome occurs when anti-Ro/SSA antibodies, anti-La/SSB antibodies, or both are transferred across the placenta from the mother's circulation into the developing fetus. The autoantibodies have the potential to cause transient skin rashes and low white blood cell counts in the fetus. A rare but potentially serious and permanent complication is congenital complete heart block, which can be diagnosed in the fetus before birth and may require treatment with a pacemaker (Buyon et al., 1988). Antiphospholipid antibodies are antibodies directed against negatively charged phospholipids. These antibodies are important in SLE pregnancy because they may be associated with recurrent fetal loss. Other problems related to antiphospholipid antibodies are vascular occlusion and thrombocytopenia. Women with antiphospholipid antibodies may require special treatment with corticosteroids, low-dose aspirin, heparin, or a combination of these drugs (Khamashta & Hughes, 1995).

Course and Prognosis

The course of SLE is highly variable, and outcome depends on the organs involved. Early detection and aggressive medical intervention before major organ damage occurs have dramatically improved the life expectancy of persons with SLE (Bertino & Lu, 1993; Hahn, 1997). Physical therapists and occupational therapists can help patients to develop a realistic but optimistic outlook. Patients have reported that the first few years after diagnosis are the most difficult. Learning about the disease and its effects on the body takes time, as does understanding and adjusting to the various medications. After several years, adjustment is easier for many patients. The prognosis for patients with SLE continues to improve.

Drug Therapy

Drug therapy, which is individualized and directed at specific clinical problems, ranges from moderate doses of aspirin to the use of drugs designed to create an immunosuppressed state (Gladman & Urowitz, 1997).

Arthralgias and arthritis can be suppressed with aspirin or other NSAIDs. Ibuprofen is usually avoided because it has been reported to cause aseptic meningitis, rash, fever, and abdominal pain in patients with SLE.

Photosensitivity and skin rashes may be mitigated by using sunscreens with a sun protection factor (SPF) of 15 or higher, ultraviolet-protective clothing, and antimalarial drugs. Hydroxychloroquine in doses of 200 to 400 mg/day is often used. Although the occurrence of retinal toxicity due to hydroxychloroquine is very low, ophthalmological examinations at 6-month intervals are recommended (Wallace, 1994).

Fever, severe rashes, and serositis are treated with a low dose of a corticosteroid preparation. Prednisone, the most commonly used steroid drug in SLE, is given at the level of 0.5 mg/kg/day or less in one or two daily doses. Alternate-day therapy seldom suppresses the symptoms of active disease. After a disease flare-up is controlled and the prednisone dose is tapered to a maintenance level of 5 or 10 mg/day, the dose may be changed gradually to an every-other-day schedule.

SLE crisis, neuropsychiatric disease, severe hemolytic anemia, thrombocytopenia, and severe SLE renal disease are customarily treated with high doses of prednisone of 1.0 mg/kg/day (for a 140-lb. woman, the dose would be 60 mg/day). Intravenous methylprednisolone may be used for severely ill patients. After high-dose corticosteroid treatment is started, the initial dose is usually maintained for 4 weeks. As a favorable clinical response occurs, the dose is tapered gradually over a period of months and even years. It is often not possible to discontinue prednisone completely.

Complications of Corticosteroid Therapy

Corticosteroids are used commonly to treat SLE, and patients and therapists must have a good understanding of their potential complications. This class of drugs is effective in resolving most manifestations of SLE and can be lifesaving.

Most patients who take corticosteroids will eventually experience a change in body habitus referred to as *cushingoid features* that involve truncal obesity, facial fullness ("moon facies"), and stretch marks on the abdomen and thighs. These changes are reversible after reduction or discontinuation of the drug. Other possible adverse reactions are cataracts, hypertension, myopathy, osteoporosis, osteonecrosis, alterations in mood or personality (including mood swings), psychosis, thin fragile skin, and increased susceptibility to infections. Laboratory tests may show elevations of blood glucose and serum cholesterol concentrations (Stein & Pincus, 1997). In some cases, treatment with potent immunosuppressive drugs such as methotrexate, azathioprine, or cyclophosphamide (Cytoxan) afford better control of the disease and permit the use of lower doses of corticosteroids (Klippel, 1997).

Rehabilitation

Earlier diagnosis and more effective medical intervention have resulted in increased survival for persons with SLE. Therefore, intervention by allied health professionals for persons affected by SLE is important. Patient education, arthritis and symptom self-management, joint protection, pain control, fatigue management, stress management, fitness exercise, and social and psychiatric interventions may be required during the course of the illness. Occupational therapists and physical therapists can usually obtain insurance reimbursement for patient education in self-management.

It is crucial for therapists working with patients with SLE to be aware of the spectrum of potential health problems that this disease can cause. Complications of the disease can delay the achievement of rehabilitation goals. Physical therapy referrals for persons with SLE are made frequently for management of pain and fatigue, strengthening exercises, aerobic conditioning, osteoporosis prevention, treatment of avascular necrosis (AVN), postoperative joint surgery, or rehabilitation after a cerebrovascular accident (CVA) (see Table 1).

Occupational therapy referrals are most often for hand or upper-extremity therapy, hand orthoses, joint protection training, ergonomic education, energy conservation and fatigue management, activities of daily living (ADL) evaluation, ADL training and assistive technology, education about Raynaud's phenomenon, and postoperative hand surgery. Patients with neuropsychiatric symptoms may require psychiatric occupational therapy intervention.

Evaluation

Evaluation is a major component of rehabilitative management. Objective evaluations must be repeated over time to document rehabilitation changes and possible disease fluctuation (Gall, 1988). The evaluation should include a thorough medical history, objective pain evaluation,

Table 1. Indications for Occupational Therapy and Physical Therapy Intervention in Systemic Lupus Erythematosus

Problems	Interventions
Arthralgias, arthritis, myalgias, and stiffness	Training in self-management of symptoms
Hand and upper-extremity arthritis	ADL training and assistive technology
Muscle weakness and atrophy	Joint protection training
Deconditioning	Gait training
Impaired ability for self-care, ADL, and instrumental ADL	Therapeutic exercise (ROM, strengthening)
	Fitness exercise
Fatigue	Hand therapy and splinting
Stress and depression	Foot orthoses
CVA	Fatigue management (e.g., energy conservation,
AVN	ergonomic education, work simplification, sleep
Raynaud's phenomenon	hygiene)
Osteoporotic risk or fracture	Weight control education
	Sleep hygiene training

Note: ADL=Activities of daily living, CVA=cerebrovascular accident, AVN=avascular necrosis, ROM=range of motion.

musculoskeletal evaluation, fatigue evaluation (including sleep pattern and quality), and functional ADL evaluation. Documentation should include the presence of cutaneous manifestations (e.g., rashes, thin skin, ulcerations), Raynaud's phenomenon, and information about neuropsychiatric status (e.g., depressed affect, frequent headaches) or steroid euphoria (manifested by difficulty with focusing, concentration, and retention). Additional information regarding the person's social support system; home, work, and school status; knowledge about SLE and its treatment; and previous treatments is valuable.

Health status assessments are a valuable source of information. Many are valid and reliable in SLE populations. The most commonly used tools for SLE include the Health Assessment Questionnaire (HAQ) (Milligan et al., 1993), the modified HAQ (Callahan, Brooks, Summey, & Pincus, 1987), and the Arthritis Impact Measurement Scales (AIMS) (Joyce, Berkebile, Hastings, Yarboro, & Yocum, 1989). The shortened form of the HAQ includes eight functional tasks (dressing, standing, eating, walking, hygiene, reaching, gripping, and errands and chores) plus visual-analog pain and fatigue scales. Valid and reliable, the HAQ's brief completion time and easy scoring have made it a popular clinical tool (Callahan et al., 1987; Hawley, 1998).

All physical therapy and occupational therapy intervention should result from a thorough evaluation of the patient's condition, the goals of the patient and therapist, the patient's support network, and sound therapeutic principles. It is imperative to recognize that, for persons with SLE, changes in disease status are inevitable, and programs will extend far beyond the discharge date. All program instruction should be provided in writing. Family members should be involved early. Patients and family members need education in self-management and methods for modifying the program when SLE is active.

Implications for Managed Care

In the current managed health care environment, visits to physical therapists and occupational therapists are allocated according to the primary condition and are strictly limited by number or length of time. This has increased the need for physical therapists and occupational therapists to coordinate care so that all necessary treatment is covered. Good communication becomes essential to optimize an effective treatment plan.

- Documentation, communication, and early education of the health insurer are important. SLE has an unpredictable course, and patients often have disease complications and comorbid health problems that compromise the ability to achieve treatment goals.
- Provide persons with SLE with the necessary written information about the entire spectrum of their rehabilitation process, and involve their family members. Education should focus on self-management and independent functioning, with specifics on home programs, setting goals, managing flare-ups, self-monitoring and modifying their home program, and public and community programs and other resources available for education and support (Boutaugh & Brady, 1998; Haralson-Ferrell, 1998). (See Box 2 and volume 1, chapter 17, of this series.)
- As always, early and ongoing communication with the referring physician is vital.

Patient Education

The importance of comprehensive patient and family member education cannot be overemphasized (Klippel, 1998). Ongoing support, education, and programming make an important difference in health status and quality of life for persons with chronic diseases (Boutaugh & Brady, 1998; Braden, McGlone, & Pennington, 1993). Patients in one survey (White, 1977 as cited in Sutton, Navarro, & Stevens, 1984) wanted to know

- what SLE is, how it affects the body, and what laboratory studies mean;
- the emotional effects of SLE and drug treatment;
- the warning signs of and how to avoid flare-ups;
- how to use medication, what the side effects are, and how to reduce them;
- how to avoid fatigue and pace activities; and
- how to educate family members about SLE.

In this same survey, 40% of the respondents identified physical problems as their main concern, and 38% identified psychosocial problems as their main concern.

The Arthritis Foundation has developed an SLE self-management course modeled after the successful course for persons with arthritis. This course consists of seven weekly 2.5-hr sessions designed for groups of 8 to 18 literate adults of all ages. The classes are offered throughout the country (Box 2). Health professionals interested in teaching these courses should contact their state Arthritis Foundation chapter. Braden (1991) evaluated the changes that 291 course participants demonstrated in "learned response to chronic illness" during the course and 2 months after the course and found that "uncertainty" and "depression" decreased over time and "enabling skill," "self-efficacy," and "self-worth" increased. The participants demonstrated an increased knowledge about SLE and management skills such as use of rest, relaxation, heat, and exercise.

Rest, avoidance of agents that may trigger an exacerbation (e.g., ultraviolet light, infection, certain drugs, stress, fatigue), and education are important. The patient with SLE should be encouraged to learn about the disease and to adopt an attitude of realistic optimism, empowerment, and control over the life situation. The Arthritis Foundation is an excellent source of information about SLE. The Lupus Foundation of America has many resources for the patient with SLE, and local chapters of this organization provide educational seminars and invaluable peer group support (Box 2).

Fitness Exercise

Most persons with SLE who are referred to therapy have not been able to exercise for quite some time due to arthritis, fatigue, or systemic manifestations. The challenge for therapists is to get these patients into a regular fitness exercise program without increasing symptoms. Research on exercise in the rheumatic diseases has demonstrated the value of low-impact aerobic conditioning. In clinically stable patients, conditioning programs for SLE have proved effective in increasing aerobic capacity by as much as 20% without symptom exacerbation (Alpiner, Oh, Hinderer, & Brander 1995). Control of inflammation, disease process, and joint swelling should be achieved before beginning a conditioning program (Minor, 1998).

Table 2. Symptoms and Aerobic Exercise Program Modification in Systemic Lupus Erythematosus

Symptom	Modification
Fatigue, arthralgia, and myalgia	Reduce duration or intensity of aerobic session, exercise for less time but more frequently throughout the day, intersperse brief exercise (3–5 min) with rest periods (1–2 min), and gradually resume program as able.
Acute joint inflammation	Modify program to gentle ROM, treat joint with cold modalities and splint if possible, continue other exercises that do not involve the joint, and slowly restart the program as symptoms subside.
Sudden acute joint pain that persists	May indicate fracture or AVN; stop aerobics; and contact the physician. Patients may continue ROM for unaffected areas.
Difficulty rising from a chair, using steps, or using arms overhead and aching in proximal muscles	May indicate myositis; contact physician, stop fitness exercise, and continue ROM.
Chest pain with exertions and acute shortness of breath	This may indicate pleurisy or pericarditis. Stop aerobic activity and contact a physician.
Difficulty following instructions, forgetting to self-monitor heart rate, or exhibiting poor judgment during exercise	Close monitoring by a physical therapist during exercise is necessary, and involvement and careful instruction of a home support network is needed.

Source: Alpiner et al. (1995), Banwell (1988), Robb-Nicholson et al. (1989), and Schur (1993).

Note: ROM=range of motion, AVN=avascular necrosis.

Anecdotal experience of the authors suggests that persons with SLE can obtain positive results from less intense fitness programs (e.g., "stretch and tone" classes or gentle exercise or water programs). Benefits may include increased hardiness, improved functional strength, decreased inflammation, improved energy levels, decreased depression, elevated self-esteem, improved self-effectiveness, and better-quality sleep. For debilitated persons, these classes may lead to cardiovascular conditioning. Information on exercise design is included later in this chapter. Debilitated patients must begin at a low level of activity. For some, walking one block will be too much. For persons experiencing flare-ups, strenuous exercise is not recommended and, indeed, may not be possible. For patients with mild flare-ups, modifications to exercise programs may include changing the duration or intensity of the exercise, interspersing exercise and rest periods, and decreasing the number of times exercise is performed throughout the day. Symptoms such as foot or knee pain while walking can be reduced by using appropriate supportive footwear with shock-absorbing soles. Orthotic inserts or heel pads may be helpful. (See the Appendix at the end of this volume on shoes and foot orthoses.) Other symptoms that may require modification of a fitness program are described in Table 2.

The fitness activity should be chosen on the basis of patient preference, accessibility, desired goals, and associated factors such as photosensitivity. The goal is maximum long-term patient adherence. Possibilities for fitness conditioning in SLE include walking (indoors if photosensitive), stationary or moving bicycles, treadmills, jogging, non- or low-impact aerobics, and aquatic exercise. Persons with knee and foot arthritis generally do better with varied exercises rather than repetitive exercises such as walking or pedaling. Persons with hand arthritis must be cautious about holding onto bicycle or equipment handles. Persons with polyarthritis often do well in warm-water pool exercise programs, but the pool must have easy access for persons who cannot manage a pool ladder. Pool shoes help cushion the feet. Pool activity is contraindicated if the warm water increases fatigue.

Aerobic Conditioning

Fatigue in SLE has been ascribed, in part, to lowered aerobic capacity (Alpiner, et al., 1995). Compared with healthy age- and gender-matched populations, persons with SLE perform at about 45% of their expected aerobic capacity, a level similar to that found in patients with RA (Robb-Nicholson et al., 1989). In clinically stable patients, conditioning programs for SLE were effective in increasing aerobic capacity by as much as 20% without symptom exacerbation (Alpiner et al., 1995). When the patient is ready for an advanced program, aerobic conditioning can provide benefits in the presence of deconditioning (Alpiner et al., 1995), weight gain, and osteoporosis. Aerobic conditioning can likewise help prevent bone demineralization (Hahn & Mazzaferri, 1995) and assist in management of fatigue (Robb-Nicholson et al., 1989) and depression (Alpiner et al., 1995; Robb-Nicholson et al., 1989).

Before beginning an exercise program, persons with SLE should have their physician's approval, undergo a physical therapy evaluation, and receive exercise education specific to their needs. Guidelines in one study excluded persons from aerobic conditioning programs who had elevated creatine phosphokinase (CPK) levels, hematocrit levels less than or equal to 30%, previous myocardial infarction or CVA, severe cognitive impairments (e.g., cerebritis), resting diastolic blood pressure greater than or equal to 100 mmHg, severe arthritis of three or more weight-bearing joints, or who received beta-blocker therapy (Robb-Nicholson et al., 1989). Lung and cardiac involvement could likewise be a restriction.

In the absence of these parameters, an aerobic conditioning program should begin at approximately 60% of maximum heart rate. Gradual progression can continue toward achieving 60% to 80% of the maximum heart rate. A person with clinically stable SLE could begin with a 5-min warm-up (e.g., range of motion [ROM], slow walking), 3 to 5 min of aerobic exercise, and 5 min of cool-down and then add 3 to 5 min of the aerobic program per week until the goal of 30 min for the total program (three times per week) is achieved (Alpiner et al., 1995).

Instruction in self-monitoring heart rate, perceived exertion, and use of the "talk test" is an essential part of physical therapy management. An exercise diary is helpful for monitoring long-term programs (Lorig & Fries, 1990). Written instructions for all exercise activities must be provided. Exercise success and maintenance appear to be enhanced by using time, rather than distance, as the aerobic exercise goal (Minor, 1998).

Symptoms and Management

Arthritis and Pain

Arthralgias or arthritis are the most common presenting manifestation of SLE, and up to 53% of patients develop frank arthritis (Figure 2) (Fries & Holman, 1975). The arthritis associated with SLE has the same distribution as that in RA (i.e., it is symmetrical and affects the small peripheral joints more frequently than the larger joints). Unlike RA, the arthritis associated with SLE typically does not erode the cartilage but primarily affects the capsule and supporting structures (Labowitz & Schumacher, 1974). Hand deformities are not as common as in RA, but they do occur. Approximately 5% of persons with SLE develop deforming arthropathy (e.g., swan-neck deformities, metacarpophalangeal [MCP] subluxation, ulnar drift, thumb deformities, and occasional carpal collapse) (Nalebuff & Melvin, in press). The deformities in SLE are primarily due to capsular and ligamentous

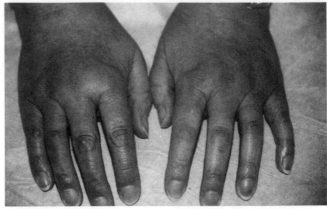

Figure 2. A woman (47 years of age) had SLE for 13 years with fever, photosensitivity, malar rash, arthritis, and proteinuria. She had positive tests for ANAs, anti-SSA/Ro, anti-dsDNA, and anti-Sm. Her disease flared up, and she developed painful, swollen MCP joints. The arthritis resolved after treatment was begun with prednisone 20 mg/day. (Photo courtesy of Sara Walker, MD)

laxity rather than erosive cartilage and bone changes. Therefore, joint instability and subluxation are common sequelae; contractures and ankylosis are unusual (Cronin, 1988). Joints most commonly involved are the proximal interphalangeal, MCP, wrist, and metatarsophalangeal joints; the interphalangeal joints of the feet; and the knee (Alpiner et al., 1995; Feldman, Zuckerman, & Buyon, 1992).

Conditions That Mimic Arthritis

Complications of corticosteroid therapy that can be misinterpreted as arthritis include AVN that is found frequently in the femoral head and less frequently in the shoulders, proximal femurs, and distal tibial areas. It is rare in the scaphoid bone in the wrist. AVN presents with pain, small effusions, and decreased ROM and function of the affected joint. Another complication misinterpreted as arthritis is accelerated osteoporosis resulting in compression fractures, especially in postmenopausal women, that can present as acute back or rib pain (Stein & Pincus, 1997). Therapists should be alert for these symptoms and have the patient report them to the physician.

Systemic Lupus Erythematosus and Fibromyalgia Syndrome

One study of 102 persons with SLE indicated that 22% showed signs of FMS when using the American College of Rheumatology diagnostic criteria for FMS, which suggests that FMS is not uncommon in persons with SLE (Middleton, McFarlin, & Lipsky, 1994). FMS is associated with the following symptoms: diffuse pain or tenderness throughout the body, fatigue, subjective sense of muscle weakness, muscular aching and pain, headaches, tenderness at specific tender points, impaired cognitive skills, increased depression or anxiety, and sleep disorders. Frequently, the symptoms of FMS are misinterpreted as SLE symptoms. Therapists working with patients with SLE should be aware of the diagnostic, evaluative, and treatment approaches for FMS. (See chapter 6 in this volume.) There appears to be a subset of women who developed a malar rash, sun sensitivity, Raynaud's phenomenon, borderline positive ANA, arthralgias, and FMS. Further symptoms of SLE never developed, and FMS became the primary problem. The patients with and without FMS did not differ in measures of SLE activity (Middleton et al., 1994).

Treatment of pain and fatigue in persons with both SLE and FMS is challenging and requires careful monitoring, an understanding of each diagnosis, and a blend of management techniques.

Rehabilitation Management of Arthritis and Pain

Chronic arthritis and pain are best managed in a holistic, self-management approach that includes good sleep, excellent nutrition, regular exercise, stress management, and joint protection techniques.

The program emphasis should be on providing the patient with the tools needed to gain a sense of control over the symptoms and the ability to function. Specific physical measures include the application of superficial thermal modalities and ROM exercise. Cold application must be used with caution, especially in the small joints of the hands and feet, because Raynaud's phenomenon is frequently present. Cold can be successfully used in a limited fashion for acute large-joint inflammation and pain. Joint pain or arthritis with laxity should be treated with functional orthotic support, counteractive muscle strengthening exercise, and thermal agents. Persons with SLE may experience both acute and chronic pain. When managing chronic pain, biofeedback, stress management and relaxation techniques, and routine conditioning exercise programs are useful.

Treatment for the acute, subacute, and chronic stages of arthritis is the same as outlined for inflammatory joint disease in RA. (See chapter 7 in this volume.)

Therapeutic exercise. Indications for exercise programs in SLE are numerous. Exercise, when applied to persons with rheumatic disease, is generally described in three categories: ROM, strengthening, and aerobic conditioning (Banwell, 1988). For patients with SLE, exercise combats depression and helps to counteract three undesirable side effects of corticosteroid medications: osteoporosis, weakness of the shoulder and hip girdle muscles (steroid myopathy), and weight gain.

ROM. ROM exercises are indicated to maintain or improve joint ROM in persons with arthralgias, arthritis, and joint stiffness. Myalgias, muscular weakness, and postural problems benefit from specifically designed ROM exercises. These exercises are traditionally used as part of the warm-up and cool-down phases of aerobic programs. Active ROM should be used on days when the person's fatigue level prohibits participation in a more vigorous exercise routine or aerobic program. Keep in mind that persons with SLE tend to have joint laxity, so patients often must be cautioned not to "overrange" a joint because excessive stretching can be detrimental.

Active ROM is encouraged at all times except in acute myositis with acutely elevated CPK levels. Active assisted ROM or therapist-dispensed passive ROM may be indicated until the inflammation is controlled to avoid muscle tissue damage.

Two ROM video programs appropriate for persons with SLE and arthritis are useful: *P.A.C.E. Level I* and *II* (*People with Arthritis Can Exercise*) and the *ROM Dance*. Although none is a substitute for individually designed physical therapy programs, any one of them may improve the person's adherence to home programs by providing easily accessible activities (Box 2).

Strengthening. Exercise to improve muscle strength may be performed isometrically and isotonically. When using isometric exercise, it is important to be aware of any limiting conditions such as cardiopulmonary involvement or hypertension. Similarly, isotonic exercise may require modification in persons with joint changes, AVN, or myositis.

Even in the presence of acute joint pain and inflammation, isometric exercise can generally be performed with minimal risk of exacerbating joint symptoms. Subacute or chronic joint pain allows for gradual progression of isotonic and resistive exercise. The preferred application of these exercises is single-joint short-arc motion. Resistive exercises on several joints increase the likelihood that deforming forces may develop.

Therapists must keep in mind that persons with SLE may experience daily fluctuations in their ability to perform exercise. Programs must involve methods to modify exercise without quitting. This information is crucial for home programs and should always be given verbally and in writing.

Strengthening of the hands. The hands are unique, in part, because of the functional demands placed on a kinetic chain of joints controlled by long tendons. Inflammation or laxity in any joint in the chain can alter the biomechanical forces on all the joints in the chain. In most joints, strong muscles improve stability and help protect the joints. This is not necessarily true in the hands, however, where a combination of strong muscles and fragile joints can be a formula for deformity and dislocation. Persons with arthritis in their hands must use their hands gently. Over a period of time, this will naturally reduce hand strength; this is not necessarily harmful, as long as patients are able to perform self-care and basic daily activities. Weakness itself is not an automatic indication for strengthening exercises. Patients often complain that their hands are so weak that they cannot open a jar or car door, and this usually generates a referral to occupational therapy for hand strengthening. In these cases, it is critical to determine whether the problem is a result of true weakness or of pain inhibiting muscle strength. If it is the latter, then the treatment should be joint protection training, not strengthening. If it is true weakness, then a determination must be made regarding whether strengthening grip muscles will increase deforming forces on the hand. If so, then adaptive devices and joint protection techniques may be the best solution (Melvin, 1989; Melvin, in press; Nalebuff & Melvin, in press).

Fatigue and systemic manifestations. Fatigue is almost universal in patients with active SLE, and many patients consider it to be their most disabling problem (Krupp, LaRocca, Muir, & Steinberg, 1990). Systemic symptoms include fever, malaise, fatigue, weight loss, anorexia, and weakness. Systemic manifestations (except for fever) must be distinguished from the symptoms of depression.

Fatigue is a symptom of SLE that can be the most influenced by rehabilitation. There is no universally accepted definition of fatigue (Goldenberg, 1995). One suggested definition is "an overwhelming sense of exhaustion with decreased capacity for physical and mental work that is sustained and not relieved by rest" (Carpenito, 1993, p. 316). In 80% to 100% of persons with SLE, fatigue is present even when there are no other symptoms (Goldenberg, 1995; Schur, 1993). For practical purposes, the fatigue of SLE can be defined as decreased endurance and stamina.

Fatigue can be disruptive to the patient's lifestyle, interfere with gainful employment and family responsibilities, and detract from social activities. Fatigue is usually present to some degree in all patients with SLE, regardless of their disease activity. An increase in the usual level of fatigue can be an early indicator that the disease is becoming more active. Fatigue may be intensified by depression, which is often associated with SLE. Poor sleep patterns and sleep disruption from corticosteroids predispose patients to FMS, which often coexists with SLE. (See chapter 6 in this volume.) In some instances, SLE disease activity may regress or respond to therapy, but FMS may remain and become the primary problem that requires treatment.

Factors that increase the level of fatigue in persons with rheumatic diseases include flare-up of illness, associated medical disorders, sleep disturbances, minor or major mood disturbances, psychosocial stressors, and cardiovascular deconditioning (Goldenberg, 1995). Several fatigue scales are available, but there is no agreement on which one is most useful for fatigue evaluation (Goldenberg, 1995; McNair, Lorr, & Droppleman, 1971; Schwartz, Jandorf, & Krupp, 1993). An example of an analog scale used to document fatigue is shown in Figure 3 (Robb-Nicholson et al., 1989).

Instructions: For questions 1–4, circle the number that best describes you on the following scales. Each scale is different. Be sure to read each question carefully.

1. In the last 7 days, how would you describe your stamina?

0   1   2   3   4   5   6   7   8   9   10

Can't do anything   I'm able to do everything
without getting   I want to do and still have
tired or pooped.   some energy left over for other things.

2. Compared with others of my age and gender, I have

0   1   2   3   4   5   6   7   8   9   10

Less energy   More energy

3. All in all, my energy level is

0   1   2   3   4   5   6   7   8   9   10

Not enough for   More than enough
what I want to do   for what I want to do

4. I am tired

0   1   2   3   4   5   6   7   8   9   10

All of the time   Never

Figure 3. Scale of fatigue. *Note:* From "Effects of aerobic conditioning in lupus fatigue: A pilot study," by L. C. Robb-Nicholson, L. Daltroy, H. Eaton, V. Gall, E. Wright, L. H. Hartley, P. H. Schur, and M. H. Liang, 1989, *British Journal of Rheumatology, 28*(6), pp. 500–505. Copyright 1989 by Oxford University Press. Reprinted with permission. For patient use the scales must be 10 cm long.

Rehabilitation management of fatigue. Treatment depends on whether the underlying disease is active or inactive. If the patient with SLE is experiencing increased fatigue because the disease is active, some improvement is expected after the flare-up of disease is treated with medications. During a flare-up, rest is required, and conditioning exercise is not beneficial. Patients with inactive SLE continue to require sufficient rest. Some patients perform best when they have 10 hours of sleep per night; others may need 8 or 9 hours at night plus a nap during the day. Physical therapists and occupational therapists provide fatigue management through development of aerobic exercise plans, pain management programs, sleep hygiene training, and instruction in energy conservation, time management, and relaxation techniques. Other possible interventions, many of which can be applied directly by the patient, are outlined in the fatigue care wheel shown in Figure 4 (Systemic Lupus Erythematosus Self-Help Course, 1994). (See volume 1, chapter 12, of this series for information on fatigue management.)

Level of fatigue is affected by sleep and rest patterns. Some patients taking high doses of corticosteroids may have a great deal of difficulty sleeping at night, which results in greater fatigue and pain amplification during the day. (See chapter 3 in this volume.) (Patients with disturbed sleep or who awake exhausted should follow the guidelines for sleep enhancement recommended for persons with FMS in chapter 6 in this volume.)

Muscle involvement and management. SLE can produce inflammatory myositis with proximal muscle weakness. True inflammatory myopathy is relatively rare in SLE and occurs in 5% to 10% of patients (Cronin, 1988). The most common cause of muscle weakness in SLE is corticosteroid treatment (Klippel, 1997). Steroid myopathy is not inflammatory and is usually painless and insidious in onset. The initial complaints are difficulty doing activities at shoulder height or stepping up onto a curb. The proximal muscles are weak initially, and weakness may progress to involve distal muscle groups. Steroid myopathy is treated by reducing the drug. Antimalarial drugs such as

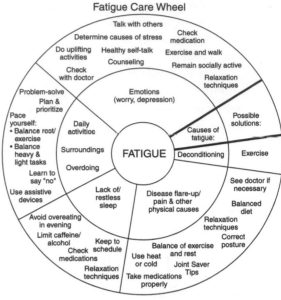

Figure 4. Fatigue interventions in SLE (fatigue care wheel). *Note:* From *Systemic lupus erythematosus self-help course*, 1994, Atlanta, GA: The Arthritis Foundation. Copyright 1994 by the Arthritis Foundation. Reprinted with permission.

hydroxychloroquine can cause vacuolar myopathy and muscle weakness. When hydroxychloroquine-induced myopathy occurs, the medication is discontinued (Cronin, 1988).

In SLE-related muscle inflammation (myositis), physicians monitor serum CPK levels. CPK is elevated when muscle tissue breaks down or is damaged by inflammation. When CPK is elevated, weak muscles must be protected. In the acute phase, exercise is restricted, and passive ROM is used to prevent contractures. Timing for active and resistive exercise is determined by CPK levels. Physical therapy and occupational therapy for this type of myositis is the same as for polymyositis. (See chapter 12 in this volume.)

The therapist should be alert to signs of proximal muscle weakness in all patients with SLE, especially if treatment includes corticosteroids or hydroxychloroquine. Typical signs of involvement include difficulty in stabilizing the neck, drooping of the shoulders, difficulty rising from a chair without assistance (not resulting from joint involvement), a waddling gait, or difficulty stepping onto a step or curb. Sometimes the problem presents as a dramatic reduction in muscle strength. If these signs are observed, a group muscle test should be performed to detect actual proximal weakness, and the findings should be reported to the physician as soon as possible.

In the presence of myositis, as in any situation involving acute inflammation, deep modalities such as ultrasound, diathermy, and laser therapy are contraindicated.

Raynaud's Phenomenon and Management

Raynaud's phenomenon is present in 18% to 20% of persons with SLE (Hodges, 1995). Affected persons have digital coldness, aching, and reduced sensation and function. Symmetrical digital pallor (white) appears with exposure to cold or stress followed by cyanosis (blue) and hyperemic rubor (red) (Hodges, 1995.) Physical examination should include pulses, documentation of trophic skin changes, and presence of digital ulcers. Raynaud's phenomenon associated with SLE differs from that seen with systemic sclerosis (scleroderma) in that it often resolves if the SLE goes into prolonged remission. Intervention should involve education in prevention of occurrences. (See Table 7 on self-management of Raynaud's phenomenon in chapter 9 in this volume.) Skin temperature biofeedback has been used with some success in long-term management (Hodges, 1995).

Cardiopulmonary Involvement and Management

Cardiac involvement in SLE may consist of inflammation of the pericardium with accumulation of pericardial fluid (pericarditis). This complication of SLE is manifested by sharp pain under the anterior chest wall, and the patient may experience shortness of breath. The heart muscle itself may become involved, which leads to myocarditis. This is a very severe manifestation of SLE; the heart may become enlarged, and congestive heart failure may develop. Patients with myocarditis are usually quite ill and experience shortness of breath and extremely limited exercise tolerance. Active exercise is contraindicated until pericardial and myocardial inflammation are controlled by treatment, which usually consists of high-dose corticosteroids.

In addition, the pleura and lungs may be involved. Pleural fluid may collect around the lungs (pleurisy), and this complication is often associated with pleuritic chest pain (i.e., sharp pain made worse by taking a deep breath or coughing). The lungs themselves may become inflamed, a condition known as *lupus pneumonitis*. The pneumonitis makes patients quite ill, and many require assisted breathing and high doses of corticosteroids (Gladman & Urowitz, 1997).

In general, pericarditis and pleurisy are more common, more painful, and less harmful than deeper involvement of the heart and lungs. The therapist must watch carefully for limitation of work tolerance in patients with SLE. Shortness of breath and chest pain should be reported promptly to the physician.

Avascular Necrosis and Management

AVN occurs in 3% to 52% of persons with SLE (Schur, 1993). Persons treated with long-term high-dose corticosteroids (e.g., more than 20 mg/day of prednisone) are at greatest risk for developing AVN; however, it can occur in patients who are not taking corticosteroids. Rehabilitative measures depend on the method of management.

It is important to carefully monitor for AVN. AVN in SLE most commonly involves the femoral head and less frequently involves the shoulder and distal tibia (Schur, 1993). In the hip, AVN may present as vague aching in the groin, or the pain may develop suddenly. Initially, the pain may respond to treatment with aspirin or other NSAIDs, but the pain tends to persist.

The therapist can be helpful by bringing complaints of hip pain in a corticosteroid-treated patient with SLE to the attention of the physician. It is extremely important to make the diagnosis of AVN early before the femoral head has begun to collapse. The most accurate noninvasive test for making the diagnosis is magnetic resonance imaging (MRI). MRI can confirm the diagnosis in the earliest stage when hip radiography is still normal. Patients with early (stage 1) AVN of the hip may be treated with surgical decompression, in which an orthopedic surgeon drills a hole through the femoral head. Patients are then not weight bearing for a prolonged period (up to 6 months) (Warner, Philip, Brodsky, & Thornhill, 1987). Patients with early collapse of the femoral head may not be weight bearing in an attempt to arrest progress of femoral head destruction. Most persons with femoral head collapse have total hip arthroplasty (Feldman, Zuckerman, & Buyon, 1992). Patients usually need training with assistive devices to accomplish ADL while not weight bearing.

Renal Lupus and Management

Some patients have SLE for many years and never develop clinical involvement of the kidneys, but about 25% of patients develop severe renal disease. The type and severity of renal involvement is usually determined by a needle biopsy of the kidney. Patients with the more severe forms of lupus nephritis and diffuse proliferative glomerulonephritis (Class IV) have severe inflammation and destruction of renal glomeruli. They traditionally receive treatment with high-dose corticosteroids such as prednisone (60 to 80 mg/day). Prednisone is often given in combination with intravenous doses of cyclophosphamide (Cytoxan). Kidney involvement can lead to hypertension, leg edema, fatigue, and renal failure. Rehabilitation goals may therefore be limited when the renal disease is active.

Neuropsychiatric Involvement and Management

Functional changes are common in SLE. Patients may react to the disease with depression, anxiety, and increased psychological needs. SLE may affect the CNS directly and produce various signs and symptoms, and the therapist should be alert for neuropsychological involvement. Headaches, memory loss, diminished cognitive ability, confusion, psychosis, paralysis, movement disorders, and motor and sensory neuropathies may indicate CNS involvement (Calabrese & Stern, 1995; Denburg, Denburg, Carbotte, Fisk, & Hanly, 1993; Gladman & Urowitz, 1997). Corticosteroids are potent drugs that may induce insomnia, cause the patient to feel hyperactive, and decrease mood stability. In addition, corticosteroids can produce a confusing clinical picture that mimics SLE of the CNS. Corticosteroids can produce depression, confusion, or even psychosis. Because psychological and neurological changes can indicate disease activity or drug toxicity, it is extremely important to report observed neurological or personality changes to the referring physician (Box 3).

Transverse cord myelopathy is rare but has been reported. It can result in quadriplegia or paraplegia.

Skin and Hair Manifestations and Management

An erythematous skin eruption may involve the sun-exposed areas of the face to form a characteristic malar or "butterfly" rash. Other rashes may occur over the face, neck, extremities, hands, and elbows. The rash may be episodic or chronic and may involve scarring. In some cases, the rash appears to be a healthy-looking blush. Exposure to sunlight or ultraviolet light frequently causes the rash or systemic manifestations to flare up, which is referred to as *photosensitivity*. Ulceration

---

Box 3
High-Dose Corticosteroids and Patient Education

A word of caution is needed regarding instruction for patients taking high-dose corticosteroids. This medication can produce a wide range of side effects, including euphoria and a false sense of well-being. This does not occur in all patients, but when it is present, even in a mild form, patient instruction is extremely difficult. When a patient is euphoric, he or she cannot perceive the seriousness of the condition or the need for instruction. Many of these patients are in the process of having their medications stabilized. If possible, patient education should be delayed until the medication is reduced. All education for patients on high-dose corticosteroids should be reinforced with written instructions.

---

of the mouth and nasal mucosa is possible. Nasal ulcers are painless but may be painful and make talking uncomfortable for the patient. These lesions resolve with corticosteroid therapy.

The patient with SLE skin involvement should be advised to avoid sun exposure, wear protective clothing, and use a sunscreen daily that has a SPF of at least 15. These precautions should be considered regardless of whether the rash flares up on exposure to the sun. Antimalarial drugs such as hydroxychloroquine are used commonly to treat cutaneous manifestations of SLE. The drug has a good safety record, but side effects may include noninflammatory myopathy, emotional changes, and the rare occurrence of retinal pigmentation with diminished visual acuity (Klippel, 1997). The use of concealing facial cosmetics may have a major positive effect on self-esteem.

Alopecia is a common manifestation of SLE. Although alopecia is usually not permanent, bald patches are seen with discoid lupus erythematosus. Hair loss may involve diffuse loss of head hair. When the disease becomes inactive, hair growth becomes normal. Some patients with active disease have "lupus hair," which is a collection of thin, broken hairs at the hair line. Most patients with SLE do not become completely bald. For patients with thinned hair, wearing a wig may have positive effects on self-confidence and social functioning (Callen, 1997; Drake et al., 1996; Sontheimer & Provost, 1997).

Joint Surgery: Postoperative Rehabilitation

The most common reason for joint arthroplasty in SLE is AVN. Rehabilitation of a person with SLE who has had total joint arthroplasty surgery follows commonly applied protocols and programs. (See volume 5 of this series.) However, each patient will present with complications from the disease itself that will provide challenges in accomplishing functional rehabilitation.

Postoperative rehabilitation will likely involve treatment of the SLE as well as treatment aimed at the operative site. Lightweight ambulation aids with adapted hand grips, use of modalities for pain management, and individualized exercise programs may be indicated. Goals established in physical therapy may be more moderate for this population than for patients without SLE.

Insurance companies and managed health care organizations must be informed early about the complicating factors involved in the patient's rehabilitation, the likely need for a longer course of physical therapy, the possibility of discharge to a rehabilitation center or nursing home, and the need for home therapy in the event of delayed independence. Close ongoing monitoring and physical therapy program modification, use of the patient's support system, and written home instructions are necessary.

Cerebral Vascular Accident Rehabilitation

CVAs occur in 5% to 15 % of persons with SLE (Schur, 1993). CVAs may be the result of the primary disease process or secondary to infection, uremia, kidney disease, or use of certain medications (Alpiner et al., 1995). These patients are likely to have comorbid medical problems.

Persons with SLE who experience a CVA are younger than the average patient with a CVA. They are more likely to have children and work responsibilities. Joint pain, stiffness, overwhelming fatigue, decreased aerobic capacity, and depression limit their ability to participate in rehabilitation. The rehabilitation approach will require a great deal of knowledge about the patient's condition, modification at many phases of rehabilitation, and treatment of the symptoms of SLE separate from those attributed to the CVA.

Conclusion

SLE is a complex illness that provides daily challenges for affected persons and their health care providers. Physical therapists and occupational therapists can have a positive effect on the quality of life of these persons by furnishing them with the tools necessary for successful symptom management, coping strategies, and improved health status through exercise conditioning.

References

Alarcon-Segovia, D. (1988). Systemic lupus erythematosus: Pathology and pathogenesis. In H. R. Schumacher (Ed.), *Primer on the rheumatic diseases* (9th ed., pp. 97–100). Atlanta, GA: Arthritis Foundation.

Alpiner, N., Oh, T. H., Hinderer, S. R., & Brander, V. A. (1995). Rehabilitation in joint and connective tissue diseases: 1: Systemic diseases. *Archives of Physical Medicine and Rehabilitation, 76,* S32–S40.

Andonopoulos, A. P., Skopouli, F. N., Dimou, G. S., Drosis, A. A., & Moutsoupoulos, H. M. (1990). Sjögren's syndrome in systemic lupus erythematosus. *Journal of Rheumatology, 17,* 201–204.

Arden, N. K., Lloyd, M. E., Spector, T. D., & Hughes, G. R. (1994). Safety of hormone replacement therapy (HRT) in systemic lupus erythematosus (SLE). *Lupus, 3,* 11–13.

Arnett, F. C., Jr. (1993). The genetic basis of lupus erythematosus. In D. J. Wallace, B. H. Hahn, F. P. Quismorio, Jr., & J. R. Klinenberg (Eds.), *Dubois' lupus erythematosus* (4th ed., pp. 13–36). Philadelphia: Lea & Febiger.

Banwell, B. F. (1988). Exercise for arthritis. In B. F. Banwell & V. Gall (Eds.), *Physical therapy management of arthritis* (pp. 43–66). New York: Churchill Livingstone.

Bertino, L. S., & Lu, L. C. (1993). The bite of the wolf: Systemic lupus erythematosus. *Rehabilitation Nursing, 18,* 173–178.

Boutaugh, M. L., & Brady, T. (1998). Patient education for self-management. In J. L. Melvin & G. Jensen (Eds.), *Rheumatologic rehabilitation series: Volume 1: Assessment and management* (pp. 219–258). Bethesda, MD: American Occupational Therapy Association.

Braden, C. J., McGlone, K., & Pennington, F. (1993). Specific psychosocial and behavioral outcomes from the Systemic Lupus Erythematosus Self-Help Course. *Health Education Quarterly, 20*, 29–41.

Braden, C. J. (1991). Patterns of change over time in learned response to chronic illness among participants in a systemic lupus erythematosus self help course. *Arthritis Care and Research, 4*, 158–167.

Buskila, D., & Schoenfeld, Y. (1992). Anti-DNA antibodies. In R. G. Lahita (Ed.), *Systemic lupus erythematosus* (2nd ed., pp. 205–236). New York: Churchill Livingstone.

Buyon, J., Roubey, R., Swersky, S., Pompeo, L., Parke, A., Baxi, L., & Winchester, R. (1988). Complete congenital heart block: Risk of occurrence and therapeutic approach to prevention. *Journal of Rheumatology, 15*, 1104–1108.

Calabrese, L. V., & Stern, T. A. (1995). Neuropsychiatric manifestations of systemic lupus erythematosus. *Psychosomatics, 36*, 344–359.

Callahan, L. F., Brooks, R. H., Summey, J. A., & Pincus, T. (1987). Quantitative pain assessment for routine care of rheumatoid arthritis patients using a pain scale based on activities of daily living and a visual analogue scale. *Arthritis and Rheumatism, 30*, 630–636.

Callen, J. P. (1997). Management of skin disease in lupus. *Bulletin on the Rheumatic Diseases, 46*, 4–7.

Carpenito, L. J. (1993). *Nursing diagnosis: Application to clinical practice* (5th ed.). Philadelphia: Lippincott.

Cronin, M. E. (1988). Musculoskeletal manifestations of systemic lupus erythematosus. *Rheumatic Disease Clinics of North America, 14*, 99–106.

Denburg, S. D., Denburg, J. A., Carbotte, R. M., Fisk, J., & Hanly, J. C. (1993). Cognitive deficits on systemic lupus erythematosus. *Rheumatic Disease Clinics of North America, 19*, 815–831.

Drake, L. A., Dinehart, S. M., Farmer, E. R., Goltz, R. W., Graham, G. F., Hordinsky, M. K., Lewis, C. W., Pariser, D. M., Skouge, J. W., Webster, S. B., Whitaker, D. C., Butler, B., Lowery, B. J., Sontheimer, R. D., Callen, J. P., Camisa, C., Provost, T. T., & Tuffanelli, D. L. (1996). Guidelines of care for cutaneous lupus erythematosus: American Academy of Dermatology. *Journal of the American Academy of Dermatology, 34*, 830–836.

Dubois, E. L. (1966). *Lupus erythematosus*. New York: McGraw-Hill.

Feldman, D. S., Zuckerman, J. D., & Buyon, J. P. (1992). Articular manifestations of systemic lupus erythematosus. In R. G. Lahita (Ed.), *Systemic lupus erythematosus* (2nd ed., pp. 823–844). New York: Churchill Livingstone.

Fox, D. A., & McCune, W. J. (1994). Immunosuppressive drug therapy of systemic lupus erythematosus. *Rheumatic Disease Clinics of North America, 20*, 265–299.

Fox, R. I. (1997). Sjögren's syndrome. In J. H., Klippel, C. M. Weyand, & R. L. Wortmann (Eds.), *Primer on the rheumatic diseases* (11th ed., pp. 283–288). Atlanta, GA: The Arthritis Foundation.

Fries, J., & Holman, H. (1975). *Lupus erythematosus: A clinical analysis*. Philadelphia: Saunders.

Friou, G. J. (1957). Clinical application of lupus serum-nucleoprotein reaction using the fluorescent antibody technique [Abstract]. *Journal of Clinical Investigation, 36*, 390.

Gall, V. (1988). Patient evaluation. In B. F. Banwell & V. Gall (Eds.), *Physical therapy management of arthritis* (pp. 43–66). New York: Churchill Livingstone.

Gladman, D. D., & Urowitz, M. B. (1997). Systemic lupus erythematosus: Clinical and laboratory features. In J. H. Klippel, C. M. Weyand, & R. L. Wortmann (Eds.), *Primer on the rheumatic diseases* (11th ed., pp. 251–257). Atlanta, GA: The Arthritis Foundation.

Goldenberg, D. L. (1995). Fatigue in rheumatic disease. *Bulletin on the Rheumatic Diseases, 44*, 4–8.

Hahn, B. H. (1997). Management of systemic lupus erythematosus. In W. N. Kelley, E. D. Harris, S. Ruddy, & C. B. Sledge (Eds.), *Textbook of rheumatology* (5th ed., pp. 1040–1056). Philadelphia: Saunders.

Hahn, B. H., & Mazzaferri, E. L. (1995). Glucocorticoid-induced osteoporosis. *Hospital Practice, 30*, 45–49, 52–56.

Haralson-Ferrell, K. M. (1998). Community resources in comprehensive rehabilitation. In J. L. Melvin & G. Jensen (Eds.), *Rheumatologic rehabilitation series: Volume 1: Assessment and management* (pp. 393–408). Bethesda, MD: American Occupational Therapy Association.

Hargraves, M. M., Richmond, H., & Morton, R. (1948). Presentation of two bone marrow elements: The "tart" cell and the "L. E." cell. *Proceedings of Staff Meetings of the Mayo Clinic, 23*, 25–28.

Harvey, A. M., Shulman, L. E., Tumulty, P. A., Conley, C., & Schoenrich, E. H. (1954). Systemic lupus erythematosus: Review of the literature and clinical analysis of 138 cases. *Medicine, 33*, 291–437.

Hawley, D. J. (1998). Clinical outcomes: Issues and measurements. In J. L. Melvin & G. Jensen (Eds.), *Rheumatologic rehabilitation series: Volume 1: Assessment and management* (pp. 65–92). Bethesda, MD: American Occupational Therapy Association.

Hochberg, M. C. (1992). Epidemiology of systemic lupus erythematosus. In R. G. Lahita (Ed.), *Systemic lupus erythematosus* (2nd ed., pp. 103–117). New York: Churchill Livingstone.

Hodges, H. (1995). Raynaud's disease: Pathophysiology, diagnosis and treatment. *Journal of the American Academy of Nurse Practitioners, 7*, 159–164.

Illei, G. G., & Klippel, J. H. (1999). Why is the ANA result positive? *Bulletin on the Rheumatic Diseases, 48*(1), 1–4.

Joyce, K., Berkebile, C., Hastings, C., Yarboro, C., & Yocum, D. (1989). Health status and disease activity in systemic lupus erythematosus. *Arthritis Care and Research, 2*, 65–69.

Kallenberg, C. G. (1993). Overlapping syndromes, undifferentiated connective tissue disease, and other fibrosing conditions. *Current Opinion in Rheumatology, 6*, 650–654.

Khamashta, M. A., & Hughes, G. R. V. (1995). Antiphospholipid antibodies and antiphospholipid syndrome. *Current Opinions in Rheumatology, 7*, 389–394.

Klippel, J. H. (1997). Systemic lupus erythematosus: Treatment. In J. H. Klippel, C. M. Weyand, & R. L. Wortmann (Eds.), *Primer on the rheumatic diseases* (11th ed., pp. 258–262). Atlanta, GA: The Arthritis Foundation.

Klippel, J. H. (1998). Systemic lupus erythematosus: Management. In J. H. Klippel & P. Dieppe (Eds.), *Rheumatology* (2nd ed., pp. 7.7.1–7.7.8). St. Louis, MO: Mosby.

Koffler, D., Schur, P. H., & Kunkel, H. G. (1967). Immunological studies concerning the nephritis of systemic lupus erythematosus. *Journal of Experimental Medicine, 126*, 607–624.

Krupp, L. B., LaRocca, N. G., Muir, J., & Steinberg, A. D. (1990). A study of fatigue in systemic lupus erythematosus. *Journal of Rheumatology, 17*, 1450–1452.

Labowitz, R., & Schumacher, H. R. (1974). Articular manifestations of systemic lupus erythematosus. *Annals of Internal Medicine, 74*, 911–921.

Lahita, R. G. (1992). Sex, age, and systemic lupus erythematosus. In R. G. Lahita (Ed.), *Systemic lupus erythematosus* (2nd ed., pp. 527–542). New York: Churchill Livingstone.

Liang, M. H., Stern, S., & Esdaile, J. M. (1988). Systemic lupus erythematosus activity: An operational definition. *Rheumatic Disease Clinics of North America, 14*, 57–66.

Lorig, K., & Fries, J. F. (1990). *The arthritis helpbook* (3rd ed.). Reading, MA: Addison-Wesley.

McNair, D. M., Lorr, M., & Droppleman, L. F. (1971). *Profile of Mood States manual*. San Diego, CA: Educational and Instructional Testing Services.

Melvin, J. L. (1989). Systemic lupus erythematosus. In J. L. Melvin (Ed.), *Rheumatic disease in the adult and child: Occupational therapy and rehabilitation* (3rd ed., pp. 99–105). Philadelphia: F. A. Davis.

Melvin, J. L., (in press). Therapeutic exercise and thermal modalities in the management of arthritis of the hand. In J. L. Melvin & E. A. Nalebuff (Eds.), *Rheumatologic rehabilitation series: Volume 4: The hand: Evaluation, therapy, and surgery*. Bethesda, MD: American Occupational Therapy Association.

Middleton, G. D., McFarlin, J. E., & Lipsky, P. E. (1994). The prevalence and clinical impact of fibromyalgia in systemic lupus erythematosus. *Arthritis and Rheumatism, 37*, 1181–1188.

Milligan, S. E., Horn, D. L., Ballou, S. P., Persse, L. J., Svilar, G. M., & Coulton, C. J. (1993). An assessment of the Health Assessment Questionnaire Functional Ability Index among women with systemic lupus erythematosus. *Journal of Rheumatology, 20*, 972–976.

Minor, M. (1998). Exercise for health and fitness. In J. L. Melvin & G. Jensen (Eds.), *Rheumatologic rehabilitation series: Volume 1: Assessment and management* (pp. 351–367). Bethesda, MD: American Occupational Therapy Association.

Mintz, G., Niz, J., Gutierrez, G., Garcia-Alonso, A., & Karchmer, S. (1986). Prospective study of pregnancy in systemic lupus erythematosus: Results of a multidisciplinary approach. *Journal of Rheumatology, 13*, 732–739.

Mukerji, B., & Hardin, J. G. (1993). Undifferentiated, overlapping, and mixed connective tissue diseases. *American Journal of Medical Sciences, 305*, 114–119.

Nalebuff, E. A., & Melvin, J. L. (in press). Systemic lupus erythematosus in the hand. In J. L. Melvin & E. A. Nalebuff (Eds.), *Rheumatologic rehabilitation series: Volume 4: The hand: Evaluation, therapy, and surgery*. Bethesda, MD: American Occupational Therapy Association.

Pisetsky, D. S. (1997). Systemic lupus erythematosus: Epidemiology, pathology, and pathogenesis. In J. H. Klippel, C. M. Weyand, & R. L. Wortmann (Eds.), *Primer on the rheumatic diseases* (11th ed., pp. 246–251). Atlanta, GA: The Arthritis Foundation.

Robb-Nicholson, L. C., Daltroy, L., Eaton, H., Gall, V., Wright, E., Hartley, L. H., Schur, P. H., & Liang, M. H. (1989). Effects of aerobic conditioning in lupus fatigue: A pilot study. *British Journal of Rheumatology, 28*, 500–505.

Schur, P. H. (1993). Clinical features of systemic lupus erythematosus. In W. N. Kelley, E. D. Harris, S. Ruddy, & C. B. Sledge (Eds.), *Textbook of rheumatology* (4th ed., pp. 1017–1042). Philadelphia: Saunders.

Schwartz, J. E., Jandorf, L., & Krupp, L. B. (1993). The measurement of fatigue: A new instrument. *Journal of Psychosomatic Research, 37*, 753–762.

Sequeira, J. H., & Balean, H. (1902). Lupus erythematosus: A clinical study of seventy-one cases. *British Journal of Dermatology, 14*, 367–379.

Shoenfeld, Y. (1992). Autoimmunity and autoimmune diseases like systemic lupus erythematosus. In R. G. Lahita (Ed.), *Systemic lupus erythematosus* (2nd ed., pp. 3–14). New York: Churchill Livingstone.

Smith, C. D., & Cyr, M. (1988). The history of lupus erythematosus. *Rheumatic Disease Clinics of North America, 14*, 1–14.

Sontheimer, R. D., & Provost, T. T. (1997). Cutaneous manifestations of lupus erythematosus. In D. J. Wallace & B. H. Hahn (Eds.), *Dubois' lupus erythematosus* (5th ed., pp. 569–623). Baltimore: Williams & Wilkins.

Stein, C. M., & Pincus, T. (1997). Glucocorticoids. In W. N. Kelley, E. D. Harris, Jr., S. Ruddy, & C. B. Sledge (Eds.), *Textbook of rheumatology* (5th ed., pp. 787–803). Philadelphia: Saunders.

Sutton, J. D., Navarro, A., & Stevens, M. B. (1984). Systemic lupus erythematosus XI: Nonpharmacological management. *Maryland State Medical Journal, 33,* 469–472.

Systemic lupus erythematosus self-help course. (1994). Atlanta, GA: Arthritis Foundation.

Tan, E. M., Cohen, A. S., Fries, J. F., Masi, A. T., McShane, D. J., Rothfield, N. F., Schaller, J. G., Talal, N., & Winchester, R. J. (1982). The 1982 revised criteria for the classification of systemic lupus erythematosus. *Arthritis and Rheumatism, 25,* 1271–1277.

Wallace, D. J. (1994). Antimalarial agents and lupus. *Rheumatic Disease Clinics of North America, 20,* 243–263.

Warner, J. J., Philip, J. H., Brodsky, G. L., & Thornhill, T. S. (1987). Studies of nontraumatic osteonecrosis: The role of core decompression in the treatment of nontraumatic osteonecrosis of the femoral head. *Clinical Orthopedics, 225,* 104–125.

SYSTEMIC SCLEROSIS (SCLERODERMA)

Jeanne L. Melvin, MS, OTR, FAOTA, E. Carwile LeRoy, MD, and Cathy S. Elrod, MS, PT

Systemic sclerosis (SSc) is a generalized disorder of the small blood vessels and the diffuse connective tissues. It is characterized by fibrotic, ischemic, and degenerative changes in the skin and internal organs. The systemic nature of SSc is evidenced by frequent involvement of the digestive tract, synovium, lungs, heart, and kidneys in addition to the skin. (SSc is the preferred abbreviation because "SS" is commonly used for Sjögren's syndrome.)

Scleroderma is an umbrella term for a group of disorders that include sclerosis of the skin as a predominant feature. SSc is the generalized or systemic form. Morphea or linear scleroderma are the localized forms. Patients often prefer the term *scleroderma* because it is easier to say and to understand. Therefore, scleroderma is often used as the common term for SSc.

Etiologic Factors

SSc is the result of excess deposition of fibrous tissue and microvascular occlusion; these processes occur in all involved organs, but the cause is unknown (Smith & LeRoy, 1994). The two current theories on pathogenesis (vascular and immunological) are complementary and not mutually exclusive. Some believe the primary event is vascular damage resulting from endothelial cell injury (LeRoy, 1982). This is supported by the early presence of Raynaud's phenomenon, capillary and renal vascular changes, and a serum factor toxic to endothelial cells (LeRoy, 1982; Sternberg, 1985). The immune theory holds that the initial event is T and B lymphocyte immunity to previously unrecognized tissue antigens (Postlethwaite & Kang, 1984). The activated lymphocytes produce lymphokines that stimulate fibroblast migration, proliferation, and collagen production (fibrosis). Products from activated lymphocytes and macrophages can cause endothelial cell injury and lead to intimal proliferation, vascular scarring, obliteration of the microvasculature, fibroblast activation, and ultimately fibrosis. These changes activate the T lymphocyte response and perpetuate the cycle (LeRoy, 1985; LeRoy & Lomeo, 1989; Sternberg, 1985). For example, if a retrovirus suppressed since birth reappeared and was expressed in endothelial cells, immune cells would interact, activate, and injure those cells that could in turn activate fibroblasts, which would lead to capillary obliteration and scar tissue formation. This scenario could create a unified hypothesis explaining the immune, vascular, and interstitial events seen in SSc.

Although the etiology is unknown and genetic predisposition is still uncertain, major strides have been made in early detection and prediction of who will develop SSc. Virtually all cases of diffuse SSc occur in adults who have biphasic, episodic Raynaud's phenomenon (*biphasic* means they have pallor or cyanosis as well as suffusion in response to cold) (LeRoy, 1981; LeRoy & Lomeo, 1989). There are two diagnostic procedures capable of predicting 95% of the persons destined to develop SSc.

1. Nailfold capillary microscopy to detect characteristic capillary dilation and or vascular areas in the nailfold

2. Serum antinuclear antibody determinations of anticentromere and antinuclear antibodies (LeRoy et al., 1988)

Raynaud's phenomenon (biphasic) affects 3% to 5% of the population worldwide across all ethnic groups. In selected populations, such as women in their childbearing years, the prevalence of Raynaud's phenomenon may be as high as 40%. A total of 10% to 15% of all persons with Raynaud's phenomenon are diagnosed with SSc by using one or both of the above diagnostic procedures. This means that nearly all patients with the potential for severe sclerosis and organ failure can be detected before irreversible scarring occurs. When effective treatments are developed, early intervention and prevention should be possible (LeRoy et al., 1988).

Population Affected

SSc is found in all racial groups and usually occurs during the third to fifth decades. Onset is uncommon in elderly persons and is rare in children, although linear and localized scleroderma can occur in childhood (LeRoy, 1981). SSc affects women three to four times more frequently than men and affects African-Americans slightly more than other racial groups (Medsger, 1988). It is estimated that there are about 300,000 persons with all forms of scleroderma, of which 100,000 to 200,000 have SSc.

Classification and Diagnosis

Systemic Sclerosis (SSc)

When SSc is classified by clinical and laboratory features, five distinct subtypes become evident (LeRoy et al., 1988). Diagnosis is made on the basis of characteristic clinical and laboratory findings as described below.

Diffuse cutaneous systemic sclerosis (dcSSc). In this subset, there is often rapid progression of skin thickening

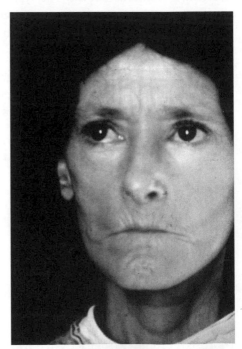

Figure 1. Classic facial changes seen in dcSSc. Note tight skin, loss of wrinkles and subcutaneous fat, and fissuring around lips. This patient is still capable of lip closure, a critical function to maintain. Reprinted from *Assessment and Management of the Rheumatic Diseases: The Teaching Slide Collection for Clinicians and Educators.* Used with permission of the American College of Rheumatology.

beginning as edema distally in the extremities (acral) and progressing proximally to include the trunk. Figure 1 illustrates the taut facial skin of a patient with dcSSc. Raynaud's phenomenon occurs within 1 year of the onset of skin changes. Tendon friction rubs are palpable, polyarthritis is common, and the serum can be positive for antibodies to Scl-70 (which is topoisomerase I) and antibodies to RNA polymerases (Medsger, 1988). These patients are at a higher risk for developing early and often severe visceral involvement, such as renal crisis, myocardial failure, interstitial lung disease, and gastrointestinal involvement (Medsger, 1988). dcSSc produces the most severe hand deformities. It is important to keep in mind that even though the name *scleroderma* refers to "hard skin," in dcSSc, the fibrosis affects all of the soft tissue: skin, fat, fascia, muscles, tendons, ligaments, and joint capsules. The patient is figuratively "encased in steel" (Osler, 1898).

Limited cutaneous systemic sclerosis (lcSSc). This is the most common form of SSc. There is limited involvement of the skin confined to the distal extremities and face (i.e., the trunk is spared). The skin changes may be stable or slowly progressive, and Raynaud's phenomenon is present long before skin thickening occurs. There is a prominence of digital telangiectasia (dilated capillaries) and subcutaneous calcinosis, although the latter may be microscopic or occur late. Approximately 70% to 80% of whites in this subtype have circulating anticentromere antibodies. Persons with this subtype rarely develop interstitial pulmonary, myocardial, or renal disease but are prone to late (after 10 or more years) appearance of visceral involvement, including primary pulmonary arterial hypertension, intestinal malabsorption, biliary cirrhosis, and Sjögren's syndrome with vasculitis. CREST (calcinosis, Raynaud's phenomenon, esophageal dysmotility, sclerodactyly, and telangiectasia) syndrome is synonymous with lcSSc. These features can occur in dcSSc. Overall, patients with lcSSc have a better prognosis and lower mortality rate than patients with dcSSc (LeRoy & Lomeo, 1989).

Sine scleroderma. There is no apparent skin thickening in this subtype, but there are characteristic internal organ changes and vascular and serological features. (*Sine* means without.)

Overlap syndrome. Patients fulfill the criteria for SSc, usually lcSSc, and meet the diagnostic criteria for other rheumatic diseases such as systemic lupus erythematosus (SLE), dermatomyositis, rheumatoid arthritis (RA), or Sjögren's syndrome.

Undifferentiated connective tissue disease. Raynaud's phenomenon is present with features of serum anticentromere antibody, abnormal nailfold capillaroscopy, finger edema, and ischemic injury but no skin thickening. These patients may develop lcSSc or an overlap syndrome.

Localized Scleroderma

Scleroderma can occur as a localized disease in which fibrotic lesions occur in a single patch (morphea), multiple patches (guttate morphea), confluent patches (generalized morphea), or linear bands. There is no associated systemic or visceral involvement (Seibold, 1993). Localized scleroderma primarily affects mostly female children and young adults. Morphea begins with an area of erythematous or violaceous discoloration of the skin that progresses to a waxy or ivory-colored sclerotic patch surrounded by an inflammatory border. The lesions frequently soften after a few months or years. New lesions usually stop after 35 years of age (Seibold, 1993). In children, morphea affects all of the associated soft tissue and can retard bone growth. Linear scleroderma that crosses a joint may lead to a severe contracture and fibrotic distortion of the nearby neurovascular compartment.

When linear scleroderma occurs in the hand, usually only one or two digits are involved. This form of scleroderma is very resistant to treatment (Rudolph, Leyden, & Berger, 1974; Seibold, 1993). Hand therapy can be modeled on the program outlined in this chapter for dcSSc, except that the precautions for Raynaud's phenomenon, swelling, and deformity patterns do not apply.

Course and Prognosis

The course of SSc is extraordinarily variable. Although usually gradual and indolent in onset (Raynaud's phenomenon and "puffy" fingers and face), SSc can be almost explosively rapid. Involvement is symmetrical, beginning in the fingers, nose, toes, ears, or other acral parts and may spread centrally. When limited to the skin, SSc is usually not fatal, and such patients may expect a normal life span. When internal involvement is present, the quality and duration of life is determined by the site and degree of organ failure. Renal SSc used to be the most common disease-related cause of death, but this can now be controlled by antihypertensive medication, especially angiotensin-converting enzyme (ACE) inhibitors introduced in 1980. Lung SSc is now the most common disease-related cause of death in patients with SSc.

Drug Therapy

No single drug or combination of agents has proven valuable for renal disease except for ACE inhibitors. Current drug therapy is symptomatic. Steroids such as prednisone are usually contraindicated except in those patients with inflammatory complications such as polymyositis. Antihypertensive drugs should be used to control hypertension, which may presage renal SSc.

Medications for Raynaud's phenomenon fall into two categories: those that prevent vascular spasm (e.g., prazosin, reserpine, guanethidine, and methyldopa) and calcium-channel blockers that induce vasodilation (e.g., nifedipine and diltiazem). The newer delayed-release formulations of nifedipine (Procardia XLs, Adalat CCs) require only a single daily dose and are preferred for patients with SSc because these formulations have fewer side effects. Medsger (1988) reported that nifedipine and prazosin have been the most successful in controlling symptoms and preventing the progression of skin ulcers. These last two medications, however, are used only after all behavioral methods have failed because they can cause serious cardiac, gastrointestinal, and psychological side effects. Fortunately, some patients only need to take the medications during the winter or trips to cold climates (Freedman, Ianni, & Wenig, 1984).

The presence of digital, ulnar, or elbow ulcers should be treated aggressively with regional nerve blocks, nitroglycerine paste locally over digital arteries, and treatment of skin and bone infection including hospitalization, epidural cervical blocks, and parenteral antibiotics when indicated (Goodfield, Hume, & Rowell, 1988; Goodfield & Rowell, 1988).

Characteristic Skin and Musculoskeletal Involvement

For most persons, the first symptom of SSc is swelling (pitting or nonpitting edema) and tightness in the hands, feet, and possibly the face. Raynaud's phenomenon may be present for years

Table 1. Stages of Skin Changes (LeRoy, 1985)

Early	Classic	Late
Hands, feet, and possibly the face are puffy, especially in the morning. This evolves into a nonpitting edema that fills the fingers, toes, and dorsal hand and foot skin. The epidermis remains intact. (Figure 2)	Puffiness subsides and is replaced by tight, hidebound skin that feels dry and coarse and often itches. Hypo- or hyperpigmentation is common. The epidermis becomes thin and atrophic. Hair disappears, and sweating is noticeably impaired. (These changes are considered diagnostic.) (Figure 3)	About 3 to 15 years after the beginning of the classic skin changes, the skin softens and becomes more pliable, but epidermal atrophy and loss of epidermal appendages remain. This may be part of a more general remission or can occur while other symptoms (e.g., finger ulcers) continue to be active.

with lcSSc or occur 1 year before the onset of dcSSc. For some persons, swelling and Raynaud's phenomenon may be the only symptoms, whereas others develop the simultaneous onset of polyarthritis with associated malaise, joint pain, and fatigue (LeRoy, 1985; Table 1).

Edema is the expression of several pathological factors, including abnormal vascular permeability, increased extracellular connective tissue deposition in the dermis, local inflammation, poor lymphatic return, and microvascular disruption (Clements & Medsger, 1996). It is *not* similar to other forms of edema encountered in rehabilitation, and routine interventions to treat edema are not effective because it is the underlying vascular pathology that is the source of the edema. Gradually edema is replaced by fibrosis, which gives the skin a tight, hard, smooth appearance, and hair disappears or becomes coarse. Itching can be episodic and severe and is a problem if scratching leads to further skin damage. Topical 1% hydrocortisone is recommended to reduce itching for short periods of time. The skin likewise becomes dry because of damage to sweat glands. Dry skin can cause fissuring, scaling, and ulceration. Patient education on management of dry skin is as important as any other topic (Figure 2). Table 2 contains suggestions for reducing dry skin.

Hyper- or hypopigmentation may occur in spots or blotches. The changes are often symmetrical and progress proximally to include the arms, neck, face, trunk, and lower extremities. Another common skin condition is telangiectasia, which appears as small reddish spots on the skin. This results from chronic dilation of capillaries and small arterial branches. The condition usually is benign

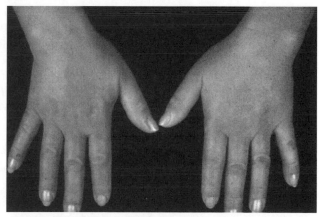

Figure 2. dcSSc with early-stage skin changes of nonpitting edema and taut skin that cannot be pinched over the dorsum of the proximal phalanx. Patient still has near full range of motion. Reprinted from *Assessment and Management of the Rheumatic Diseases: The Teaching Slide Collection for Clinicians and Educators.* Used with permission of the American College of Rheumatology.

Table 2. Suggestions for Reducing Dry Skin Problems

1. In the winter, use a humidifier in the house.
2. Keep the body warm with clothes, but keep the house air as cool as is reasonable and comfortable.
3. Use creamy sunscreens before outings.
4. Use gentle soaps such as glycerin (Neutrogena®) or face soaps and rinse thoroughly.
5. Use moisturizing lotions (e.g., Aquaphor®, Eucerin®, Lubriderm®, Vaseline Dermatology Lotion®, Theraplex, or Lac-Hydrin 12% lotion) after bathing or washing hands.
6. Use mild cleansing lotions for sensitive skin or lipid-free moisturizing lotions to cleanse the face of dirt and excess oil.
7. Avoid the use of astringents and aftershave lotions.
8. Avoid handling dirt (it is high in acid and is detrimental to the skin). Use rubber gloves when gardening, potting, or cleaning vegetables. If gloves make hands sweat excessively, try wearing thin cotton gloves under the gardening gloves.
9. For severe dry skin cracks (but not open ulcers), a petroleum product (e.g., Bag Balm®) on the hands at night covered with loose cotton gloves can be effective (albeit a little medicinal smelling).

and is indicative of internal vascular changes, although in the fingertips, telangiectasia may be tender or sensitive (Postlethwaite & Kang, 1984). All of these changes can be unsightly, and many patients can benefit from a consultation with a cosmetic specialist who is skilled in working with facial disfigurement and concealing makeup (Murray, 1972; Trust, 1981).

Patients usually are referred to therapy when they begin to lose range of motion (ROM), particularly in the hands. In mild cases, it is possible that the skin is the primary or only tissue involved. In most cases, ROM limitations are secondary to a combination of decreased skin mobility, edema, arthritis, and fibrosis of the subcutaneous tissues, muscles, tendons, synovium, and joint capsules (LeRoy, 1985; Medsger, 1988). The patient usually perceives any and all of these changes as stiffness. For evaluation purposes, this must be distinguished from morning stiffness, which tends to wear off. As fibrosis progresses, structures become bound down, and the potential for joint contractures increases. Joint contractures may be unavoidable or develop as a result of disuse, inappropriate or lack of ROM exercise, and improper positioning. Contractures that develop from these later processes are often preventable.

Leathery creaking is often audible where tendons pass over joints and is due to fibrinous deposits on the surfaces of the tendon sheaths and overlying fascia. These are called *tendon friction rubs*, and patient often reports hearing them when moving at night. There is no specific treatment for this problem.

Pain in SSc can result from four sources. First, arthritis causes pain in the joints at rest and with movement. Second, ulcers can be quite painful; the most common are fingertip ischemic ulcers and dorsal proximal interphalangeal (PIP) ulcers that are sensitive to touch such as a paper cut. Third, calcium deposits cause pain when pressure is applied. Fourth, Raynaud's phenomenon can cause aching and pain in the hands of the "pins and needles" variety.

Pain has serious secondary consequences. Fear of pain from hand or foot ulcers encourages a guarded posture during ambulation. Patients often walk with their hands held in front of them to avoid accidentally brushing them against something. This posture encourages elbow flexion deformities, tightness in the shoulders, and altered gait. Pain can make an otherwise healthy person tense and stressed. This process occurs in persons with SSc, which further encourages shallow breathing and inactivity. Pain reduction is a primary goal in rehabilitation of SSc.

Arthralgias or arthritis occur in 90% of SSc cases at some time. About one third of the patients have articular symptoms first (LeRoy, 1982). Typically, the arthritis is a polyarticular, inflammatory, small-joint, symmetrical arthritis of the same pattern as RA. The arthritis is usually mild, nonerosive, nondeforming, and self-limited. However, arthritis may prevent effective ROM and encourage flexion contractures. The arthritis may be more difficult to perceive and evaluate because the diffuse edema, periarticular fibrosis, and tight

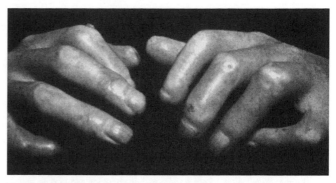

Figure 3. dcSSc with classic-stage skin changes of tight hidebound, atrophic skin, hypo- and hyperpigmentation, loss of hair, and impaired sweat gland function. This patient has a characteristic deformity pattern of MCP joint extension and PIP joint flexion. Note resorption of distal tuft of index finger and an ulcer on the tip of the right thumb and dorsum of the left middle PIP joint. Fortunately, the patient is still able to do a lateral pinch, an essential function to maintain in persons with dcSSc. Reprinted from *Assessment and Management of the Rheumatic Diseases: The Teaching Slide Collection for Clinicians and Educators*. Used with permission of the American College of Rheumatology.

skin may mask the swelling and warmth associated with joint inflammation. Pain may be the only symptom of arthritis. Figure 3 illustrates the hand deformities of dcSSc.

Digital ischemic ulcers have three typical forms of presentation. The most common are small ulcers over the fingertips or palmar surface that are often the size of a pinhead or smaller. They are attributed to cutaneous ischemia; the inadequate blood supply causes painful tissue necrosis. Then, as the ulcer forms scar tissue, the ratio of viable tissue to the available blood supply comes into balance, the ulcer appears healed, and the pain stops (LeRoy, 1985). Unfortunately, new ulcers tend to appear, and patients usually have several at one time. They are painful and limit the person's ability to manipulate objects and perform daily activities. This is comparable to having multiple paper cuts on your fingertips. The effect of these ulcers on function and the need for specific adaptive measures is part of the hand evaluation for these patients (Melvin, 1989) (Table 3).

The second type of ulcers includes those occurring over the dorsum of the PIP joints as a result of ischemia and mechanical pressure from PIP joint flexion contractures. They tend to be larger and appear more like a classic ulcer. They are different from deep fingertip ulcers in that they are not a result of arterial occlusion. In the early stages, they appear as a demarcated, tender area that may remain for a long time or develop an open necrotic center. Some ulcers remain open; others develop thick scabs. The PIP joints are prone to these ulcers because they develop flexion contractures that stretch the taut skin over the dorsum of the joint. Active flexion reduces the blood supply to this area (which is evident by dorsal blanching during grip) and impedes wound healing and closure. Additionally, the dorsum of these joints is vulnerable to trauma during activities.

The third form of ulcer is a classic ischemic ulcer that can occur on the sides of the hand, the ends of the fingers, or the elbows as a result of a more generalized ischemia to the area. These ulcers are the result of arterial occlusion and can become gangrenous (Jones, 1996). Often the digit

Table 3. Methods for Reducing Pain of Ulcers and Calcinosis

Ulcers	
Fingertip ulcers	Cotton laboratory gloves or a finger sleeve cut from a cotton stretch glove
Thumbs	Cica Care® or T-foam® pads held in place with Tubiton® (tan stretch style)
Dorsal PIP ulcers	Cotton stretch gloves, splints, or Tubiton® digit sleeves
Calcinosis	
Digits	Donut-type pads over the deposit, gel pad sleeves, or padding handles to reduce pressure
Elbows	Heelbo® or other elbow protector pads
Knees	Sew a foam pad or shoulder pad into an elastic knee support to reduce the pain of kneeling or use commercial knee pads
Ischial bones	T-foam® cushions or convoluted cushions may help relieve pressure and discomfort
Ankle malleoi	Cica Care® or T-foam® pads held in place with an elastic support (not tight) or Ace® wrap

is allowed to autoamputate to preserve the maximal amount of digit length possible; otherwise, surgical amputation is indicated. Ischemic ulcers are likewise found on the lateral malleoli. These large, deep, painful ulcers are usually the result of vasculitis (Clements & Medsger, 1996).

For all open ulcers, meticulous wound and skin care is important. This includes soaking in warm water or a whirlpool a couple of times a day and application of topical antibiotics (e.g., silver sulfadiazine, zinc bacitracin) (Jones, 1996; Wigley & Matsumoto, 1995). Protective splinting is helpful. These patients are vulnerable to developing *Staphylococcus* infections that can quickly progress to osteomyelitis. All patients should be taught the signs of infection and to report them to their physician promptly.

Calcinosis refers to the deposition of calcium salts under the skin and is a common phenomenon in both SSc subtypes (see Figure 4). It is found in about 15% of the patients with dcSSc and 44% of patients with lcSSc (Jones, Raynor, & Medsger, 1987; Seibold, 1993). There are two types of subcutaneous calcification. The more common one occurs as localized subcutaneous deposits (calcinosis circumscripta) around joints or near bony prominences and feels like pebbles under the skin. In the upper extremity, deposits tend to occur over functional pressure areas such as the volar aspect of the thumb interphalangeal (IP) joint, the heel of the hand, the lateral surface of the index finger, the medial edge of the palm, the ulnar wrist, and the elbow. In the lower extremity, they occur over the prepatellar area, lateral malleoi, and ischial tuberosities. Deposits can occur in the tendon sheaths and the thoracic outlet (Seibold, 1993). In general, localized deposits are painless, but their stiffness makes the skin and

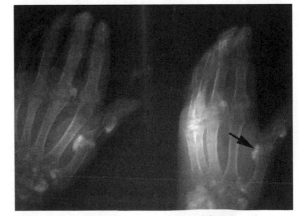

Figure 4. X-ray showing subcutaneous calcium deposits. Deposits on the volar aspect of the thumb MCP joint are painful and limit grasp ability. Photo courtesy of Edward Nalebuff, MD.

tissue over and under them even more sensitive to pressure. They are an annoying problem for patients and may be so tender that they make it impossible for patients to sit in a hard chair, to kneel, or to use their elbows for support or mobility in bed.

The second type of subcutaneous calcification is a diffuse, encasing calcification (calcinosis universalis) that may contribute to severe joint contractures. (See Table 3 for methods of reducing pain from ulcers and calcinosis.) The skin can break down over the deposits, which allows white, chalky calcium to extrude. Patients often mistake the calcium for pus, but unless there are obvious signs of infection such as heat, redness, and pain, this is a noninfectious process. However, any skin breakdown should be cleaned three times a day with hydrogen peroxide and kept protected and clean. Particularly troublesome deposits can be surgically removed; because these deposits occur frequently, surgery is done only in selected cases (Mendelson, Linscheid, Dobyns, & Miller, 1977). Several medications have been reported to help reduce calcinosis, but none are considered to be a reliable treatment (Wigley & Matsumoto, 1995).

Osteolysis or bony resorption is another potential sequela of dcSSc (Figure 3). It is attributed to ischemia secondary to chronic vasospasm and intimal proliferation of the blood vessels. Osteolysis is most common in the distal tuft of the distal phalanx and results in shortening of the digit with the tip becoming rounded versus tapered as the soft tissue contracts (LeRoy et al., 1988). Detection of tuft resorption is done by comparing the digit lengths of both hands. Osteolysis can occur in other bones such as the distal ulna, radius, clavicle, cervical spine, mandible, and ribs (Osial et al., 1981). There is no treatment for this condition.

Raynaud's phenomenon is defined as an episodic ischemia characterized by three phases: cyanosis (vasoconstriction), blanching (vasospasm), and erythema (suffusion) as the blood returns. Raynaud's phenomenon occurs in between 90% and 98% of persons with SSc and is the first symptom in 70% of patients (Seibold, 1993). It occurs in the hands, feet, nose, ears, and tip of the tongue. Raynaud's phenomenon is said to be elicited by cold or stress, but in SSc, it may occur without any perceivable trigger. True Raynaud's phenomenon must have at least two phases. Cyanosis by itself reflects sensitivity to cold, and continual ischemia is not considered Raynaud's phenomenon (LeRoy & Lomeo, 1989).

Distinctions between triphasic (cyanosis, blanching, and erythema) and biphasic (blanching and erythema) Raynaud's phenomenon seem to depend on whether there is sufficient venous blood visible through thickened skin to demonstrate the blue color of deoxygenated hemoglobin. Because SSc digits are relatively bloodless, cyanosis is uncommon in SSc Raynaud's phenomenon, and the distinction does not appear to have clinical or prognostic importance.

Jones (1996) proposed that Raynaud's phenomenon in SSc is caused by three different mechanisms.

1. An exaggerated sympathetic vasoconstrictive response to cold
2. Segmental occlusions of the common digital and proper digital arteries due to proliferation of the intima or inner lining of the arteries
3. External compression of the common digital arteries and proper digital arteries as a result of the adventitia or outer covering of the arteries

These mechanisms usually act in concert.

Muscle weakness may result from disuse, atrophy, ischemic atrophy, myositis, or muscle sclerosis. During the active phase of SSc, disuse of the involved muscles occurs because the patient avoids painful movements. Joint effusion, joint contracture, ulcer pain, and joint pain can influence the amount of active movement around the joint. With continued disuse, the muscle begins to atrophy, and the sarcomeres begin to adjust to the limited movement patterns. Pathological changes in the muscle include atrophy and necrosis of muscle fibers, fibrosis of the fiber sheaths with increased production of connective tissue, a diminished number of capillaries with perivascular infiltrates of lymphocytes, and plasma cells early and fibrosis and capillary obliteration later (Blocka, 1996).

Myositis occurs in persons with SSc as one of two types. The most common is described by Clements and associates (1978) as a "simple myopathy" and is characterized by mild proximal muscle weakness and mild elevations of serum muscle enzymes that may have an ischemic basis. Symptoms tend to wax and wane or be slowly progressive and are not responsive either to corticosteroids or other medications. A small percentage of patients develop an inflammatory myositis indistinguishable from polymyositis, which can be treated with corticosteroids. The early clinical signs of acute polymyositis to monitor are a sudden or new inability to hold the arms overhead (shoulder girdle weakness) or to climb steps or a curb, a waddling gait (pelvic girdle weakness), an inability to hold one's head up, and pain in the proximal muscles. All of these symptoms should be reported to the patient's physician immediately.

Occupational and Physical Therapy

Philosophy and Approach

When the patient begins to lose function due to joint limitations, it is easy for the patient, physician, and therapist to become focused solely on physical treatment of the joints. However, holistic treatment requires a broad, integrative approach that addresses all aspects of a person's life that can influence his or her health: exercise, nutrition, attitude, interpersonal relationships, response to stress, productive work, social roles, leisure, and enjoyment (Melvin, 1989). Table 4 outlines a

Table 4. Comprehensive Care for Patients With SSc

1. Provide counseling to help the patient explore and work through the psychological, family, social, and vocational ramifications of an uncommon disease with visible deformities.
2. Educate the patient about symptoms and treatment, both those that are effective and those that are not.
3. Use specific medications and modalities (e.g., biofeedback) to control symptoms, relieve pain, and improve function.
4. Provide the patient with an effective ROM program to maintain joint mobility and chest excursion.
5. Counsel the patient about nutrition and dental care.
6. Instruct the patient in adaptive methods of compensating for functional loss.
7. Instruct the patient in methods to reduce pain and protect skin during activities.
8. Instruct the patient in fatigue management. (See chapters 6 and 8 in this volume.)
9. Educate the patient on maintaining or regaining physical fitness appropriate to the medical condition.

comprehensive holistic team approach to care for the person with SSc (Melvin, Brannan, & LeRoy, 1984). It is helpful to advise patients that the taut skin may partially subside after 3 to 5 years, but joint contractures tend to be permanent. This way, their efforts can be seen as an investment to maintain function until some natural regression occurs.

Rehabilitative treatment of joint involvement in SSc is different from treating RA, in which the variability in inflammation, swelling, stiffness, and medication effectiveness can create fluctuating ROM on a daily basis. Persons with SSc have an insidious loss of ROM. Deformities occur secondary to uncontrolled fibrosis, inactivity, and the lack of an objective way for patients to determine their maximal ROM on a daily basis. (Recovery of motion is rare, except with remission.) Prevention of loss is the key to successful treatment. Can we prevent all of the deformities? No. Some occur despite good therapy, especially if pain, arthritis, illness, or ulcers prevent adequate ROM exercise. Can you prevent some of the deformities? Yes. In the experience of one author (J.M.), some of the most dysfunctional contractures (e.g., loss of mouth aperture, thumb abduction, and lateral pinch) can often be prevented or function preserved (Melvin, 1989).

To help dispel the myth that therapy cannot influence SSc, Askew, Beckett, An, and Chao (1983) carefully evaluated ROM, function, and skin compliance before and 2 hr after a single hand therapy session consisting of a paraffin bath, friction massage, and active ROM exercises. Their results showed a statistically significant improvement in hand function after a single session of therapy. Maintaining clinical gains depends on an effective home ROM and self-evaluation program.

Research has not identified a model evaluation or treatment program for SSc. The approach described here is one that has been used for more than 20 years by one of the authors (J.M.). It can best be described as a precise ROM program. The following are the premises of the program.

- Objective self-evaluation techniques allow the patient to determine which motions they are maintaining well and those they need to work on.
- Pretreatment ROM reveals the mobility the patient can maintain with her or his current home program.
- Posttreatment ROM determines the daily self-ROM goal.
- It is only necessary to achieve a ROM goal once a day to maintain the motion. (By definition, if you achieve 90° once every day, you have maintained that motion.)
- Maintaining as much mobility as possible is important, even if the specific motion is not essential for function, to help compensate for current and future losses (especially in the hand).

ROM exercises are focused on mobilizing soft tissue in all directions, not simply achieving increased ROM in a single plane. (For example, the therapist must ask, "What can be done to mobilize the dorsal metacarpophalangeal [MCP] structure or shoulder girdle?" not just "How can we increase flexion?")

The primary goals in treatment are to preserve motion, prevent contracture, and promote independence in daily activities. It is imperative to maintain maximal ROM because it is difficult to increase ROM. The ideal situation is to have the patient referred to therapy before he or she loses ROM. This allows the therapist to determine the patient's normal measurements and use them as the baseline or objective for treatment (Melvin, 1989).

The patient must be aware of these realistic objectives so that he or she does not have false expectations or false guilt if limitations develop. It is imperative that the patient realizes that he or she must take an active role in achieving goals.

Evaluation

Goniometric measurements should be taken of all joints in all planes of motion. Encourage the patient to take an active role in the measurement of ROM. Not only does daily self-evaluation minimize the potential for loss of motion, but also it provides a form of biofeedback and positive reinforcement that the exercises are beneficial and effective. In addition, patients may not be able to achieve their goals during a flare-up, but afterward they have an objective goal for regaining function.

Box 1
Resources

Organization Resources

Scleroderma Foundation
(A merger of the Scleroderma Federation and the United Scleroderma Foundation)
89 Newbury Street
Suite 201
Danvers, MA 01923
800-722-HOPE
Internet address: www.scleroderma.com

The Arthritis Foundation
1330 West Peachtree Street
Atlanta, GA 30309
404-872-7100 or 800-283-7800
Internet address: www.arthritis.org

Scleroderma International Foundation
704 Gardner Center Road
New Castle, PA 16101
This organization publishes a newsletter for patients.

American Occupational Therapy Association
1-800-SAY-AOTA
This organization publishes a patient education and home program guide, *Scleroderma: Caring for your hands and face* (Melvin, 1994).

Internet Resources

- A search for "scleroderma" on www.hotbot.com will link you to all Web sites related to this topic.

- The Amazon Bookstore (www.amazon.com) lists numerous books published on scleroderma.

- Abledata is a national database for adaptive equipment and assistive devices (www.abledata.com).

Adaptive Equipment and Clothing Resources

Guide for Independent Living (available from the Arthritis Foundation, see address above)

Damart Catalogue (warm undergarments)
1811 Woodbury Avenue
Portsmouth, NH 03801

Winter Silks
(warm undergarments, clothes, and socks)
2700 Laura Lane
P.O. Box 620130
Middleton, WI 53562

Use of Thermal Modalities

Selected heat modalities can be used safely to increase flexibility of the skin and soft tissues before ROM exercises. All heat modalities must be used with caution because the blood supply to the skin is compromised, and the systemic capacity to dissipate heat is diminished. For some patients, "warm" is sufficient. The patient's tolerance for heat must be determined before its application. Cold modalities are usually contraindicated because of Raynaud's phenomenon (Michlovitz, 1986). Moisturizing lotions should be used after heat applications.

When determining the appropriate method for heat application, keep in mind the time frame you have to treat the patient and your goal to begin the patient on a daily home program for maintaining ROM. Heat should be used in conjunction with the ROM activities, not instead of them. If heat is a part of the program, then the ideal situation is to use the same method in the clinic that you want the patient to use at home (e.g., a heating pad rather than a hydrocollator pack). Patients do their exercises at home in or after a warm bath or shower and should be advised not to become chilled after bathing and to use a water-based lotion (not oils) afterward to lubricate the skin. (See Table 2 on skin care.)

The normal heat of a paraffin bath and hydrocollator packs may be tolerated by some persons with SSc, but generally it is too hot for persons with vascular compromise. For the hands, one alternative is to put the hand in a plastic disposable glove before dipping it in paraffin or soaking it in hot water. This reduces the temperature on the skin and prevents the water from drying out the skin. Hot packs with extra towels often work well to increase circulation and thus help reduce edema and stiffness and increase mobility before exercise. Fluidotherapy is not recommended because it dries the skin, and it is a clinic-based treatment that does not facilitate self-management at home (Poole, 1996).

Massage and Joint Mobilization

Massage, especially deep massage, is used to increase circulation, reduce adhesion to the fascia, decrease edema, and improve flexibility. When used in conjunction with lotions, massage can deliver moisture to the skin. Water-based lotions such as Lubriderm® and Eucerin® are recommended versus oils for improving skin hydration. (See Table 2 on skin care.)

Massage can be used before ROM activities if the patient is unable to tolerate heat applications or after a heat application. The techniques can be specific to the particular area surrounding the joint or generalized to the whole body to promote relaxation and increased blood flow. If the patient reports comfort or relief from the massage, then caregivers can be taught the appropriate massage techniques to use at home. Massage should be used in conjunction with and not instead of daily ROM exercises.

In specific situations, joint mobilization techniques as defined by Maitland (as cited in Trelkeld, 1992) can be helpful in restoring the subtle motion between joint surfaces in stiff joints. These mobilizations are applied by the therapist by using small-amplitude passive motions that are intended to produce gliding or traction at the joint (Trelkeld, 1992). They can be particularly beneficial in the early stages of SSc. The value of this technique must be documented. Caution should be used with these techniques to ensure that trauma is not occurring at the joint, which could further exacerbate edema, pain, and stiffness. Mobilization is contraindicated for painful or inflamed joints.

Exercises for Mobility

Passive, assisted, and active exercises can be useful tools to maximize function and minimize loss of ROM. Please note that the type of ROM program used with other patients is not sufficient for scleroderma patients. Patients must always be aware of the maximal movement available at the joint and continually exercise to achieve that same amount of range. Patients seem to maintain mobility more effectively when they have objective goals that provide encouragement and a means to measure their progress. Table 5 provides some examples of objective ROM self-evaluation measures. Specific joints can be targeted if the patient has minimal deficits or complains of occasional stiffness; a general program encompassing all the major joints should be provided. It is important that the patient or caregiver demonstrate the recommended exercises because he or she will be performing them at home without a therapist's guidance.

The challenge to the therapist is to help the patient develop a system of applying sustained, gentle, passive stretch to all affected joints if the patient is unable to achieve full motion actively. This is often difficult for patients with sensitive painful fingertip ulcers because they are unable to apply pressure with their fingers. Arthritis can be a limiting factor. Swollen painful joints should be ranged gently, and nonsteroidal anti-inflammatory drugs, if used, should be taken

Table 5. Precise Range of Motion System: Objective Self-Evaluation Techniques

Hands	
Finger Flexion	Distance between fingertips and proximal palmar crease marked on an index card (goal: to touch marks every day)
MCP Flexion	Use of templates
PIP Joint Extension	In the early stages, achieve a prayer position with all digit joints touching
Digit Abduction	Hand tracing on paper in maximal abduction
Shoulder Abduction	Stand with the side of the body next to a wall, raise the arm closest to the wall, walk fingers up the wall, and mark the wall (or use a Post-It™) at the tip of the middle finger
Flexion	Stand facing a wall, raise one arm, walk fingers up the wall, and mark the wall at the tip of the middle finger
External Rotation	Stand with the back up against a wall, with hands behind the neck, bring elbows back to touch the wall, and measure distance lacking or bring elbows back in line with the shoulders or another landmark
Elbow Flexion–Extension	Stand against a wall with the back of the upper arms touching the arm on a flat surface (e.g., a table) with the arm out straight and measure the distance between the hand and the table
Mouth Aperture	Mark the distance between upper and lower teeth on an index card
Rib Cage Excursion	Measure the rib cage during inhalation and exhalation with a tape measure
Knee Extension	Sit on a flat surface with legs straight in front and have the back of the knee on a flat surface

before exercising. A maintained stretch for 15 to 30 sec or longer is recommended because it is less likely to cause microtrauma than ballistic or quick stretching (Kisner & Colby, 1990). Specific guidelines should be given regarding proper hand placement and the amount of force used during the stretch (i.e. "tolerable discomfort but no pain"). (Precaution: If range limitation is a result of active synovitis, forceful stretching should not be done. It will increase inflammation and subsequent fibrosis.)

The ROM program and instructions can be simplified if the patient has already developed an effective method for exercising certain joints. Whatever the patient is doing effectively to maintain motion should be reinforced and incorporated into the formal home program. The therapist can present the objective of the exercise program to the patient and let the patient determine the exercise he or she prefers to perform to achieve the goal. Compliance is less of a problem if the patient takes an active role in shaping his or her specific regimen.

Therapists should define the rate and frequency of the exercises. To help strengthen your argument for adherence to a daily program, review with the patient the benefits of therapeutic and fitness exercise (see Table 6). *Daily exercise is a must during active or acute phases of the disease.* The joint should be moved through the full ROM. Five or more repetitions of each exercise is recommended. If the joint is painful, advise the patient to perform at least one repetition for each joint. It would be detrimental for the patient to get into the habit of avoiding movement because the goal is to preserve motion throughout the progression of the disease to minimize the effects of skin changes. SSc is active or acute when there is edema and progressive tightness. During remissions or when ROM seems stable, patients who have objective methods for monitoring self-ROM can reduce exercises to two to three times a week as long as they are able to achieve objective goals on this schedule.

Exercises for Strengthening

Isometric exercises are recommended for strengthening because they cause the least amount of shear forces across the joint and address strength and endurance limitations. A single 6-sec isometric contraction daily at two thirds or maximal effort has been shown to increase strength in healthy persons (Hicks, 1990). It is important to avoid isotonic exercise for a patient with active myositis or restrictive lung disease (Blom-Bulow, Jonson, & Bauer, 1983; Casale, Buonocore, & Matucci-Cerinic, 1997).

For endurance, an aerobic exercise program should be designed for the patient to improve or maintain energy levels and cardiopulmonary function. Pulmonary or cardiac involvement will compromise aerobic capacity; therefore, physician approval is imperative before designing a specific aerobic program.

An aquatic therapy program can incorporate both strengthening and endurance activities in a relatively pain-free environment because of the buoyancy of the water. Working in a warm pool

Table 6. Benefits of Fitness and Therapeutic Exercise

1. Improved circulation to the skin, including oxygenation and nutrition
2. Maximal skin pliability to reduce taut skin contractures
3. Increased strength, energy, and endurance
4. Improved function and ability to care for self
5. Positive self-image
6. Decreased stress and anxiety
7. Improved mood and sleep

with a therapist is recommended until a program has been designed for the patient to perform independently. Chlorine can burn ulcers, and pool therapy is contraindicated when open ulcers are present.

Hands

The characteristic early hand deformities (Rodnan, Jablonska, & Medsger, 1979) that occur in dcSSc are loss of flexion of the MCP joints; loss of extension of the PIP joints; loss of thumb abduction, opposition, and flexion; and loss of wrist motion in all planes. As involvement progresses, motion is usually lost in all joints in all planes. The distal interphalangeal (DIP) joints are often fixed in mid-range flexion. This results in a hand fixed in MCP extension and PIP flexion with the thumb adducted and the wrist in neutral (Figure 3).

To preserve hand function and prevent deformity, the primary objectives of hand therapy in the early stages are to preserve MCP joint flexion, thumb abduction, and PIP extension. Patients who are acutely ill and who have arthritis in the wrists are at risk for developing wrist flexion contractures. Prevention of wrist-drop deformity is critical.

Typical skin and vascular changes include painful small ulcerations over the fingertips and dorsum of the PIP joints and Raynaud's phenomenon (Entin & Wilkinson, 1973). These can severely limit hand function, especially for fine tasks such as writing, buttoning, sewing, and using zippers, and they impair strong grip. The ulcers may heal after sufficient atrophy has occurred and the blood flow becomes adequate for the remaining tissue (LeRoy, 1981). Calcium deposits tend to occur on the thumb and digits versus the palm. Later in the disease, bony resorption of the distal phalanges can result in shortening of the fingers.

Goniometric measurements should be taken of all joints in all planes of motion, and a tracing of the hand should be made to document digit abduction and thumb web space. Ideally, measurements should be taken before and after a heat and exercise program. Measurements taken before indicate *how much mobility the patient easily maintains*, and measurements taken afterward determine *exercise objectives*.

Patients with SSc need a detailed hand function and activities of daily living evaluation to determine adaptive methods and equipment to improve function and reduce pain from ulcers, calcium deposits, Raynaud's phenomenon, and arthritis.

Exercise and Orthotic Treatment

MCP joints. The MCP joints tend to become stiff in extension because of fibrosis of the delicate dorsal expansion (Figure 3). MCP flexion requires smooth gliding and full elongation of the dorsal expansion and collateral ligaments. MCP flexion is the most important motion to maintain because extension of the MCP joints encourages flexion of the PIP joints. The main method to preserve PIP extension is to maintain MCP flexion. Some patients can effectively maintain motion by using passive manual pressure applied to the dorsum of the proximal phalanges with the heel of the other hand. Others may need the help of a dynamic flexion assistance device (a wrist strap placed over a simple volar wrist support with leather finger cuffs that slip over the proximal phalanges). The tension on the rubber bands should allow gentle pressure for at least 30 min. If the patient can tolerate only 10 min, the bands are too tight. A device like this allows the patient to apply sustained pressure while watching television or doing other activities. Not all patients can tolerate this type of device. All splints have to be carefully monitored for their effect on edema, decreased circulation, vasospasm, and skin vulnerability (Seeger & Furst, 1987). One method for allowing patients to determine if they are achieving maximal flexion is to have them use a template with the desired degree angle cut out of it. These can easily be made out of cardboard by cutting a wedge out of a 2- to 3-in. circle of cardboard equal to the desired ROM goal. If the patient can fit the wedge over the flexed joint, he or she knows that the goal has been achieved. Many patients need only one or two templates (Melvin, 1989).

In the early stages, when ROM is near normal, MCP hyperextension is an important motion to maintain because it is often the first to be lost. With hands together in a praying position, the patient can measure hyperextension span against a ruler or by marking it on an index card.

PIP joints. Similar to the MCP joints, the PIP joints are dependent on the intricate gliding and sliding of the dorsal expansion, lumbricals, lateral bands, and central slip, all structures at high risk for sclerosis. The PIP joints are at greater risk than the MCP joints because their circulation is more distal, they have less soft tissue around them, and some portion of the collateral ligaments is always lax and at risk for contracture. In addition, this joint has the greatest amount of flexion of all the hand joints and requires considerable extensibility of the dorsal skin. Except for the position of full flexion, the dorsal skin and underlying structures are always loose and, therefore, at risk of contracture. Complicating factors include arthritis or dorsal ischemic ulcers, which may make ROM exercises impossible (Melvin, 1995).

Active, active assisted, gentle passive, and gentle sustained passive ROM with self-adhesive tape (Coban®; 3M Company, St. Paul, MN) and joint mobilization techniques are appropriate if the patient does not have ulcers or arthritis in the PIP joints. Neoprene sleeves (available in hand therapy catalogs) to encourage extension and protect ulcers may be helpful for selected patients. All treatment for the index finger should be directed toward maintaining lateral pinch. If there is limited index PIP mobility, try to encourage PIP limitations in an arc appropriate for lateral pinch. It is better to have the index finger ankylosed in a position for lateral pinch than to have motion and no pinch. Again, the best way to maintain PIP extension is to preserve MCP flexion (Melvin, 1995).

Seeger and Furst (1987) published the only study evaluating the effectiveness of a dynamic PIP extension orthosis for reducing PIP flexion contractures in patients with SSc. The orthosis was thermoplastic and custom molded with a dorsal wrist-MCP design that extended distally to the PIP joints with a high-profile wire outrigger and assists placed distal to the PIP joints. It was held in place with two volar forearm straps and one volar palm strap. The protocol was to wear the orthosis 8 hr a day for 2 months on a randomly selected hand. The nonsplinted hand served as a control. Nineteen patients entered the study, and 8 completed it. Of the original 19, 4 (21%) patients dropped out because the orthosis exacerbated their Raynaud's phenomenon. The results in the final 8 patients varied widely. Only 1 patient gained statistically significant ROM (43° in total PIP extension in the splinted hand and a loss of 21° in the control hand). Another patient gained equally in both hands, and others lost ROM in both hands. The conclusion was that this specific orthosis and protocol could not be recommended because it helped only 1 out of 19 patients. Some clinicians refer to this study as proof that dynamic splinting does not work. This, however, is not a valid conclusion because the study involved only one specific orthosis and protocol.

DIP joints. These joints frequently become limited in a functional position and, therefore, do not require much treatment. Palmar ulcers are common; dorsal ones are rare. In the early stages, joint mobilization techniques may be helpful.

Thumb. The main treatment for the thumb is to maintain the web space and the ability for lateral pinch. The MCP and IP joints tend to become stiff in a mid-range functional position.

Finger–thumb abduction. One of the most severe deformities that has the potential for prevention is the loss of thumb abduction. This motion requires full elongation of the adductor pollicis muscle and the web space. Unless a person is actively abducting the thumb, these structures are slack and vulnerable to contracture. Patients can monitor their abduction and thumb web space by having a copy of their hand tracing at home. They should do active and passive abduction and adduction of each MCP joint until they achieve their span goal each day. If the fingers are tight, passive stretch can be achieved by wedging a folded tissue or piece of cloth between all fingers a pair at a time for 5 min or longer (Melvin, 1995). If a patient is starting to lose thumb web space, the only effective method for maintaining it is to use a thumb carpometacarpal (CMC) stabilization splint with a C-bar (short opponens splint) made out of a high-conforming material such as 1/16-in. Aquaplast (WFR/Aquaplast Corp., Wyckoff, NJ). Positioning the thumb midway between palmar abduction and extension provides maximal stretch to the web space. Wearing the splint at night is usually sufficient; however, patients in an acute episode should wear it during prolonged bed rest and during the day if necessary.

Finger intrinsic muscles. Exercising the interossei and lumbricals mobilizes the dorsal expansion. Mobilization exercises include applying resistance to PIP joint extension with the MCP joints flexed by spreading a rubber band apart with the middle phalanges and thumb, active PIP joint flexion with the MCP joints extended (classic intrinsic muscle stretching), and resistance to abduction (or trapping an index card between the fingers to provide resistance to the adductors).

Wrist. The wrist tends to become stiff in a neutral position and generally does not need treatment except for ROM exercise. In one author's (J.M.) opinion, full-hand resting splints are *not* indicated for ambulatory patients with dcSSc and certainly not lcSSc. Severely ill, bed-confined patients with wrist motion can develop wrist flexion contractures if not splinted or carefully ranged.

General Hand Therapy Guidelines

When possible, exercises should be done daily to maintain motion in all joints and in all planes. This includes flexion and extension of all the finger and thumb joints; finger and thumb abduction and adduction; thumb circumduction; wrist flexion, extension, deviation, and circumduction; and forearm supination and pronation. It is not feasible to list every possible ROM method that can be used with SSc patients. Each program must be developed with creativity and sensitivity to the patient's ability to carry out the program. Some patients can only manage 3 or 4 exercises despite the 20 or more that could be recommended. It is better that they perform 3 or 4 exercises effectively than none at all (Melvin, 1995).

Other Considerations

When patients have fixed deformities that limit function, the only recourse is to adapt equipment to accommodate the deformity. Typically this includes built-up handles and cuffs (e.g. a universal cuff utensil holder). If the patient has skin ulcers, it is important to evaluate hand function for fine tasks such as writing and buttoning.

There is likewise increased vulnerability of the skin to infection and irritation. Avoid any abrasive activities, materials, or substances that irritate the skin. Patients should be careful about traumatizing the skin over the dorsum of the finger joints. See Table 7.

Behavioral Treatment of Raynaud's Phenomenon

A range of behavioral methods can be used by patients to help control the symptoms of vasospasm. These constitute a patient education program for Raynaud's and are listed in Table 7. During the past 20 years, treatment of Raynaud's phenomenon has been limited to teaching

Table 7. Self-Management of Raynaud's Phenomenon (Melvin, 1994)

1. If you smoke or use tobacco, STOP! Nicotine narrows the blood vessels and reduces circulation. (The vasoconstrictive effects of nicotine last for days to weeks.)
2. Dress for warmth
   a. Keeping the trunk of your body warm helps increase the temperature and blood flow of the arms and legs (e.g., wearing a warm vest).
   b. Layer clothes, wear an undershirt or camisole, and wear two thin socks rather than one thick pair. (Silk is warmer than cotton.)
   c. New lightweight, high-tech fabric clothes and undergarments specifically designed to retain heat are available in camping goods stores or catalogs. (See Box 1.)
   d. Wear hats and scarves outside in the cold to retain body heat.
   e. Some patients wear inexpensive white cotton laboratory gloves at night or around the house to keep fingers warm.
   f. Wear socks to bed.
   g. Wear gloves to the grocery store, theater, mall, or places with constant air conditioning.
3. Around the house
   a. Use an electric blanket or sheet to warm the bed before getting in. If you do not like sleeping with an electric blanket, use it only to prewarm the bed. A down comforter can add warmth and is lightweight.
   b. Be careful to avoid getting chilled getting in and out of the bathtub or shower; fluffy terry cloth robes help.
   c. Eat modest meals; large meals decrease circulation in extremities.
4. When traveling
   a. On cold days, have someone preheat the car before getting in if possible.
   b. One patient reports carrying a small travel-size hair dryer to help warm her hands quickly when away from home.
5. Avoid medications that constrict blood vessels. These include certain migraine, heart, and blood pressure medications. Check with your pharmacist or physician before taking any new drugs.
6. Factors that can trigger a Raynaud's attack include a cold environment, touching something cold, air conditioning, drafts, nervousness or stress, or holding your hands down at your side for a prolonged period.

patients self-management techniques and thermal biofeedback (Table 7), but some new possibilities exist. Goodfield and Rowell (1988) conducted a controlled study in the United Kingdom that evaluated the effect of hot-water hand soaks every 4 hr during the day as a prophylactic treatment to improve blood flow in persons with SSc. The patients alternated weeks of warming with weeks of nonwarming. The results showed a notable decrease in the number and duration of Raynaud's attacks during the warming weeks. By measuring blood flow using laser Doppler flowmetry, they found that patients had at least 2 hr of improved blood flow after the warming procedure. They reported that simply having patients with SSc warm their hands before going out in the cold has been helpful for reducing symptoms (Goodfield et al., 1988).

Thermal biofeedback has been found to be effective in teaching patients how to volitionally raise digital temperature (Freedman et al., 1984; Yocum, Hodes, Sundstrom, & Cleeland, 1985). For certain patients, the ability to raise their peripheral temperature at will is helpful. It takes practice, however, to learn and maintain these skills. Biofeedback does not work for everyone with SSc because of the physical damage to the arteries described above. The specific usefulness of thermal biofeedback for severe symptoms such as debilitating pain, ulcers, or risk of gangrene needs further investigation. Arterial spasm in patients with this form of vasomotor instability can occur spontaneously or be triggered by exposure to cold, conscious emotional change (e.g., excitement, nervousness, and anger), subconscious fears, trauma, or pain. Most clients are aware of events that bring on an attack, especially if the event is associated with pain. However, the client may not relate emotional changes or the use of tobacco, caffeine, recreational drugs, or various medications to an attack. Nicotine is a major vasoconstrictor. Patients having difficulty quitting smoking may find it helpful to join a community organization devoted to assisting smokers to quit. (Call the lung or cancer association in your state for information.)

Face

Facial mobility may be lost early in the disease. The skin becomes taut, and the lips may atrophy and recede. The face takes on a characteristic masklike appearance (Figure 1). Facial involvement is one of the most devastating aspects of the disease. It robs patients of the ability to project their personality and unique individuality in an unparalleled manner. Facial changes can create a communication problem between patient and therapist, in that one cannot always rely on facial expressions as a cue to the patient's emotions or understanding of instructions.

One of the major consequences of facial involvement is the limitation of mouth aperture (microstoma) and temporomandibular joint excursion secondary to sclerosis of the skin, subcutaneous tissues, and facial muscles. Limited excursion restricts oral hygiene, dental care, and the ability to chew solid foods and reduces verbal articulation.

Therapy

If lack of facial expression is causing a communication problem, discuss it with the patient. He or she usually is aware of facial changes, but the loss of nonverbal communication may be unsuspected. Having the patient bring in a photograph taken before the onset of SSc is helpful. A photograph may facilitate discussion about the psychological effects of the facial changes and help the therapist to appreciate the individuality of the patient and the changes the patient has experienced.

When there is decreased jaw mobility, teach the patient how to measure the mouth aperture (the distance between upper and lower teeth) in front of a mirror at least once a day to monitor the excursion. The distance can be marked on an index card and kept handy for measuring to ensure that the patient attains maximal aperture every day. This method provides visual feedback so that stretching exercises can be increased if ROM is lost. It is important to evaluate the patient's oral hygiene habits and to educate the patient about the importance of maintaining dental health. If the patient has marked limitations, determine what assistive equipment would facilitate better hygiene (e.g., electric toothbrushes, water-jet pics, small brush heads, and dental floss applicators [devices that loop the floss around the tooth]).

Maintaining Facial Mobility Through Exercise

When planning therapy for facial involvement, it is important to keep in mind that fibrosis and atrophy take place in all the soft facial structures, including the skin, subcutaneous fat, and muscles. Table 8 provides a series of facial exercises designed to move a specific muscle or group of muscles to mobilize the fluid in the tissue and stretch the facial structures.

Patients who use this program daily report one or more of the following outcomes: an increase in the number of different exercises performed over time, an increase in

Table 8. Facial Exercise Program for Scleroderma (Melvin, 1977)

Instructions to the patient
1. Do exercises in front of a mirror.
2. Massage (firm touch) the entire face using small circular motions with the fingertips, a warm washcloth, or a vibrator. Then massage each specific area again just before exercising that part.
3. The number of repetitions necessary to get maximal mobility depends on the person. One approach is to do the exercise quickly two or three times as a warm-up and then do five repetitions holding each stretch position to the count of five. Sustained stretch is more effective for increasing mobility than rapid motions.

Exercises
These directions are designed to isolate, contract, and stretch the major facial muscles.
1. Raise the eyebrows as high as possible, then return to the normal position.
2. Bring the eyebrows down and together as hard as possible, as if frowning, then raise the eyebrows as high and wide as possible.
3. Wrinkle the bridge of the nose by raising the upper lip and then frowning (as if smelling something bad).
4. Close the eyes tightly, then release the squeeze slowly and raise the eyebrows as high as possible before opening the eyes.
5. Flare the nostrils, then narrow the nostrils down while pushing the upper lip out.
6. Make an exaggerated tight wink with each eye separately and use the cheek muscles to help close the eye.
7. Cover the teeth with the lips, then open the mouth as wide as possible keeping the teeth covered with the lips. Close lips and press hard (as if blotting lip gloss).
8. Open the mouth with the lips as wide apart as possible.
9. Open the mouth so that the teeth are as far apart as possible.
10. Push the jaw forward to create an underbite (bottom teeth in front of the upper teeth).
11. Make as wide a grin as possible without showing the teeth.
12. Pucker the chin by pushing the lower lip upward.
13. Stick the tongue out as far as possible.
14. Push the lower lip down and outward (as in an exaggerated pout).
15. Keep the mouth closed and puff the cheeks out with air; hold to the count of five and then release the air and suck the cheeks inward.
16. Lean the head back as far as possible and open and close the mouth five times.
17. Turn the head to look over one shoulder. Then look over the other shoulder.
18. Bend the ear down to the side to touch the shoulder. Repeat with the other ear.

the ability to perform the exercises, and a subjective sense of increased flexibility and suppleness after the exercises.

A patient should not be instructed in these exercises unless there is definite evidence of sclerosis (skin changes or hardness) in the face. If there is sclerosis only in the hands or arms, however, there is no way of predicting the course of the disease. In some patients, the disease may affect only the hands, but these patients should be monitored for disease progression.

All of the facial and neck muscles should be exercised, regardless of the stage of involvement. Obviously, many of the muscles will not move in the moderate or severe stages of sclerosis, let alone respond to exercise; therefore, the program must be individually tailored for each patient. A patient with severe involvement may be able to do only a couple of the prescribed exercises. The lip and mouth exercises are the most important because a limited mouth opening interferes with eating and oral hygiene (Rodnan et al., 1979; Yocum et al., 1985) (Table 8).

Feet

Complications in the feet, although uncommon, can be caused by Raynaud's phenomenon or fibrosis of the skin and surrounding structures. "Ram's horn nail," a thick twisted toenail, can occur as a result of vascular insufficiency to the nailbed (Wright, 1988). Corns may develop over joints where contractual deformities cause rubbing of the skin against the top of the shoe (Wright, 1988). The services of a pedorthotist to provide special modifications to a shoe to minimize complaints of pain may be beneficial. Hidebound ankle skin can adversely affect walking.

Thoracic Area

Chest expansion may decrease as a result of fibrosis of the skin, subcutaneous tissues, and intercostal muscles. The therapy objective is to maintain normal chest excursion. Treatment includes instructing the patient in deep breathing exercises. Evaluation of progress can be made by measuring the chest circumference during inspiration and expiration at the nipple line or below the breasts. Mobility is enhanced by having the patient perform total body, upper trunk, and chest stretching exercises.

Gastrointestinal Involvement

Involvement of the alimentary tract most frequently results in a slowing or absence of the peristaltic waves throughout the tract. The esophagus is usually involved first. The effects of this hypomotility are more pronounced in the recumbent position. Hypomotility results in difficulty swallowing (dysphagia), reflux esophagitis, heartburn, bloating, nausea, vomiting, and regurgitation with the risk of aspiration (LeRoy, 1982). More extensive involvement of the bowel may lead to malabsorption with consequent severe weight loss and weakness (Sternberg, 1985). Alternating constipation and diarrhea are common.

Patients with gastrointestinal symptoms are at high risk for developing nutritional deficiencies directly from the symptoms, from a decreased interest in food, or from difficulty in planning or preparing full meals. Patients often start omitting foods that are difficult to eat without making appropriate substitutions for the nutritional loss. Blockade of acid secretion usually improves reflux, and promotility agents improve motility.

The symptoms of hypomotility, reflux, and dysphagia can be reduced or alleviated by having the patient do the following: sit erect while drinking or eating to optimally align the esophagus and to allow gravity to assist motility; eat smaller and more frequent meals; cut food, especially meat, into small pieces; avoid dry food and sip beverages frequently during meals; and chew food well and concentrate on the chewing and swallowing process. Natural enzyme tablets (available in health food stores) can aid digestion and reduce gas.

Antireflux measures include sleeping with the head of the bed elevated 4 to 6 in. by placing blocks or telephone books under the legs to allow gravity to assist motility (this can be achieved with a foam wedge for the top half of the bed) and not eating large meals for 3 hr before bedtime. All patients who have difficulty eating or who cannot eat certain foods should receive counseling from a nutritionist.

Pulmonary Involvement

The two major clinical manifestations of lung involvement are fibrosing alveolitis (which occurs in 75% of the patients with SSc) and pulmonary vascular disease (which occurs in 50% of the patients with SSc) (Black & du Bois, 1996). Pulmonary disease is currently considered to be the major cause of death in SSc. Patients with dcSSc often have early pulmonary fibrosis and subsequent secondary pulmonary hypertension. Patients with lcSSc often present with primary pulmonary hypertension 10 or more years after onset; pulmonary fibrosis, if present, progresses at a slow rate. Patients may have pulmonary disease long before they have clinical symptoms because of the reserve capacity of the lungs (Silver, 1994). As much as one third to one half of the lungs may be involved before symptoms are evident (Black & du Bois, 1996). The most common symptom of pulmonary fibrosis is dyspnea initially on exertion and later at rest. The next most common symptom is a nonproductive cough. Pulmonary involvement diminishes oxygen uptake, decreases vital capacity, and involves dyspnea (Black & du Bois, 1996).

Dyspnea is described as a result of two factors: (1) a ventilation–perfusion mismatch and (2) the loss of alveolar compliance triggers stretch receptors, which results in reflex hyperpnea. This adds to the sensation of breathlessness because of the thickened interstitium (Black & du Bois, 1996). One study suggested that failure of the circulatory system is the limiting factor for exercise in SSc (Sudduth et al., 1993).

The patient should be instructed in energy conservation methods. Training in adaptive self-care methods should be provided along with diaphragmatic breathing principles. If the patient experiences severe dyspnea with exertion, the physician should be contacted immediately to evaluate the extent of pulmonary involvement. The restrictive pulmonary disease with associated fibrosis will affect the patient's ability to perform aerobic activities. The patient should be monitored carefully to minimize complaints of dyspnea and ensure adequate oxygen perfusion during his or her aerobic exercise program.

Before the development of pulmonary symptoms, deep breathing exercises can improve the health of the lungs and facilitate use of full lung capacity. For patients with dcSSc, exercises to improve and maintain rib cage excursion are essential for maintaining thoracic mobility and full lung capacity.

Cardiac Involvement

The most common forms of cardiac involvement include pericardial effusion, myocardial necrosis with fibrosis, and involvement of the large and small vessels of the coronary arteries. Myocardial infarctions are usually related to the usual risk factors, including family history, age, lipids, and stress (LeRoy, 1982).

The symptoms of cardiac involvement are similar to those of pulmonary involvement (e.g., shortness of breath at rest and dyspnea on exertion). The combination of orthopnea, cardiomegaly, and dependent edema usually indicates primary cardiac disease. Pitting edema can be a clue to unsuspected cardiac disease.

It is important to determine the condition of the heart from the patient's physician because the overall treatment program should reflect the ability of the heart to accommodate the stresses demanded of it during exercise. The therapist must observe work simplification principles in the clinic.

Renal Involvement

Renal failure was formerly the most common cause of death in SSc. Patients with proteinuria, hypertension, azotemia, or hyperreninemia are at high risk for developing renal failure (LeRoy, 1982). Deaths from scleroderma renal crisis continue to decrease in frequency, which is due primarily to effective antihypertensive therapy.

Patients with renal failure are treated with aggressive antihypertensive therapy by using ACE inhibitors and with renal support measures of dialysis. Kidney transplantation has been used successfully with selected patients (LeRoy, 1982).

Surgery for Systemic Sclerosis

Surgeries specific for SSc can be categorized based on purpose (Jones, Raynor, & Medsger, 1987). Surgeries to improve circulation and ulcer management include digital artery sympathectomy, microsurgery revascularization of the radial and ulnar arteries, PIP resection and arthrodesis, amputations, and excision of calculi. Surgeries to reduce deformities and improve hand function include MCP excisional arthroplasty, MCP capsulotomies, PIP arthrodesis, and thumb–IP arthrodesis. In addition, surgeries for specific secondary problems include carpal tunnel release, extensor tenolysis and relocation, and the Darrach procedure (removal of the distal ulna).

Surgeries to treat ulcers, calcinosis, and infections are specific and well documented (Gahos, Ariyan, Frazier, & Cuono, 1984; Jones et al., 1987; Jones, Imbriglia, Steen, & Medsger, 1987; Mendelson et al., 1977; Norris & Brown, 1985). Surgery to improve function in severely deformed hands has not been adequately discussed in the literature and is described by Nalebuff and Melvin (in press) in this series.

Figure 5. This is a woman 55 years of age who had dcSSc for 6 years; the disease went into remission in the third year, but deformities progressed because of bio-mechanical forces. Skin changes are late stage. The hand on the left looked identical to the one on the right with fixed MCP hyperextension before having MCP excision arthroplasty and PIP fusions. She has 45° of MCP flexion and is able to do a lateral pinch. When the patient stopped therapy, the MCP joints were fixed in 15° hyperextension. They progressed to 65° hyperextension as she used her palms to accomplish daily activities. Photo courtesy of Edward Nalebuff, MD.

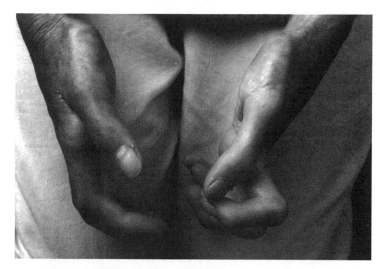

Hands with fixed, severe, classic deformities of MCP extension and PIP flexion can often benefit from PIP arthrodesis in a more functional position (especially to allow lateral pinch) and MCP excisional arthroplasty (silicon implants are generally not needed for stability) (Figure 5). The postoperative goal for the MCP arthroplasty is often a functional arc of motion in 30° to 50° of motion and the ability to grasp objects unilaterally. All surgery and therapy for the index finger should be directed toward maintaining or restoring lateral pinch.

References

Askew, L. J., Beckett, V. L., An, K. N., & Chao, E. Y. (1983). Objective evaluation of hand function in scleroderma patients to assess effectiveness of physical therapy. *British Journal of Rheumatology, 22*(4), 224–232.

Black, C. M., & du Bois, R. M. (1996). Organ involvement: Pulmonary. In P. J. Clements & D. E. Furst (Eds.), *Systemic sclerosis* (pp. 299–331). Baltimore: Williams & Wilkins.

Blocka, K. (1996). Organ involvement: Musculoskeletal. In P. J. Clements & D. E. Furst (Eds.), *Systemic sclerosis* (pp. 409–424). Baltimore: Williams & Wilkins.

Blom-Bulow, B., Jonson, B., & Bauer, K. (1983). Factors limiting exercise performance in PSS. *Seminars in Arthritis and Rheumatism, 13*(2), 174–181.

Casale, R., Buonocore, M., & Matucci-Cerinic, M. (1997). Systemic sclerosis (scleroderma): An integrated challenge in rehabilitation. *Archives of Physical Medicine and Rehabilitation, 78*(7), 767–773.

Clements, P. J., Furst, D. E., Campion, D. S., Bohan, A., Harris, R., Levy, J., & Paulus, H. E. (1978). Muscle disease in progressive systemic sclerosis: Diagnostic and therapeutic considerations. *Arthritis and Rheumatism, 21*(1), 62–71.

Clements, P. J., & Medsger, T. A. (1996). Organ involvement: Skin. In P. J. Clements & D. E. Furst (Eds.), *Systemic sclerosis* (pp. 389–407). Baltimore: Williams & Wilkins.

Entin, M. A., & Wilkinson, R. D. (1973). Scleroderma hand: A reappraisal. *Orthopedic Clinics of North America, 4,* 1031.

Freedman, R. R., Ianni, P., & Wenig, P. (1984). Behavioral treatment of Raynaud's phenomenon in scleroderma. *Journal of Behavioral Medicine, 7*(4), 343–353.

Gahos, F., Ariyan, S., Frazier, W. H., & Cuono, C. B. (1984). Management of sclerodermal finger ulcers. *Journal of Hand Surgery, 9*(3), 320–327.

Goodfield, N. J. D., & Rowell, N. R. (1988). Hand warming as a treatment for Raynaud's phenomenon in systemic sclerosis. *British Journal of Dermatology, 119*, 643–646.

Goodfield, N. J. D., Hume, A., & Rowell, N. R. (1988). The effect of simple warming procedures on finger blood flow in systemic sclerosis. *British Journal of Dermatology, 118*, 661–668.

Hicks, J. E. (1990). Exercise in patients with inflammatory arthritis and connective tissue disease. *Rheumatic Disease Clinics of North America, 16*(4), 845–870.

Jones, N. F. (1996). Surgical treatment of the hand in systemic sclerosis. In P. J. Clements & D. E. Furst (Eds.), *Systemic sclerosis* (pp. 569–579). Baltimore: Williams & Wilkins.

Jones, N. F., Imbriglia, J. E., Steen, V. D., & Medsger, T. A. (1987). Surgery for scleroderma of the hand. *Journal of Hand Surgery, 12*, 391–400.

Jones, N. F., Raynor, S. C., & Medsger, T. A. (1987). Microsurgical revascularization of the hand in scleroderma. *British Journal of Plastic Surgery, 40*, 264–269.

Kisner, C., & Colby, L. A. (1990). *Therapeutic exercise: Foundations and techniques*. Philadelphia: F. A. Davis.

LeRoy, E. C. (1981). Scleroderma (systemic sclerosis). In W. M. Kelley, E. D. Harris, S. Ruddy, & C. B. Sledge (Eds.), *Textbook of rheumatology* (pp. 1183–1205). Philadelphia: Saunders.

LeRoy, E. C. (1982). Pathogenesis of scleroderma (systemic sclerosis). *Journal of Investigative Dermatology, 79*(Suppl. 1), S87–S89.

LeRoy, E. C. (1985). Scleroderma (systemic sclerosis). In W. M. Kelley, E. D. Harris, Jr., S. Ruddy, & C. B. Sledge (Eds.), *Textbook of rheumatology* (2nd ed., pp. 1183–1205). Philadelphia: Saunders.

LeRoy, E. C., Black, C., Fleischmajer, R., Jablonska, S., Krieg, T., Medsger, T. A., Jr., Rowell, N., & Wollheim, F. (1988). Scleroderma (systemic sclerosis): Classification subsets and pathogenesis. *Journal of Rheumatology, 15*, 202–205.

LeRoy, E. C., & Lomeo, R. (1989). The spectrum of scleroderma: Part I. *Hospital Practice, 24*, 33–42.

Medsger, T. A., Jr. (1988). Systemic sclerosis and localized scleroderma. In R. Schumacher, Jr. (Ed.), *Primer on the rheumatic diseases* (pp. 111–117). Atlanta, GA: Arthritis Foundation.

Medsger, T. A., Jr. (1985). Systemic sclerosis (scleroderma), localized forms of scleroderma, eosinophilic fasciitis, and calcinosis. In D. J. McCarty & W. J. Koopman (Eds.), *Arthritis and allied conditions: A textbook of rheumatology* (10th ed., pp. 994–1036). Philadelphia: Lea & Febiger.

Melvin, J. L. (1977). *Rheumatic disease: Occupational therapy and rehabilitation*. Philadelphia: F. A. Davis.

Melvin, J. L. (1989). Systemic sclerosis. In *Rheumatic disease in the adult and child: Occupational therapy and rehabilitation* (3rd ed., pp. 106–122). Philadelphia, F. A. Davis.

Melvin, J. L. (1994). *Scleroderma: Caring for your hands and face*. Rockville, MD: American Occupational Therapy Association.

Melvin, J. L. (1995). Scleroderma (systemic sclerosis): Treatment of the hand. In J. M. Hunter, E. J. Mackin, & A. D. Callahan (Eds.), *Rehabilitation of the hand: Surgery and therapy* (4th ed., pp. 1385–1397). St. Louis: Mosby.

Melvin, J. L., Brannan, K. L., & LeRoy, E. C. (1984). Comprehensive care for the patient with systemic sclerosis (scleroderma). *Clinical Rheumatology in Practice, 2*(3), 112.

Mendelson, M. B., Linscheid, R. L., Dobyns, J. H., & Miller, S. A. (1977). Surgical treatment of calcinosis cutis in the upper extremity. *Journal of Hand Surgery, 2*(4), 318–324.

Michlovitz, S. L. (1986). *Thermal agents in rehabilitation*. Philadelphia: F. A. Davis.

Misra, R., Darton, D., Jewkes, R. F., Black, C. M., & Maini, R. N. (1995). Arthritis in scleroderma. *British Journal of Rheumatology, 34,* 831–837.

Murray, R. L. (1972). Principles of nursing interventions for the adult patient with body image changes. *Nursing Clinics of North America, 7,* 697.

Nalebuff, E. A., & Melvin, J. L. (in press). Systemic sclerosis in the hand. In J. L. Melvin & E. A. Nalebuff (Eds.), *Rheumatologic rehabilitation series: Volume 4: The hand: Evaluation, therapy, and surgery.* Bethesda, MD: American Occupational Therapy Association.

Norris, R. W., & Brown, H. G. (1985). The proximal interphalangeal joint in systemic sclerosis and its surgical management. *British Journal of Plastic Surgery, 38,* 526–531.

Osial, T. A., Avakian, A., Sassouni, V., Agarwal, A., Medsger, T. A., Jr., & Rodnan, G. P. (1981). Resorption of the mandibular condyles and coronoid processes in progressive systemic sclerosis (scleroderma). *Arthritis and Rheumatism, 25,* 729.

Osler, W. (1898). Scleroderma. *Journal of Cutaneous and Genito-Urinary Diseases, 16,* 49, 127.

Poole, J. L. (1996). Occupational and physical therapy. In P. J. Clements & D. E. Furst (Eds.), *Systemic sclerosis* (pp. 581–590). Baltimore: Williams & Wilkins.

Postlethwaite, A. E., & Kang, A. H. (1984). Pathogenesis of progressive systemic sclerosis. *Journal of Laboratory and Clinical Medicine, 103,* 506–510.

Rodnan, G. P., Jablonska, S., & Medsger, T. A., Jr. (1979). Classification and nomenclature of progressive systemic sclerosis (scleroderma). *Rheumatic Disease Clinics of North America, 5,* 5–13.

Rudolph, R. I., Leyden, J. J., & Berger, B. J. (1974). Efficacy of physiatric management of linear scleroderma. *Archives of Physical Medicine and Rehabilitation, 55,* 428–431.

Seeger, M. W., & Furst, D. E. (1987). Effects of splinting in the treatment of hand contractures in progressive systemic sclerosis. *American Journal of Occupational Therapy, 41,* 118–121.

Siebold, J. R. (1993). Scleroderma. In W. N. Kelley, E. D. Harris, Jr., S. Ruddy, & C. B. Sledge (Eds.), *Textbook of rheumatology* (4th ed., pp. 1113–1143). Philadelphia: Saunders.

Silver, R. M. (1994). Systemic sclerosis (scleroderma). In M. M. Frank, K. F. Austen, H. N. Claman, & E. R. Unanue (Eds.), *Samter's immunological diseases* (5th ed., pp. 805–822). Boston: Little, Brown.

Smith, E. A., & LeRoy, E. C. (1994). Connective tissue diseases: Systemic sclerosis: Etiology and pathogenesis. In P. A. Klippel & J. M. Dieppe (Eds.), *Rheumatology* (pp. 9.1–9.10). London: Mosby-Year Book.

Sternberg, E. M. (1985). Pathogenesis of scleroderma: The interrelationship of the immune and vascular hypotheses. *Survey of Immunologic Research, 4*(1), 69–80.

Sudduth, C. D., Strange, C., Cook, W. R., Miller, K. S., Baumann, M., Collop, N. A., & Silver, R. M. (1993). Failure of the circulatory system limits exercise performance in patients with systemic sclerosis. *American Journal of Medicine, 95,* 413–418.

Trelkeld, A. J. (1992). The effect of manual therapy on connective tissue. *Physical Therapy, 72*(12), 61–70.

Trust, D. (1981). Disfigurement: Something to face up to. *Medical Times, 109*(7), 88–92.

Wigley, F. M., & Matsumoto, A. (1995). Scleroderma. In M. A. Weisman & M. E. Weinblatt (Eds.), *Treatment of rheumatic disease* (pp. 172–191). Philadelphia: Saunders.

Wright, N. D. (1988). Footcare in scleroderma: Part 1. *Newsletter of the Scleroderma International Foundation, 16*(2), 1–3.

Yocum, D. E., Hodes, R., Sundstrom, W. R., & Cleeland, C. S. (1985). Use of biofeedback training in treatment of Raynaud's disease and phenomenon. *Journal of Rheumatology, 12*(1), 90–93.

10

Psoriatic Arthritis

Proton Rahman, MD, FRCPC, MSC, Dafna D. Gladman, MD, FRCPC, Victoria Gall, MEd, PT, and Jeanne L. Melvin, MS, OTR, FAOTA

Psoriatic arthritis (PsA) is an inflammatory form of arthritis associated with psoriasis. It is a disease with diverse heterogeneous clinical features associated with relapsing and remitting symptoms that have classically been described in five different clinical patterns. As a result, there is some debate about the group of arthritides to which PsA belongs. Currently, it is classified with seronegative spondylarthropathies because the disease is characterized by a peripheral arthritis, spondylitis in 40% of patients (one subtype), association with human lymphocyte antigen (HLA) B-27, and a lack of rheumatoid factor (RF) and antinuclear antibody (ANA) activity in the sera of most patients. (PsA is presented as a separate chapter in this volume because therapists frequently see patients with subsets that do not have spinal involvement.)

Background

The first reported case of PsA was described by Baron Jean Luis Aubert in 1818, and the term *psoriasis arthritique* was first coined by Pierre Bazin in 1860 (Wright, 1956). The American College of Rheumatology (ACR) (formerly the American Rheumatism Association) recognized PsA as a distinct clinical entity in 1964. Since then, epidemiological studies have shown that PsA is a separate disease entity with its characteristic demographic, clinical, and radiological features.

Classification

The currently accepted definition for PsA was developed by Moll and Wright (1973), who described it as the presence of psoriasis with inflammatory arthritis and classified it into five subtypes (Moll & Wright, 1973). Other classification systems have been described by Bennett (1979), Vasey & Espinoza (1984), and the European Spondyloarthropathy Study Group (Dougados et al., 1991), but these have not been widely used (Gladman, 1995). Despite the fact that there are no formally accepted criteria for the diagnosis of PsA, most clinicians and investigators use the working definition that it is an inflammatory arthritis associated with psoriasis and is usually seronegative for RF.

Population Affected

The true incidence of PsA in the general population is unknown, and its prevalence can only be estimated. Psoriasis is a common disorder that affects between 1% and 3% of the population (Goodfield, 1994). The frequency of inflammatory arthritis in the general population has been reported to be between 2% and 3%. About 6% to 42% of patients with psoriasis develop arthritis; this is higher than the rate of arthritis in the general population (O'Neill & Silman, 1994). The wide range of the frequency of PsA may be due to the lack of validated criteria for PsA and to variability in the selection bias in various studies. Thus, the estimated prevalence of PsA varies between 0.5% and 1.2% in European and North American studies (Hellgren, 1969; van Romunde, Valkenburg, Swart-Bruinsma, Cats, & Hermans, 1984).

Overall, PsA affects both genders almost equally (Gladman, 1990; Jones et al., 1994; Moll & Wright, 1973; Veale, Rogers, & Fitzgerald, 1994). In terms of its prevalence, however, there is a slightly higher number of male patients with distal arthritis and spinal disease and a slightly higher number of female patients with polyarthritis. The disease usually occurs in the third or fourth decades of life, although pediatric PsA has been recognized. (See volume 3 of this series.) The psoriasis usually precedes the arthritis, but in 15% of patients, the psoriasis occurs after the onset of articular features (Gladman, 1990). There is little data concerning racial and ethnic differences in PsA.

Etiologic Factors

The etiology of psoriasis and PsA remains unknown but is believed to be a complex interaction among genetic, immunological, and environmental factors (Abu-Shakra & Gladman, 1994).

Genetic Factors

There is convincing evidence of a genetic basis for both psoriasis and PsA. Family history of either psoriasis or PsA is evident in more than 40% of patients with PsA. Psoriasis is increased threefold in the offspring of a parent with psoriasis, and there is a high incidence of psoriasis if both parents have the condition. In addition, concordance between monozygotic twins is 73% versus 20% between dizygotic twins (Abu-Shakra & Gladman, 1994; Eastmond, 1994). The discovery of the major histocompatibility locus on chromosome 6 in humans (HLA locus) has provided further evidence of genetic predisposition for this disease (Eastmond, 1994). HLA B-27 has clearly been associated with spine disease in PsA, thus lending further credence to its grouping with B-27–associated spondylarthropathy (Abu-Shakra & Gladman, 1994; Eastmond, 1994). HLA DR-4 appears to be associated with the peripheral articular pattern of PsA.

Immunological Factors

Evidence is progressively accumulating that the immune response plays an important role in the initiation or perpetuation of the inflammatory process in PsA (Abu-Shakra & Gladman, 1994; Panayi, 1994). However, its precise role has yet to be defined. Support for an immunological theory in PsA results from the presence of lymphocytic infiltrate in both the skin and joint lesions, the presence of circulating immune complexes in the serum, and abnormalities noted in cytokines, growth factors, and adhesion molecules.

Although the number of B lymphocytes in the peripheral blood of patients with PsA has been found to be normal, increased production of autoantibodies has been reported (Gladman, 1985). About 10% to 15% of patients with both uncomplicated psoriasis and PsA have both RF and ANA activity in their sera, and elevated levels of circulating immune complexes have been reported (Gladman, Anhorn, Schacter, & Mervati, 1986). Impaired suppressor cell function and a decreased T lymphocyte subpopulation in PsA despite normal total cell counts have likewise been detected (Abu-Shakra & Gladman, 1994).

Environmental Factors

Because there is not a complete concordance in identical twins (i.e., only one may have PsA), one must consider the role of environmental factors in the pathogenesis of PsA (Abu-Shakra & Gladman, 1994). Infection and trauma have long been recognized as potential triggering factors in psoriasis and PsA (Reveille, 1993). The temporal relationship between certain viral and bacterial infections and the exacerbation or development of psoriasis and PsA is well established. *Streptococcus* has been isolated in 26% to 79% of throat cultures and in patients with psoriasis. Similar trends have been noted in patients with PsA. There is an increase in prevalence of *Chlamydia trachomatis* as well (Silveira et al., 1993).

Both psoriasis and PsA are associated with HIV infection. Solinger and Hess (1993) found that 9 out of 1,100 HIV-infected patients had psoriasis, which is a higher frequency than expected. (See the section on HIV and PsA in chapter 13 in this volume.)

There are no detailed epidemiological studies describing the role of trauma in triggering the development of PsA (Abu-Shakra & Gladman, 1994). It is theorized that both microtrauma and major trauma may direct activated inflammatory cells to the site of the injured joint or tendon (Vasey, Seleznick, Fenske, & Espinoza, 1989). When psoriasis appears at the site of an injury such as a cut or surgical incision, it is referred to as a *positive Koebner phenomenon*. A reverse Koebner response occurs when the psoriasis clears at the injury site. This response suggests that there is a systemic mechanism controlling Koebner reactivity (Breathnach, 1993). A few studies have noted the occurrence of arthritis and acro-osteolysis after physical trauma (Scarpa et al., 1992). Whether this represents a deep Koebner phenomenon is not known.

Clinical Features

PsA is an inflammatory disease with articular and extra-articular features. The onset of arthritis is usually insidious, but up to one third of cases may have an acute presentation with sudden onset of joint pain, swelling, and intense periarticular erythema.

Constitutional symptoms are more prevalent with active polyarticular disease and can occur in up to 20% to 25% of patients with PsA. These symptoms include morning stiffness, fatigue, malaise, and weight loss. High fevers are uncommon and occur in less than 5% of patients. On the basis of clinical observations, Moll and Wright (1973) divided PsA into five different subsets. (They are reordered herein by decreasing frequency.)

Oligoarthritis

Oligoarthritis or pauciarticular arthritis is a pattern of arthritis involving only a few joints often in an asymmetrical distribution (Figure 1). Traditionally, this pattern has been considered to be the most

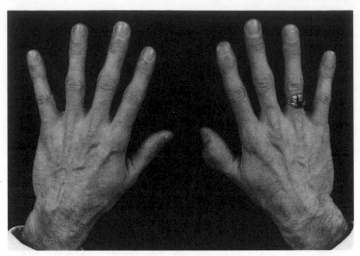

Figure 1. Oligoarticular pattern (asymmetrical involvement of a few joints). Photo courtesy of Proton Rahman, MD and Dafna Gladman, MD.

common form of PsA and accounts for approximately 70% of cases. However, more recent studies suggest that this pattern is less common, and its frequency may be related to disease duration (Gladman, 1990; Jones et al., 1994; Veale et al., 1994). Thus, although patients may initially present with an oligoarthritis, during the course of their illness, this evolves into a polyarthritis. Indeed, in reports where the disease duration was short (e.g., less than 5 years), the oligoarticular pattern was more common, but in studies that included patients with longer disease duration (e.g., greater than 10 years), the polyarticular pattern was more common (Gladman, 1994). Like other patterns of PsA, the oligoarticular presentation commonly involves the distal interphalangeal (DIP), proximal interphalangeal (PIP), metacarpal phalangeal (MCP), metatarsal phalangeal (MTP), and knee joints. Dactylitis (inflammation of the entire digit) is a frequent occurrence in this form of PsA.

Symmetrical Polyarthritis

It was once noted that symmetrical polyarthritis occurred in approximately 15% to 25% of patients with PsA (Gladman, 1994). More recent large published trials show that more than 40% of cases of PsA manifest with polyarthritis (Gladman, 1990; Jones et al., 1994; Veale et al., 1994). As noted above, the exact frequency of this pattern is related to the disease duration in the study population. Joints frequently involved are the PIPs, MCPs, shoulders, and knees. When presenting with a polyarticular distribution, PsA must be distinguished from RA. Patients with PsA tend to be less tender than patients with RA. It is often difficult to detect effusions in these patients because they tend to be tight and not as "juicy" as rheumatoid effusions.

Distal Arthritis

Arthritis involving the DIP joints is typical of PsA. This was considered a classic form of PsA and occurs in approximately 12% of patients with PsA, although some investigators have not been able to identify isolated DIP disease. Moreover, DIP joint involvement is additionally found in the other clinical subsets because it occurs in 53% of all patients with PsA, and thus its definition has been difficult (Gladman, 1990).

Arthritis Mutilans ("Opera Glass Hand" or "La Main Lorgnette")

Mutilans deformity involves severe osteolysis of the bone ends that shortens the ends and leaves the joint completely unstable (Figure 2). This deformity occurs most commonly at the digit joints in the hands and feet and at the radiocarpal and radioulnar joints in the wrist (Nalebuff & Garrett, 1976). When it occurs in the digits, the ends of the bones resorb and shorten. The overlying redundant skin give a telescoping appearance to the fingers, hence the name "opera glass hand." This deformity can severely impair function, dexterity, and grip, although it is usually painless. This is the most destructive and devastating outcome in PsA. Although frequently emphasized due to its erosive nature, mutilans deformity fortunately occurs in less than 10% of patients with PsA. It has been suggested that this form of PsA is associated with an earlier age of onset and with spondylarthropathy.

Spondylarthropathy

Spondylarthropathy develops in 20% to 40% of patients but is rarely detected at the onset of PsA (Figure 3). It consists of sacroiliitis with or without spondylitis. Most commonly, spondylarthropathy occurs together with another pattern of peripheral arthritis. In a small number of the patients, spondylarthropathy occurs without peripheral joint involvement. Sacroiliitis in patients with PsA tends to be asymmetrical, whereas the syndesmophytes (ossification of the anterior and lateral vertebral ligaments) tend to be coarse. It should be noted that spondylarthropathy in PsA is not as severe as that seen in ankylosing spondylitis. Spondylarthropathy in PsA presents at a later age and is associated with less pain and less restriction in the range of back movements than that in ankylosing spondylitis.

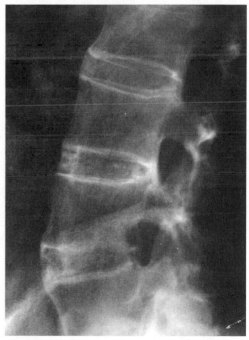

Figure 3. Spondylarthropathy. Soft-tissue calcification within the outer fibers of the annulus of the vertebral disc and the fibers of the anterior and lateral vertebral ligaments create a bony bridge between the separate vertebral bodies that gives the spine a "bamboo" appearance. This anterior and lateral new bone is called a *syndesmophyte* and is characteristic of spondylitis. Photo courtesy of Proton Rahman, MD and Dafna Gladman, MD.

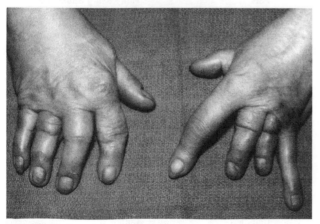

Figure 2. Mutilans deformity. The shortening of the digits can be prevented by surgical fusion (Nalebuff & Garrett, 1976). The length of the left little finger has been maintained because it ankylosed before mutilans started. Photo courtesy of Proton Rahman, MD and Dafna Gladman, MD.

In addition to these subsets, it is possible to have PsA on the basis of classic X-ray and clinical findings without any apparent signs of psoriasis. This is referred to as *PsA sine* (without) *psoriasis* (Barth, 1994).

Other Clinical Features of Psoriatic Arthritis

Other clinical features of active PsA include dactylitis (an inflammatory process involving the whole digit) and enthesitis (inflammation at sites of tendon insertions, especially around the heel). PsA is often associated with spur formation. These features are common to all seronegative spondylarthropathies. These features and the clinical subsets described above help distinguish PsA from rheumatoid arthritis (RA) and ankylosing spondylitis (Table 1).

Extra-Articular Features

Extra-articular features common to seronegative spondylarthropathy include ocular involvement (particularly iritis or uveitis), aortic insufficiency, mucous membrane lesions, and colitis, and these features may be seen in patients with PsA. On the other hand, rheumatoid nodules, vasculitis, and pulmonary and renal manifestations that may be seen in RA are not seen in patients with PsA.

Psoriasis

Most patients with PsA have the classic form of psoriasis vulgaris. Pustular psoriasis and erythroderma have been reported in PsA. Usually psoriasis precedes the onset of arthritis in approximately 70% of cases, with 15% having simultaneous onset of skin and joint involvement. The time

Table 1. Clinical Features in Psoriatic Compared With Rheumatoid Arthritis and Ankylosing Spondylitis

	RA	PsA	Ankylosing Spondylitis
Peripheral Joint Involvement	Common	Common	Uncommon
Pattern of Joint Involvement	Symmetrical	Often asymmetrical	Asymmetrical
DIP Involvement	Uncommon	Common	Occasionally
Spondylitis	N/A	Common	Always
Classic Syndesmophytes	N/A	Uncommon	Common
Paramarginal Syndesmophytes	N/A	Common	Common
Sacroiliitis	N/A	Common	Common
Bilateral Sacroiliitis	N/A	Uncommon	Common
Iritis	N/A	Uncommon	Common
Psoriasis	Uncommon	Common	Uncommon
Nail Lesions	Uncommon	Common	Common
Rheumatoid Nodules	Common	N/A	N/A

N/A = not applicable.

interval between the onset of psoriasis and arthritis is extremely variable. When arthritis precedes psoriasis, spondylitis appears to be the most common subset of PsA noted (Gladman, 1994). Simultaneous flare-ups between skin and joint manifestations are reported in 35% of patients. Nail lesions (including pitting and ridges) and onycholysis are associated with the development of PsA. These changes occur in 90% of patients with PsA and only in 41% of patients with psoriasis without arthritis. Another extra-articular manifestations of PsA is SAPHO (synovitis, acne, pustulosis [neutrophilic abscess], hyperostosis [bone hypertrophy], and osteitis [sterile bone inflammation]). SAPHO is a group of diseases with extra-articular osseous patterns (i.e., excess bone growth unrelated to a joint) and severe acne and pustulosis.

Laboratory Features

There are no specific laboratory investigations that are diagnostic for PsA. The abnormalities noted are compatible with any chronic inflammatory process. Acute-phase reactants such as erythrocyte sedimentation rate (ESR) are elevated in approximately 40% to 60% of patients. Serum protein electrophoresis reveals a polyclonal hypergammaglobulinemia with statistically significant levels of immunoglobulin A (IgA) and IgG but not IgM. Most patients are IgM negative and RF negative. Recent studies have noted that 5% to 16% of patients have a low titer of RF, and 2% to 16% of patients are ANA positive (Gladman, 1990).

Radiologic Findings

The key radiographic features of PsA include soft-tissue swelling, minimal osteopenia, bone erosions, resorption of the distal phalanx, prominent new bone formation, asymmetrical distribution, and paravertebral ossification. There is a predilection for hands, feet, sacroiliac joints, and the spine.

Although similar peripheral joints may be involved, radiographs of patients with PsA usually do not demonstrate the same degree of periarticular osteopenia as patients with RA. Indeed, PsA is associated with periosteal reaction and bone formation. As noted above for the clinical distribution, PsA tends to be asymmetrical compared with RA, although in almost 50% of patients with PsA, the distribution is symmetrical. In addition, the involvement of the DIP joints that is common in PsA is unusual in patients with RA.

Certain pertinent radiographic features help to confirm the diagnosis of PsA. PsA usually has normal bone density despite marked erosions. Erosions may be marked and lead to "pencil-in-cup" deformities (i.e., osteolysis of the proximal digit bone and hyperosteosis of the adjacent distal bone) (Figure 4). New bone formation is a striking feature of PsA and often leads to ankylosis. Indeed, patients may demonstrate a pencil-in-cup deformity in one joint, whereas another may be totally ankylosed. Tuft resorption of the distal phalanx can often be quite prominent and similar to that seen in scleroderma. The enthesitis noted above may be associated with spur formation. Thus, patients with PsA commonly present with calcaneal spurs both at the insertion of the plantar fascia and at the insertion of the Achilles' tendon. Similar "whiskering" (fine new bone formation) may be noted at the insertion of the tendons into the pelvic bones.

Drug Treatment

The aim of therapy in PsA is to induce remission of the skin lesions, alleviate articular symptoms, and prevent joint destruction. PsA should no longer be considered a benign nondisabling arthritis because up to 20% of patients may develop a destructive form of arthritis. Thus, if nonsteroidal anti-inflammatory drugs (NSAIDs) do not control the arthritis, a disease-modifying antirheumatic drug (DMARD) should be strongly considered. When starting a second-line agent, one should evaluate the extent of psoriasis because certain DMARDs such as methotrexate, cyclosporin, and sulfasalazine may help both the skin and joint manifestations (Abu-Shakra & Gladman, 1993).

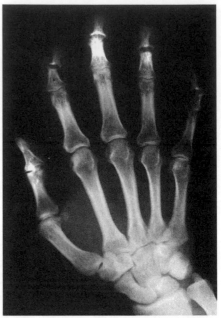

Figure 4. "Pencil-in-cup" deformity of the DIP joints. Erosive arthritis causes the proximal bone end to become conical and the distal bone to enlarge like a saucer (saucerized distortion) or cup. Photo courtesy of Proton Rahman, MD and Dafna Gladman, MD.

NSAIDs are the initial drugs selected for PsA, and most patients will settle on this treatment, even though all the NSAIDs have a similar effectiveness when given in equivalent therapeutic doses. It has been suggested that enteric coated acetylsalicylic acid, ibuprofen, naproxen, and diclofenac sodium are preferred for patients with peripheral arthritis. Indomethacin and tolectin are indicated for patients with axial disease. On occasion, certain NSAIDs such as indomethacin and phenylbutazone have been implicated in worsening psoriasis (Reshad, Hargreaves, & Vickers, 1983). Corticosteroids are usually avoided if possible. One special problem in PsA is that the skin disease may exacerbate when the steroid is discontinued.

The same second-line drugs used for the treatment of RA have been used for the treatment of PsA. These include gold, chloroquine, sulfasalazine, penicillamine, methotrexate, imuran, and cyclosporin A. Currently, chloroquine and sulfasalazine are considered to be safer second-line agents in the treatment of rheumatic diseases. Thus, these drugs are often used for milder cases that do not improve with an NSAID. The same principle can be extended for PsA. However, when treating patients with PsA, the treatment of both skin and joint disease must be considered, and medications that control both components of the disease are favored.

Both oral and intramuscular gold salts have been used to treat PsA. Intramuscular gold has been shown to be more effective than oral gold (Abu-Shakra & Gladman, 1993). In our experience, 50% of patients had at least 40% improvement in joint count. However, there was no slowing in the progression of joint damage as measured by radiographs over 2 years (Mader, Gladman, Long, Gough, & Farewell, 1995).

Antimalarials have traditionally been avoided in PsA due to possible exacerbation of skin lesions (Abu-Shakra & Gladman, 1993). More recent studies (Bruce & Gladman, 1998), however, have suggested that the prevalence of worsening skin disease is quite low and that there is no longer a contraindication in using chloroquine to treat PsA. One must be aware of the potential for erythroderma and exfoliative skin reactions that have been noted with antimalarials. Neither gold nor chloroquine has been shown to be effective against the skin disease.

There are recent trials that suggest that sulfasalazine is beneficial in the treatment of PsA (Dougados et al., 1995; Gupta et al., 1995). These studies showed a major reduction in morning stiffness and pain scores as measured by the visual analog scale and the ESR. These patients received a maximum dose of 3.0 g/day for approximately 8 weeks. There is a suggestion that sulfasalazine may be effective in treating the skin psoriasis as well. If this is confirmed, then sulfasalazine will become a drug of choice for PsA.

Methotrexate was the first drug shown to be effective in suppressing synovitis and controlling psoriasis in PsA. It appears to be a safe and effective agent for PsA as long as it is monitored carefully. Methotrexate is commonly preferred by rheumatologists for patients with persistent synovitis with or without skin lesions. Despite its popularity, there are no convincing controlled trials of low-dose methotrexate in PsA that show a benefit. Espinoza and associates (1992), in a retrospective uncontrolled trial of 40 patients followed on average for 34 months, showed a good or excellent response to methotrexate in 95% of patients. That study used a mean dose of 11.2 mg/week. However, the long-term effect of methotrexate in preventing erosions was recently questioned when it was shown in a case-control study that radiological progression was not reduced by the use of methotrexate during a 2-year period (Abu-Shakra et al., 1995).

Penicillamine has been shown to be effective, but it is toxic and takes a long time to become effective. It has not been particularly effective for the skin disease. Imuran was beneficial in one controlled study. Although it may be effective for the skin disease, it has not been widely used (Abu-Shakra & Gladman, 1993).

Cyclosporin A is highly effective for psoriasis, and its effect in PsA is derived from open studies, but it has notable toxicity that precludes its routine use. Its toxicity mainly affects the kidneys and can lead to nephrotoxicity and hypertension. Its use is reserved for patients with extremely resistant psoriasis and PsA.

Oral psoralen followed by ultraviolet A radiation (PUVA) has been used effectively for the treatment of PsA. There is only one trial with PsA that showed that PUVA had an effect on the peripheral arthritis but not on the spondylarthropathy (Perlman, Gerber, & Roberts, 1985). Because psoralen has been linked to malignancies, its use has been restricted. The effect of PUVA on the arthritis has not been tested. Recent studies (Wilfert, Honnigsmann, Steiner, Smolen, & Wolff, 1990) have suggested that there may be a role for photopharesis (i.e., using PUVA on lymphocytes removed by pharesis) in the treatment of PsA.

Artificial short-wave ultraviolet light (UVB) can be used alone or in combination with tar therapy to treat psoriasis. Although UVB is an effective treatment for psoriasis, there is no evidence that it improves the articular symptoms of patients with PsA.

Regarding retinoids, the Canadian Pilot Trial of tegison in 40 patients showed a mean improvement in tender joints from 22 to 11 over 24 weeks (Klinkhoff et al., 1989). This agent is toxic and causes drying of the skin and hyperlipidemia. New generations of this agent are currently under evaluation.

Because of the proposed role of leukotrienes in the pathogenesis of psoriasis and PsA, fish oil (through food and supplements) has been used to control both the skin and joint manifestations. Pilot studies suggested that there may be a therapeutic response, but this was not supported by controlled trials, at least for psoriasis (Abu-Shakra & Gladman, 1993).

Other treatments reported useful in PsA include vitamin D_3, bromocriptine, somatostatin, interferon, and peptide T, but their usefulness has been based on case reports and open trials (Abu-Shakra & Gladman, 1993), and they are not in routine use. These agents may become more popular in the future.

Rehabilitation

Physical therapy and occupational therapy interventions are directed at preventing contractures and ankylosis in a nonfunctional position and at optimizing and maintaining function in the presence of this chronic disease. Basic education in exercise, posture, and strategies to prevent dysfunction should take place soon after diagnosis, particularly if the disease is not responding to medication. Joint inflammation and sequelae in the polyarticular subset are similar to that seen in RA except that dactylitis creates unique stiffness problems, and deformity patterns are less predictable. Rehabilitative measures are the same as for RA. (See chapter 7 in this volume.) The exception is that persons with PsA are more likely to develop range of motion (ROM) limitations and ankylosis than persons with RA, and this can occur rapidly during acute episodes. Patients with spinal involvement require the same rehabilitation protocol as patients with ankylosing spondylitis. (See chapter 11 on ankylosing spondylitis.)

Hand Involvement

Nalebuff (1996) proposed a classification system for the PsA hand on the basis of radiographic and clinical findings rather than patterns of involvement.

- Type 1: patients who have primarily spontaneous ankylosis
- Type 2: patients with osteolysis or mutilans deformity
- Type 3: patients with RA-like deformities with stiffness

This classification is correlated here with the Moll and Wright (1973) classification.

Oligoarthritis (Pauciarticular or Nalebuff Type 1)

As the name implies, only a few joints are involved in this subtype, and they are in an asymmetrical pattern (i.e., an MCP joint on one hand and a PIP joint on the other hand) (Figure 1). Any of the hand joints can be affected.

Dactylitis is a common inflammatory process involving the entire digit and is often referred to as a "sausage digit." In the past, this was attributed to a combination of joint synovitis and flexor tenosynovitis, but it now appears that all of the tissues in the digit are inflamed. A recent study (Olivieri et al., 1996) used ultrasound and magnetic resonance imaging (MRI) to evaluate the role of tenosynovitis and arthritis in dactylitis. The study evaluated 12 dactylitic fingers and their contralateral normal digits in 10 patients with spondylarthropathy. MRI revealed flexor tenosynovitis in all digits but joint distention in only one joint. Physical examination identified 11 swollen joints, which reveals how difficult it is to evaluate joint swelling in the presence of dactylitis. The authors concluded that dactylitis was caused solely by flexor tenosynovitis. No one has explained why flexor tenosynovitis presents differently in the seronegative spondylarthropathies versus RA. In dactylitis, the swelling is firm or hard when palpated, and it appears to be present throughout the entire digit, not isolated to the volar aspect typical of flexor tenosynovitis in RA (Nalebuff, 1996). The periarticular swelling prevents passive PIP and DIP ROM and compresses the joint capsule, resulting in stiff joints. Dactylitis is unresponsive to normal edema reduction methods, is not as responsive to cold modalities as tenosynovitis in RA, and is a particularly vexing problem for therapist and patient.

Symmetrical Polyarthritis (Nalebuff Type 3)

Persons with this PsA subtype can have a pattern of arthritis that resembles RA (i.e., primarily wrist, MCP, and PIP involvement, or only the wrists or MCP joints are involved). The nature of hand involvement differs from that in RA. Generally, the synovitis is not as fluctuant or boggy, so the joint has a tighter feel, and overall the joints have more stiffness and limited ROM than laxity. Flexor and extensor tenosynovitis may occur, but they are less common than in RA, and consequently extensor tendon subluxation or rupture is less frequent (Nalebuff, 1996). Flexion contractures of the PIP joints are common and are seen without the corresponding distal joint hyperextension, so boutonnière deformities are uncommon (Belsky, Feldon, Millender, Nalebuff, & Phillips, 1982; Rose & Belsky, 1989). PIP flexion deformities can result in MCP hyperextension and stiffness. Swan-neck deformities, which are common in RA, occur occasionally in PsA and usually are secondary to a mallet deformity of the DIP joint or a flexion deformity at the MCP level versus PIP joint damage (Nalebuff, 1996).

Loss of flexion in the PIP joints encourages MCP flexion and intrinsic muscle tightness that can lead to fixed flexion deformities of the MCP joints. In the thumb, the tendency toward stiffness often results in an adduction contracture and diminished web space, which reduces the ability to grasp.

"Sausage limb." Several cases of unilateral limb thickening similar to dactylitis in the digits have been reported (Vasey & Espinoza, 1984). Although rare, one author (J.M.) treated a woman with oligoarticular PsA and a 3-year history of a "sausage forearm and wrist." The left (dominant) wrist was 4 cm larger than the right uninvolved wrist. The patient was treated with a custom circumferential wrist orthosis (made of 3/32-in. Aquaplast [WFR/Aquaplast Corp., Wyckoff, NJ]) that completely immobilized the wrist and was worn day and night to reduce hypertrophied tissue. This was done in conjunction with active ROM exercises. In 1 month, her wrist circumference decreased 2 cm, and during the next 2 months, it decreased another 1 cm; then progress plateaued. Wrist ROM improved slightly. The splint was discontinued at the fourth month, and gains were maintained after 1 year of follow-up with no additional treatment.

Similar to RA, patients with PsA are at risk for ulnar and median nerve entrapment and should be screened for this.

Hand therapy. The principles of modality application, joint protection, ROM, and strengthening are the same as for RA. For patients with stiffness and limited motion, a precise daily ROM program is helpful in preventing insidious loss. When passive digit flexion is desired, wrapping the digits into flexion with Coban® (3M Company, St. Paul, MN) can help achieve full passive ROM. Patients with wrist and MCP involvement are at risk for developing MCP ulnar drift, and (similar to RA) the key to preventing this is maintaining ulnar deviation of the wrist. (See chapter 7 in this volume.)

Distal Arthritis (Nalebuff Type 1)

DIP joint involvement with psoriasis of the nails and skin around the nail are the hallmarks of this subtype (Moll & Wright, 1973). The arthritis can range from minimal to severely erosive with osteolysis of the terminal tuft. Psoriasis often limits the use of thermoplastic splinting at the DIP joint. Cold modalities are an option for acute synovitis. Patients should be taught how to do passive ROM for DIP extension and to prevent secondary limitations in the PIP joints. Painful DIP joints cause hand use in an intrinsic-plus position, which can promote an unwanted swan-neck deformity. The antideformity exercise for this process is intrinsic stretching (e.g., making a gentle fist and extending the MCP joints to neutral, keeping the PIP and DIP joints flexed).

Arthritis Mutilans (Nalebuff Type 2)

Mutilans deformities result from osteolysis in the phalanges of the hands and feet, metacarpals, metatarsals, and occasionally the distal ulna. When it occurs in the digits, the ends of the bones resorb and shorten. The overlying redundant skin gives a telescoping appearance to the fingers referred to as "opera glass hand" (Figure 2). This condition may occur in one or all of the digits (Nalebuff, 1996; Nalebuff & Garrett, 1976). It obliterates the joint and results in short floppy fingers that flex and extend but have no stability. In severe cases, the digits may be reduced to 1½ in. in length. In the early stages, osteolysis of the PIP or DIP joint creates lateral instability and may feel like a ruptured collateral ligament, but on X-ray, the ends or corners of the phalanges are clearly missing. Persons with arthritis mutilans can develop ankylosis in other digit joints (Moll & Wright, 1973).

The only treatment and prevention of this devastating problem is surgical fusion. If detected in the early stages before extensive bone loss or shortening occurs, surgical fusion can maintain the length of the digit, create a stable pain-free joint, and prevent progression of the osteolysis. This is particularly critical in the thumb and index fingers, in which stability is more important than mobility for prehension. If the digit has shortened, the surgery is more extensive and requires bone grafting to restore length (Nalebuff & Garrett, 1976).

Occupational therapy for nonsurgical candidates includes tripoint splints to provide lateral stability and adaptive equipment and handles such as a universal cuff. (The Silver-Ring Splint Company, Charlottesville, VA, makes designs that work well for this purpose.)

Foot Involvement

The toes often have a destructive arthritis and osteolysis of the interphalangeal joints similar to that seen in the fingers that results in short unstable toes. It is common to have dactylitis in the toes that results in stiff digits (Figure 5). The MTP joints can be involved. Joint involvement is not uniform and makes wearing regular shoes difficult (Gerber, 1985).

Peripheral enthesopathies, particularly of the plantar fascia and the Achilles tendon, are more common in PsA than in RA, especially when there is a spinal component to the disease. They are, however, less common than in Reiter's syndrome and ankylosing spondylitis. Calcaneal spurs at the insertions of the plantar fascia and Achilles tendon and calcaneal periostitis are characteristics of PsA and can be seen on X-ray. The spurs may be tender to palpation and weight bearing. Mechanical foot problems such as pes planus, overuse syndromes, and obesity are contributing factors to these enthesopathies and must be addressed along with treatment of the inflammatory disease (Sheon, Moskowitz, & Goldberg, 1996).

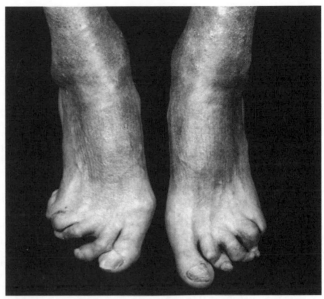

Figure 5. Toe deformities in a patient with classic distal toe involvement; the MTP joints are spared. There are mutilans deformities in several DIP joints. Photo courtesy of Proton Rahman, MD and Dafna Gladman, MD.

Foot care is essential for most persons with PsA because of the need for nail care and trimming of calluses. Self-care of the nails is extremely difficult for those with hand or spine dysfunction. Long-handled devices for bathing, applying skin lotion, and donning stockings or socks and shoes should be recommended if these activities of daily living are difficult because of limited hip or spine flexion or hand dysfunction.

Flexible footwear with a wide toe box is the first recommendation. Athletic shoes and shoes designed for walking are usually good first choices because they have soft inserts for the longitudinal arch, are in slight plantar flexion (which decreases the strain on the Achilles' tendon), and have a rubbery sole for cushioning. Running shoes provide more shock absorption than walking shoes. (See the Appendix on selecting commercial footwear for arthritis.) If a custom orthosis or heel insert is needed, it should be made of a soft resilient material such as felt, viscoelastic material, or a closed-cell thermoplastic material or polyethylene (Sheon et al., 1996). A new, open-cell material accepted by the American Podiatric Medical Association called PPT[R] (Langer Biomechanics Group, Deer Park, NY) is being used because of its "recharging" ability after compression and because it allows air circulation, which helps to keep the skin dry and cool. Semirigid or rigid orthoses may be needed to immobilize a particularly painful joint or to redistribute the weight from the metatarsal heads (Deland & Wood, 1993; Pioro & Cash, 1995). Occasionally, custom footwear is necessary.

Persistently inflamed joints or entheses benefit from rest. Ambulatory devices can decrease weight-bearing stresses and allow the person to walk with a smoother gait. An antalgic gait can place stress on other lower-extremity joints and the spine. Night splints for the foot and ankle are another method of resting the inflamed enthesis and maintaining neutral alignment at night, but they require further investigation because they are often used in conjunction with other treatments, which confuses the benefits of each (Pezzulo, 1993). Active ROM of the Achilles' tendon, toe flexors, and plantar fascia is recommended (Hurwitz, 1994). A cortisone injection, although not a common intervention, is another option for an enthesopathy not responding to conventional treatment.

A blanket cradle is helpful for preventing blankets from pulling the foot into plantar flexion during the night. (Sometimes a firm pillow between the sheets at the foot of the bed can suffice for this purpose.) Heat and cold modalities may be used in conjunction with exercise, rest, medications, and so forth, but alone they are not restorative (Guccione, 1996). Interventions with anecdotal reports of success include plantar taping, phonophoresis, iontophoresis, and icing

---

Box 1
Resources

Organization Resources

The National Psoriasis Foundation
6600 Southwest 92nd Avenue
Suite 300
Portland, OR 97223
503-244-7404 or 503-245-0626 (fax)
Internet addresses: getinfo@npfusa.org and www.psoriasis.org

This organization offers extensive resources on their Web site with links to other psoriasis resources on the Internet.

The Arthritis Foundation
1330 West Peachtree Street
Atlanta, GA 30309
404-872-7100 or 800-283-7800
Internet address: www.arthritis.org

This organization provides an excellent booklet on PsA and specific medications at no charge, aquatic and land-based exercise classes, and the Arthritis Self-Help Courses nationwide. They have a catalogue of books and videotapes for persons with RA. Some chapters offer a free video lending library.

The Arthritis Society
National Office
250 Bloor Street East
Suite 901

Toronto, ON M4W 3P2 Canada
416-967-1414 or 416-967-7171 (fax)
Internet address: www.arthritis.ca

This group offers specialized patient care programs, recreational exercise programs, resource libraries, aid in the establishment self-help groups, and consumer education material.

Internet Resources

- The Mining Company Guide to Arthritis (http://arthritis.miningco.com/msub7.htm) provides an extensive number of resources, fact sheets, interactive opportunities, and links to other Internet resources on PsA and other rheumatic diseases.

- The Amazon Bookstore (www.amazon.com) lists all the books published on psoriasis and arthritis.

- Abledata is a national database for adaptive equipment and assistive devices (www.abledata.com).

- Hot Bot is one of the best search directories for locating information on diseases by name (www.hotbot.com).

(Mooney & Maffey-Ward, 1995; Sheon et al., 1996). Some of these require 2 to 3 treatments a week for up to 5 weeks, thus incurring major costs and time commitments from the patient. Scientific scrutiny is necessary.

Spinal Involvement

Spinal involvement can occur in up to 40% of patients (McCormick & Barth, 1985). This differs from spinal involvement in ankylosing spondylitis in that it usually presents at a later age and is associated with less pain and less limitation of ROM of the spine because vertebral involvement tends to be asymmetrical. Atlantoaxial subluxation has been reported in PsA, but it is not as common as in RA. Ankylosis rather than subluxation is still the more frequent sequela, as in ankylosing spondylitis (Helliwell & Wright, 1994).

Physical therapy and occupational therapy programs are similar to those for a person with ankylosing spondylitis; however, modifications to the exercise regimen may be necessary because of peripheral symptoms. For example, weight-bearing exercises for cardiorespiratory conditioning may be hampered by foot involvement, and spinal exercises with the therapeutic gym ball may need to be altered because of difficulty with weight bearing on the hands and wrists. Pool exercise is an option only if chlorine does not aggravate the skin condition and if the patient is comfortable in a bathing suit in a public pool. Maintaining and improving posture, and thus more efficient and comfortable function, are still the goals.

Skin

Psoriasis is not a contraindication to pool therapy or recreational aquatics. Exercising in water is an excellent activity for patients with peripheral and spinal joint involvement. An appropriate moisturizer is recommended after each pool session to counteract the drying effects of water and chlorine.

Many patients believe their condition improves with exposure to sun; however, appropriate skin protection should be used. Stress has been shown to exacerbate psoriasis (Camp, 1991), and having a disease with visible cutaneous features creates additional stress for certain patients. The risk of infection from *Staphylococcus aureus* after hand or arthroplasty surgery is reported to be higher in PsA (Nalebuff, 1996).

Traditional preparations (coal tar and topical cortisone) are still in use but have no effect on the arthropathies. PUVA treatments have been beneficial for the skin and peripheral joints of some patients but not the axial joints.

Outcome Evaluation

Traditional methods for monitoring patients with PsA include clinical evaluation for joint inflammation, damage, and severity as well as radiographic evaluation. Functional and health status measures such as the ACR Revised Criteria for Classification of Global Functional Status (Stucki, Stoll, Bruhlmann, & Michel, 1991), the Arthritis Impact Measurement Scales (AIMS), the Health Assessment Questionnaire (HAQ), and the Medical Outcome Assessment Short Form (SF-36) are now widely used to evaluate outcome in clinical trials of rheumatologic diseases. We (P.R. and D.D.G.) have examined the utility of the AIMS (Duffy, et al., 1992), AIMS2 (Husted, Gladman, Farewell, & Long, 1996), HAQ (Blackmore, Gladman, Husted, Long, & Farewell, 1995), and SF-36 (Husted, Gladman, Farewell, Long, & Cook, 1997) in patients with PsA from our clinic. The results demonstrated that the original and modified AIMS questionnaires are valid for PsA. The physical function, pain, and work scales of the AIMS questionnaire correlate well with overall physical function and disease activity. In addition, the AIMS questionnaire is sensitive to changes in functional status and disease activity over time (Husted et al., 1996). The HAQ and the modified HAQ used for spondylarthropathies (HAQ-S; Daltroy, Larson, Roberts, & Liang, 1990) captured the clinical measures of function and pain in PsA. And finally, the SF-36 questionnaire is reliable and valid for use in PsA and thus can be used to compare health status across different populations. However, the AIMS did not capture the full extent of changes in the articular status or ACR functional class, and the HAQ and HAQ-S did not correlate with disease severity. Thus, it is prudent to use both traditional methods and validated health status measurements to monitor patients with PsA. (For a complete review of health status and outcome assessments, see Hawley [1998].)

Conclusion

PsA is a distinct clinical entity with its own characteristic demographic, clinical, and radiological features. The estimated prevalence of PsA in the population varies between 0.5% and 1.2% and occurs in approximately 6% to 42% of patients with psoriasis. There is no notable gender prevalence, unlike RA. The etiology is multifactorial and involves an interplay between genetic, immunological, and environmental factors. It can present with five different clinical patterns, often with overlap among the various subsets. It appears that the polyarthritis group was previously underestimated and occurs in approximately 40% of patients. Extra-articular features are present but may be not as common as in other seronegative spondylarthropathies. There are no specific laboratory investigations to confirm the diagnosis of PsA, and RF and ANAs are usually not present. A pattern of distinct radiographic changes is often suggestive of PsA. NSAIDs are the initial mainstay of therapy, and most patients respond to them. However, in the presence of active synovitis despite the use of NSAIDs, a DMARD should be used. PsA is not necessarily benign because up to 20% of patients will develop joint deformities that result in major disability.

Health care professionals should not only monitor disease activity and function, but also they should be alert to possible emotional and psychological problems that may result from a disease with notable visible external manifestations. As with other chronic diseases, self-management on the basis of knowledge and ability to modify a program according to symptoms is essential. The rehabilitation needs for the patient with severe polyarticular disease are similar to the needs of someone with RA. For patients with milder or oligoarticular involvement, physical therapy and occupational therapy may be needed episodically when new problems present such as an enthesopathy, a joint that needs splinting because of pain, or when a task becomes difficult and advice on modification is needed. But generally, the person with PsA will manage his or her medical and rehabilitation interventions with encouragement from the physician and any other team member who interacts with the patient on a routine basis.

References

Abu-Shakra, M., & Gladman, D. D. (1993). Management of refractory psoriatic arthritis. *Rheumatology Reviews, 2,* 201–206.

Abu-Shakra, M., & Gladman, D. D. (1994). Aetiopathogenesis of psoriatic arthritis. *Rheumatology Reviews, 3,* 1–7.

Abu-Shakra, M., Gladman, D. D., Thorne, J. C., Long, J., Gough, J., & Farewell, V. T. (1995). Long-term methotrexate therapy in psoriatic arthritis: Clinical and radiologic outcome. *Journal of Rheumatology, 22,* 241–245.

Barth, W. F. (1994). Psoriatic arthritis sine psoriasis. In J. H. Klippel & P. A. Dieppe (Eds.), *Rheumatology* (pp. 34.1–34.2). London: Mosby-Yearbook.

Belsky, M., Feldon, P., Millender, L. H., Nalebuff, E. A., & Phillips, C. (1982). Hand involvement in psoriatic arthritis. *Journal of Hand Surgery, 7,* 203–207.

Bennett, R. M. (1979). Psoriatic arthritis. In D. J. McCarty (Ed.), *Arthritis and allied conditions.* Philadelphia: Lea & Febiger.

Blackmore, M., Gladman, D. D., Husted, J., Long, J. A., & Farewell, V. T. (1995). Measuring health status in psoriatic arthritis: The Health Assessment Questionnaire and its modification. *Journal of Rheumatology, 22*(5), 886–893.

Breathnach, S. M. (1993). The skin immune system and psoriasis. *Clinical and Experimental Immunology, 91*(3), 343–345.

Bruce, I. N., & Gladman, D. D. (1998). Psoriatic arthritis: Recognition and treatment. *Biodrugs, 9*(4), 271–278.

Camp, R. D. R. (1991). Psoriasis. In R. Champion, J. Burton, & F. G. J. Ebling (Eds.), *Textbook of dermatology* (5th ed.,) Oxford, England: Blackwell Scientific.

Daltroy, L. H., Larson, M. G., Roberts, N. W., & Liang, M. H. (1990). A modification of the Health Assessment Questionnaire for the spondyloarthropathies. *Journal of Rheumatology, 17*(7), 946–950.

Deland, J. T. & Wood, B. (1993). Foot pain. In W. N. Kelly, E. D. Harris, Jr., S. Ruddy, C. B. Sledge (Eds.), *Textbook of rheumatology* (4th ed., pp. 459–470). Philadelphia: Saunders.

Dougados, M., Van der Linden, S., Juhlin, R., Huitfeldt, B., Amor, B., Calin, A., Cats, A., Dijkmans, B., Olivieri, I., Pasero, G., Veys, E., & Zeilder, H. (1991). The European Spondyloarthropathy Study Group's preliminary criteria for the classification of spondyloarthropathy. *Arthritis and Rheumatism, 34,* 1218–1227.

Dougados, M., Van der Linden, S., Leirisalo Repo, M., Huitfeldt, B., Juhlin, R., Veys, E., Zeidler, H., Kvien, T., Olivieri, I., & Dijkmans, B. (1995). Sulfasalazine in the treatment of spondyloarthropathy: A randomized, multicenter, double-blind, placebo-controlled study. *Arthritis and Rheumatism, 38,* 618–627.

Duffy, C. M., Watanabe-Duffy, K. N., Gladman, D. D., Brubacher, B. B., Buskila, D., Langevitz, P., & Farewell, V. T. (1992). The utility of the Arthritis Impact Measurement Scales for patients with psoriatic arthritis. *Journal of Rheumatology, 19*(11), 1727–1732.

Eastmond, C. (1994). Psoriatic arthritis: Genetics and HLA antigens. *Baillière's Clinical Rheumatology, 8,* 263–276.

Espinoza, L. R., Zakraoui, L., Espinoza, C. G., Gutierrez, F., Jara, L. J., Silveira, L. H., Cuellar, M. L., & Martinez-Osuna, P. (1992). Psoriatic arthritis, clinical response and side effects to methotrexate therapy. *Journal of Rheumatology, 19*(6), 872–877.

Gerber, L. (1985). Psoriatic arthritis: Rheumatologic, surgical and rehabilitation management. In L. H Gerber & L. H. Espinoza (Eds.), *Psoriatic arthritis.* Orlando, FL: Grune & Stratton.

Gladman, D. D. (1985). Immunological factors in the pathogenesis of psoriatic arthritis. In L. H. Gerber & L. R. Espinoza (Eds.), *Psoriatic arthritis* (pp. 33–44). Orlando, FL: Grune & Stratton.

Gladman, D. D. (1990). Psoriatic arthritis: Ankylosing spondylitis and spondyloarthropathies. *Spine: State of the Art Reviews, 4*, 637–656.

Gladman, D. D. (1994). The natural history of psoriatic arthritis. *Baillière's Clinical Rheumatology, 8*, 379–394.

Gladman, D. D. (1995). Psoriatic arthritis. *Ballière's Clinical Rheumatology, 8*, 319–329.

Gladman, D. D., Anhorn, K. A. B., Schacter, R., & Mervati, H. (1986). HLA antigen in psoriatic arthritis. *Journal of Rheumatism, 13*, 586–592.

Goodfield, M. (1994). Skin lesions in psoriasis. *Baillière's Clinical Rheumatology, 8*, 295–316.

Guccione, A. A. (1996). Physical therapy for musculoskeletal syndromes. *Rheumatic Disease Clinics of North America, 22*(3), 551–562.

Gupta, A. K., Grober, J. S., Hamilton, T. A., Ellis, C. N., Siegerl, M. T., Voorhees, J. J., & McCune, W. J. (1995). Sulfasalazine therapy for psoriatic arthritis: A double blind, placebo controlled trial. *Journal of Rheumatology, 22*, 894–898.

Hawley, D. J. (1998). Clinical outcomes: Issues and measurements. In J. L. Melvin & G. Jensen (Eds.), *Rheumatologic rehabilitation series: Volume 1: Assessment and management* (pp. 65–92). Bethesda, MD: American Occupational Therapy Association.

Hellgren, L. (1969). Association between rheumatoid arthritis and psoriasis in total populations. *Acta Rheumatologica Scandinavica, 15*, 316

Helliwell, P. S., & Wright, V. (1994). Psoriatic arthritis: Clinical features. In J. H. Klippel & P. A. Dieppe (Eds.), *Rheumatology* (pp. 31.1–31.8). London: Mosby-Year Book.

Hurwitz, S. (1994). Plantar heel pain. In J. H. Klippel & P. A. Dieppe (Eds.), *Rheumatology* (pp. 15.14–15.15). London: Mosby-Year Book.

Husted, J., Gladman, D. D., Farewell, V. T., & Long, J. A. (1996). Validation of the revised and expanded version of the Arthritis Impact Measurement Scales for patients with psoriatic arthritis. *Journal of Rheumatology, 23*(6),1015–1019.

Husted, J., Gladman, D. D., Farewell, V. T., Long, J. A., & Cook, R. S. (1997). Validating the SF-36 Health Survey Questionnaire in patients with psoriatic arthritis. *Journal of Rheumatology, 24*(3), 511–517.

Jones, S., Armas, J., Cohn, M., Lovell, C., Evison, G., & McHugh, N. (1994). Psoriatic arthritis: Outcome of disease subsets and relationship of joint disease to nail and skin disease. *British Journal of Rheumatology, 33*, 834–839.

Klinkhoff, A. V., Gertner, E., Chalmers, A., Gladman, D. D., Stewart, W. D., Schachter, G. D., & Schachter, R. K. (1989). Pilot study of etretinate in psoriatic arthritis. *Journal of Rheumatology, 16*(6), 789–791.

Mader, R., Gladman, D. D., Long, J., Gough, J., & Farewell, V. T. (1995). Injectable gold for the treatment of psoriatic arthritis (PsA): Long-term follow up. *Clinical Investigative Medicine, 18*, 139–143.

Mann, R. A., & Horton, G. A. (1996). Management of the foot and ankle in rheumatoid arthritis. *Rheumatic Disease Clinics of North America, 22*(3), 457–475.

McCormick, G. D., & Barth, W. (1985). Classification and diagnosis of psoriatic arthritis. In L. H. Gerber & L. R. Espinoza (Eds.), *Psoriatic arthritis*. Orlando, FL: Grune & Stratton.

Moll, J. M. H., & Wright, V. (1973). Psoriatic arthritis. *Seminars in Arthritis, 3*, 55–78.

Mooney, M., & Maffey-Ward, L. (1995). All heel pain is not plantar fasciitis. *Physiotherapy Canada, 47*(3), 185–189.

Nalebuff, E. A. (1996). Surgery of psoriatic arthritis of the hand. *Hand Clinics, 12*(3), 603–614.

Nalebuff, E. A., & Garrett, J. (1976). Opera-glass hand in RA. *Journal of Hand Surgery, 1*(3), 210.

Olivieri, I., Barozzi, L., Favaro, L., Pierro, A., deMatteis, M., Borghi, C., Padula, A., Ferri, S., & Pavlica, P. (1996). Dactylitis in patients with seronegative spondylarthropathy: Assessment by ultrasonography and magnetic resonance imaging. *Arthritis and Rheumatism, 39*(9), 1542–1528.

O'Neill, T., & Silman, A. (1994). Psoriatic arthritis: Historical background and epidemiology. *Baillière's Clinical Rheumatology, 8*, 245–261.

Panayi, G. (1994). Immunology of psoriasis and psoriatic arthritis. *Baillière's Clinical Rheumatology, 8*, 419–427.

Perlman, S. G., Gerber, L. H., & Roberts, M. (1985). Photochemotherapy and psoriatic arthritis: A prospective study. *Annals of Rheumatic Disease*, 189–193.

Pezzullo, D. J. (1993). Using night splints in the treatment of plantar fasciitis in the athlete. *Journal of Sports Rehabilitation, 214*, 187–197.

Pioro, M. H., & Cash, J. (1995). Treatment of refractory psoriatic arthritis. *Rheumatic Disease Clinics of North America, 21*(1), 129–149.

Reshad, H., Hargreaves, G. K., & Vickers, C. H. F. (1983). Generalized pustular psoriasis precipitated by phenylbutazone and oxyphenbutazone. *British Journal of Dermatology, 108*, 111.

Reveille, J. D. (1993). Interplay of nature versus nurture in predisposition to the rheumatic diseases. *Rheumatic Disease Clinics of North America, 19*, 15–27.

Rose, J., & Belsky, M. (1989). Psoriatic arthritis in the hand. *Hand Clinics, 5*, 137–144.

Scarpa, R., Del Puente, A., di Girolamo, C., della Valle, G., Lubrano, E., & Oriente, P. (1992). Interplay between environmental factors, articular involvement, and HLA-B27 in patients with psoriatic arthritis. *Annals of Rheumatic Disease, 51*, 78–79.

Sheon, R. P., Moskowitz, R., & Goldberg, V. M. (1996). Lower limb disorders. In *Soft tissue rheumatic pain*. Baltimore: Williams & Wilkins.

Silveira, L. H., Gutierrez, F., Scopelitis, E., Cuellar, M. I., Citera, G., & Espinoza, L. R. (1993). Chlamydia-induced reactive arthritis. *Rheumatic Disease Clinics of North America, 19*, 351–362.

Solinger, A. M., & Hess, E. V. (1993). Rheumatic diseases and AIDS: Is the association real? *Journal of Rheumatology, 20*, 678–683.

Stucki, G., Stoll, T., Bruhlmann, P., & Michel, B. A. (1991). Construct validation of the ACR 1991 Revised Criteria for Global Functional Status in Rheumatoid Arthritis. *Clinical and Experimental Rheumatology, 13*(3), 349–352.

Tomfohrde, J., Silverman, A., Barnes, R., Fernandez-Vina, M. A., Young, M., Lory, D., Morris, L., Wuepper, K. D., Stastny, P., & Menter, A., et al. (1994). Gene for familial psoriasis susceptibility mapped to the distal end of human chromosome 17q. *Science, 264*, 1141–1145.

van Romunde, L. K. J., Valkenburg, M. A., Swart-Bruinsma, W., Cats, A., & Hermans, J. (1984). Psoriasis and arthritis: I: A population study. *Rheumatology International, 4*, 55.

Vasey, F. B., & Espinoza , L. R. (1984). Psoriatic arthropathy. In A. Calin (Ed.), *Spondyloarthropathies* (p. 45). New York: Grune & Stratton.

Vasey, F. B., Seleznick, M. J., Fenske, N. A., & Espinoza, L. R. (1989). New signposts on the road to understanding psoriatic arthritis. *Journal of Rheumatology, 16*(11), 1405–1407.

Veale, D., Rogers, S., & Fitzgerald, O. (1994). Classification of clinical subsets in psoriatic arthritis. *British Journal of Rheumatology, 33*, 133–138.

Veale, D., Yanni, G., Rogers, S., Barnes, L., Bresnihan, B., & Fitzgerald, O. (1993). Reduced synovial membrane macrophage numbers: ELAM-1 expression and lining layer hyperplasia in psoriatic arthritis as compared to rheumatoid arthritis. *Arthritis and Rheumatism, 36,* 893–900.

Wilfert, H., Honnigsmann, H., Steiner, G., Smolen, J., & Wolff, K. (1990). Treatment of psoriatic arthritis by extracorporeal phototherapy. *British Journal of Dermatology, 122*(2), 225–232.

Wright, V. (1956). Psoriasis and arthritis. *Annals of Rheumatic Disease, 15,* 348.

11

ANKYLOSING SPONDYLITIS

Victoria Gall, MEd, PT, Frank C. Arnett, MD, and Dena Slonaker, MSEd, OTR, CHT

Ankylosing spondylitis (AS) is a chronic inflammatory disease primarily affecting the axial skeleton. AS has a predilection for the sacroiliac and spinal apophyseal joints as well as for the multiple entheses along the spine. An enthesis is the site of insertion for a tendon, ligament, capsule, or articular cartilage into bone (Arnett, 1996; Schweitzer & Resnick, 1994). One third of patients with AS have peripheral arthritis or enthesopathy (Cohen & Ginsburg, 1982).

Classification

AS is a member of a family of clinically, epidemiologically, and genetically related disorders that are termed *spondylarthropathies* (Dougados et al., 1991). These related diseases include reactive arthritis or Reiter's syndrome, psoriatic arthritis, enteropathic arthritis (ulcerative colitis or Crohn's disease), and Whipple's disease. AS is considered primary when only spinal symptoms are present and is considered secondary when associated with other nonskeletal conditions. Frequently, individual patients have overlapping clinical features of two or more of these entities and are then classified as having an *undifferentiated spondylarthropathy*. (AS is discussed separately to provide a clear model for rehabilitation for spinal involvement. The other spondylarthropathies are discussed in chapters 10 and 13 in this volume.)

Etiologic Factors

There is a definite genetic predisposition to AS and other spondylarthropathies (Arnett, 1996; Khan, 1994). Although environmental factors play the greater role in timing of onset, genetic factors are more important in influencing prognosis (Calin & Elswood, 1989). The inherited human lymphocyte antigen (HLA) B-27, which occurs in less than 10% of healthy persons, has been found in more than 90% of persons who develop AS. AS occurs in about 20% of the relatives of patients with AS who inherit HLA B-27. Among random HLA B-27-positive persons in the population, only about 2% will develop AS (Calin & Fries, 1975). In addition, AS shares many clinical and genetic similarities with reactive arthritis, a disorder that is triggered by certain bacterial infections, including *Salmonella*, *Shigella*, and *Chlamydia*. In fact, fragments of these bacteria can be found in the inflamed peripheral joints of patients with reactive arthritis, and some studies suggest that living but dormant microorganisms are the actual cause of the persistent inflammation. Currently, it is unknown whether similar bacterial products (or living organisms) are involved in the inflamed joints and entheses of patients with AS; however, there is increasing evidence that AS is linked to certain bacteria in the bowel.

Population Affected

Sacroiliac and spinal disease usually develops around 28 years of age in patients with primary AS, but persons of other ages are affected by the secondary forms. Juvenile spondylarthropathy usually presents with peripheral arthritis, enthesitis, or both with spondylitis developing later. Juvenile spondylarthropathy accounts for approximately 20% of all cases in the United States and Europe and a higher proportion in underdeveloped countries (Arnett, 1996). (Spondylarthropathies in children are discussed in volume 3 of this series.) There are few differences between the outcome of juvenile- and adult-onset AS. Overall, juvenile patients do well in adulthood (Bakker et al., 1994; Calin & Elswood, 1988), although some researchers believe that an age of onset less than 16 years is indicative of a poor prognosis (Amor, Santos, Nahal, Listrat, & Dougados, 1994).

The classic form of AS with severe spinal involvement primarily affects men (3 out of 4 cases). Milder and atypical forms of AS are more likely to occur in women (Arnett, 1996; Khan, 1994), many of whom tend to have less involvement of the lower spine but more peripheral joint and neck involvement. The prevalence of AS in different ethnic populations parallels the frequency of HLA B-27 (Arnett, 1996; Gran & Ostensen, 1998; Khan, 1994). The disease is most common in certain Native American and Eskimo tribes in which HLA B-27 occurs in up to 30% of the population, but the disease is quite rare in African and Japanese persons, populations that have a low frequency of the gene (1–2%). Various Caucasian groups have intermediate frequencies of both HLA B-27 (6–15%) and AS. On the basis of the 1990 U.S. Census, approximately 200,000 Americans have AS (Arnett, 1996; Khan, 1994).

Diagnosis

Calin (1985a) described the characteristic features of AS as insidious onset before 40 years of age, persistent pain or stiffness in the lower back, symptoms that last more than 3 months, and an association with morning stiffness.

Physical examination may show a restriction of spinal motion, especially lumbar flexion and decreased chest expansion, but both may be normal early in the disease. The most specific diagnostic finding is bilateral sacroiliitis on X-rays of the pelvis (Van Der Linden, Valkenburg, & Cats, 1984). In some patients with characteristic symptoms, spinal X-rays may not show typical abnormalities for many years (Mau et al., 1988). In such cases, a positive blood test for HLA B-27 indicates a high likelihood that the patient has AS, whereas a negative test nearly excludes it (less than a 10% likelihood). The classification criteria for spondylarthropathies in general (Dougados et al., 1991) are listed in Table 1 and have been helpful to clinicians. (See chapter 4 in this volume for examples of radiographic findings.)

Clinical Features

Inflammatory Enthesopathy

The distribution, character, and consequences of the inflammation in AS are fundamentally different than that in rheumatoid arthritis (RA). The AS lesions result in new bone formation and fusion around both spinal and peripheral articular structures.

Entheses are metabolically active fibers with a prominent nerve supply (Schweitzer & Resnick, 1994). They occur at four anatomically distinct locations: 1) the capsular insertion of synovial joints, 2) cartilaginous articulations (e.g., discovertebral, symphysis pubis, manubriosternal), 3) syndesmotic or fibrous articulations (e.g., radioulnar joint, tibiofibular joint), and 4) extra-articular sites (e.g., calcaneus, patella, ischial tuberosity). "Zones" of collagen fibers (e.g., tendon, ligament) blend into unmineralized fibrocartilage and then mineralized fibrocartilage, make an abrupt transition to mineralized cartilage, and then blend into the bone matrix. These fibrous connections are referred to as *Sharpey's* (perforating) *fibers*.

Inflammation from lymphocytes, plasma cells, and polymorphonuclear leukocytes releases chemicals that destroy nearby tissue and stimulate certain nerve fibers that cause pain (Bluestone, 1992). Inflammation leads to osseous erosions at sites of insertion similar to the erosions in RA.

In the healing stage, bone proliferation at sites of erosion and progressive ossification at capsular insertions can ankylose the joint. Reactive bone formation of the annulus fibrosus of the intervertebral disc is termed a *syndesmophyte* (a vertically oriented outgrowth) versus the osteophytes of osteoarthritis (OA) that occur more horizontally. It is believed that movement is needed to keep the sites mobile, although the mechanism is not clearly understood. Vigorous exercise appears to be more beneficial in this disease than in diseases involving proliferative synovitis. Diffuse idiopathic skeletal hyperostosis involves flowing calcification and ossification along the anterolateral aspect of at least four contiguous vertebrae, but sacroiliac joint ankylosis is absent (Schweitzer & Resnick, 1994).

Peripheral Arthritis

Approximately 20% of persons with AS will have some peripheral arthritis or enthesitis. Hip and shoulder symptoms are more common in primary AS, and knee

Table 1. Criteria for the Classification of Spondylarthropathy*

> Inflammatory spinal pain
> **or**
> Synovitis (asymmetrical or predominantly in the lower limbs)
> **And one or more of the following:**
>   Positive family history
>   Psoriasis
>   Inflammatory bowel disease
>   Urethritis, cervicitis, or acute diarrhea within 1 month before arthritis
>   Buttock pain alternating between left and right gluteal areas
>   Enthesopathy
>   Sacroiliitis

*This classification method yields a sensitivity of 78.4% and a specificity of 89.6%. When radiographic evidence of sacroiliitis was included, the sensitivity improved to 87.0% with a minor decrease in specificity to 86.7%. *Note.* From "The European Spondylarthropathy Study Group Preliminary Criteria for the Classification of Spondylarthropathy," by M. Dougados et al., 1991, *Arthritis and Rheumatism, 34*, pp. 1218–1227. Copyright 1991 by the American College of Rheumatology. Reprinted with permission.

involvement is more common in secondary AS. A peripheral enthesopathy can occur at the humeral tuberosities, olecranon process, temporomandibular joints (Wennenberg, Kopp, & Hollender, 1984), iliac crest, ischial tuberosities, and femoral trochanters. Plantar fasciitis and Achilles tendonitis are common in AS (Arnett, 1996) (Table 2). Small-joint peripheral arthritis tends to be transitory and seldom results in deformity; however, occasionally the wrists or isolated finger joints develop severe disease. Treatment is similar to that for RA except that joints may fuse instead of developing ulnar drift or swan-neck deformities.

Hip involvement occurs most often in patients with an earlier age of onset and is predictive of major disability. About 30% of patients develop clinically notable hip disease. Many patients develop hip flexion contractures with compensatory knee flexion contractures from attempting to stand vertically and look forward. Flexion and adduction contractures can interfere with sitting, perineal care, and sexual intercourse.

In the shoulder, tendonitis or impingement syndromes can develop from increased kyphosis, protracted scapulae, and decreased chest expansion. Inflammation of the sternoclavicular, acromioclavicular, or glenohumeral joints may lead to loss of motion or even fusion.

Table 2. Nonarticular Involvement of the Ankle and Foot in the Spondylarthropathies

Enthesitis
- Insertion of Achilles tendon to calcaneus
- Attachment of plantar fascia to calcaneus
- Attachment of plantar fascia to the base of the 1st to 5th proximal phalanges
- Attachment of the plantar fascia to the heads of the 1st to 5th metatarsals

Bursitis
- Retrocalcaneal, retroachilleal, subcalcaneal

Tenosynovitis
- Peroneal tendons
- Posterior tibial tendons
- Extensor tendons

Pain

Pain is the result of the inflammatory process and paravertebral muscle spasm. Usually the pain is episodic and may be more severe at night. Stiffness in the morning and after inactivity commonly accompanies the pain and is usually confined to the involved joints or entheses (Arnett, 1996). Pain usually lasts longer than pain from mechanical spinal problems, and it is improved by exercise, whereas mechanical symptoms are made better with rest. The patient may describe joint pain as centered in the lower back or buttocks with minimal radiation.

Fatigue

In one study, during a 2-week period, 50% of subjects with AS reported fatigue as their most important symptom. In fact, the patients with AS reported more pain and fatigue than subjects with RA (Calin, Edmunds, & Kennedy, 1993).

Fatigue can be caused by several factors: the high energy cost of inefficient locomotion and bending, chronic pain, poor sleep, depression, mild anemia, and extra-articular cardiopulmonary manifestations (Bluestone, 1992; Calin et al., 1993). Fatigue management training for AS is the same as for fibromyalgia syndrome (FMS) and systemic lupus erythematosus (SLE). (See chapters 6 and 8 in this volume, which contain education on lifestyle training to improve energy and fitness training to improve functional capacity.)

Eye Involvement

Involvement of organs is referred to as "extra-articular inflammation" in AS. Inflammation may occur in the eyes, heart, or lungs. Iritis occurs in approximately 25% of patients with AS and usually involves only one eye at a time. Symptoms include acute, painful red eyes with blurred vision or insidious and progressive visual impairment. Iritis may continue long after AS has become inactive, or it may occur before the onset of joint symptoms (Arnett, 1996).

Cardiopulmonary Involvement

Heart disease occurs more frequently in persons with more severe spondylitis. It affects 3% to 5% of patients but may not be symptomatic until 25 to 30 years after onset. Aortic valve incompetence, cardiomegaly, and conduction defects are the most common findings (Calin, 1985b). Because of the severity of their cardiac problems, some patients cannot participate in vigorous activities. New cardiovascular symptoms should be reported to the physician, and all exercise programs should consider the condition of the heart.

Some patients present with a pleuritic-like chest pain that may cause sleep disturbance. This pain, which is worse on inspiration, is due to insertional tendonitis (enthesopathy) of the costosternal and costovertebral muscles. Although a rigid chest wall may result, pulmonary ventilation is usually well maintained by the diaphragm (Calin, 1985b). Patients with severe spondylitis may develop upper-lobe pulmonary fibrosis as an uncommon late manifestation, typically in the fifth decade of life. Pulmonary fibrosis presents in a manner similar to tuberculosis and may involve cough, dyspnea, and sputum.

Course and Prognosis

The course of AS varies widely. Some persons, especially teenagers or young adults, have one or more bouts of sacroiliitis or peripheral arthritis (often involving the low back, knee, or ankle) that spontaneously resolve. Such episodes are frequently attributed to a sports- or activity-related strain or injury, and the disease is not diagnosed. Years later, the characteristic sacroiliac joint changes on X-ray are discovered incidentally or when low back pain recurs. In classic AS, the symptoms of pain and stiffness gradually progress from the sacroiliac joints into the lumbar, thoracic, and then cervical spinal segments. Spinal mobility is lost gradually, and deformities develop, including loss of normal lumbar lordosis, accentuated thoracic spinal kyphosis with loss of chest expansion, and cervical mobility. The vertebrae may fuse and resemble bamboo on radiographs. A more severe outcome is predictable by the presence of hip disease or three of the following factors within the first 2 years of diagnosis: onset less than or equal to 16 years of age, erythrocyte sedimentation rate greater than or equal to 30 mm/hr, poor effectiveness of nonsteroidal anti-inflammatory drugs (NSAIDs), dactylitis ("sausage finger" or "sausage toe" deformities), limitation of lumbar spine motion, or oligoarthritis (Amor et al., 1994).

The disease usually establishes its pattern of involvement and runs its course in the first 10 years of illness (Mau et al., 1988); however, the disease process may stop at any stage with residual pain-free deformity or limitations. Less than 1% of patients with AS who present to a rheumatologist maintain long-term remission. Some 20% of patients in remission will develop active disease 2 years later.

Peripheral arthropathy can occur after the spinal disease has become inactive (Cohen & Ginsburg, 1982). The prognosis over 2 years for those with active disease is poor (Kennedy, Edmunds, & Calin, 1993). A general disease activity index of pain and stiffness has been developed (Garrett et al., 1994).

The leading causes of death or catastrophic disability due to AS include spinal fractures, especially of a fixed and brittle neck and often after seemingly trivial trauma, or other neurological insults to the spinal cord (Hunter & Dubo, 1983). Conservative management of spinal fractures with halo traction and body casts may be adequate, or surgical intervention may be required. Another neurological condition that may occur in the late stages of the disease is cauda equina syndrome, in which entrapment of the spinal nerve roots below the first lumbar vertebra cause insidious onset of leg or buttock pain with sensory and motor impairment in association with bowel or bladder symptoms (Calin, 1985b). Cardiac involvement and amyloidosis are other causes of mortality.

Women can have a severe course as described above, but most have more cervical and peripheral joint involvement and less dramatic spinal changes, including sacroiliitis and a milder course. In a study by Chamberlain (1983), women reported difficulty with lifting, carrying, and supporting a child due to a lack of spinal flexibility, pain, and diminished muscle power and frequently are limited in recreational activities. Some have had back pain during pregnancy. Although men denied that their sex lives were affected by AS, most women in the study reported that their sexual enjoyment was impaired by pain, fatigue, or diminished libido.

Employment Issues

About 75% of patients with AS remain fully employed (Arnett, 1996). The probability of prolonged sick leave or disability is associated with peripheral joint involvement, work that involves carrying heavy loads and prolonged standing (Guillemin, Briancon, Pourel, & Gaucher, 1990), exposure to cold conditions, and associated illness (Wordsworth & Mowat, 1986). Other working conditions that patients consider to be difficult are lifting, stooping, kneeling, working in cramped positions, and jarring motions (Bruckel, 1992; Guillemin, et al., 1990; Wordsworth & Mowat, 1986).

The best work situation is one that is physically undemanding or allows duties to be restricted, provides for frequent task and position change, minimizes bending and sitting, and has an environment with a comfortable temperature.

The Americans with Disabilities Act (Public Law 101-336) legislated a change in employment practices to include the employer's responsibility to provide a "reasonable accommodation" for employees with disabilities. This may include a special chair, shock-absorbing floor mats, or even adjusting the work schedule. A state's department of vocational rehabilitation may be able to provide special equipment or job retraining and placement. The Spondylitis Association of America and the Arthritis Foundation may likewise be of assistance (see Box 1).

Medical and Surgical Management

Drug Therapy

NSAIDs are usually necessary to relieve the pain and stiffness caused by inflammation and to facilitate a patient's ability to perform appropriate exercises. The most helpful NSAIDs include indomethacin (Indocin), tolmetin (Tolectin), sulindac (Clinoril), and piroxicam (Feldene). Aspirin and proprionic acids such as ibuprofen (Motrin, Advil) and naproxen sodium (Naprosyn, Aleve) have been found to be less effective in most patients.

Box 1
Resources

Organization Resources

Spondylitis associations likewise provide information on Reiter's syndrome [reactive arthritis].

Spondylitis Association of America
P.O. Box 5872
Sherman Oaks, CA 91413
800-777-8189
Internet address: www.spondylitis.org

This organization provides consumer education, a newsletter, support groups, resources, research updates, and videotapes for persons with AS (*The Water Workout Video* and *Fight Back*).

National Ankylosing Spondylitis Society (United Kingdom)
P.O. Box 179
Mayfield
East Sussex, TN206ZL
01435 873527
Internet address:
http://web.ukonline.co.uk/nass/

This organization provides extensive support services and has an excellent on-line resource.

The Arthritis Foundation
1330 West Peachtree Street
Atlanta, GA 30309
404-872-7100 or 1-800-283-7800
Internet address: www.arthritis.org

This organization provides an excellent booklet on AS and specific medications at no charge and aquatic and land-based exercise classes nationwide.

The Arthritis Society
National Office
250 Bloor Street East
Suite 901
Toronto, ON M4W 3P2 Canada
416-967-1414 or 416-967-7171
Internet address: www.arthritis.ca

This organization offers specialized patient care programs, recreational exercise programs, resource libraries, aid in the establishment self-help groups, and consumer education material.

Internet Resources

- Chris Love's Ankylosing Spondylitis Page: This web site provides an array of information and links to other sites on the web of interest to patients with AS and professionals (www.jps.net/cwlove/as.html).

- A search for "ankylosing spondylitis" on www.hotbot.com will link you to all web sites related to AS nationally and internationally. Hot Bot is a Web directory.

- The Amazon Bookstore (www.amazon.com) lists all the books published on ankylosing spondylitis.

- Abledata is a national database for adaptive equipment and assistive devices (www.abledata.com).

Phenylbutazone, which in the past has proven highly beneficial, has the potential for serious hematological side effects and should be used only in cases of severe disease that have been unresponsive to safer agents. Recently, sulfasalazine (Azulfidine), a bowel antibiotic with added salicylate, has been shown to be highly effective in AS, especially for peripheral joint disease. Whether this long-acting drug greatly alters the natural history of the disease remains to be studied. (See chapter 3 in this volume for precautions and side effects of specific drugs.)

Nutrition

There is no evidence that a high calcium intake is related to bone fusion. Adequate daily amounts of calcium, phosphorus, magnesium, and other nutrients are important in maintaining health and preventing osteoporosis, which can be caused by decreased mobility. Iron may be necessary to counteract a side effect of some NSAIDs, which can cause anemia from mild intestinal blood loss ("Some Questions We Knew You'd Ask," 1992, p. 53). It is important to maintain ideal body weight and to avoid extra fatigue, which decreases resistance to disease. A registered dietitian can help establish a well-balanced diet.

Surgery

Hip disease is more functionally disabling than a fused spine. Hip arthroplasties, when necessary, are usually done simultaneously and may require pharmacological intervention or radiotherapy to decrease formation of heterotopic bone (Walker & Sledge, 1991). Rehabilitation protocols must be adapted for the patient with limitations in spinal mobility. Cervical and lumbar osteotomies are performed only for those patients with severe postural abnormalities that compromise respiration or the ability to see ahead of them. (See Martin, Zavadak, Noaker, Jacobs, & Poss [1999] for a comprehensive review of hip surgery and therapy.)

Rehabilitation

Because the potential for deformity is great, exercise and educational interventions should begin as soon as there is a diagnosis of a spondylarthropathy. There are no cures for these diseases, so active patient participation is necessary for a better outcome. Referrals to physical therapy for instruction in pain management, posture principles, and exercises and referrals to occupational therapy for instruction in energy conservation, stress management, and adaptive activities of daily living (ADL) strategies are essential to provide a comprehensive therapy program. The goals of therapy are to reduce and manage pain and fatigue, improve and maintain spinal and peripheral mobility, and restore maximum function.

Evaluation

Medical history questions pertinent to treatment include existence of peripheral arthritis and enthesopathies, cardiac or intestinal symptoms, iritis, psoriasis, sciatica, and other comorbid conditions. Employment and recreation histories, along with previous and current medical and alternative interventions, are likewise helpful in program planning. Expectations and goals should be elicited and clarified.

A physical evaluation is necessary for treatment planning and outcome evaluation and may follow specific physical tests listed in Table 3 (Viitanen & Suni, 1995) and seen in Figure 1.

The Bath Ankylosing Spondylitis Metrology Index (BASMI) was designed to reduce the number of measurements traditionally taken and to combine the most clinically appropriate ones into an easily understandable composite score suitable for all professions involved in AS (Jenkins et al., 1994). Measurement protocols should be standardized, including time of day and number of warm-up repetitions (Roberts, Liang, Pallozi, & Daltroy, 1988).

Functional evaluations with neck- and spine-related questions have been developed for AS. They include the Health Assessment Questionnaire modified for the spondylarthropathies (Daltroy, Larson, Roberts, & Liang, 1990), the Functional Index for AS (Dougados et al., 1988), and the Bath Ankylosing Spondylitis Functional Index (BASFI) (Calin et al., 1994). Both the Functional Index for AS and the BASFI correlate equally well with disease activity and damage (Spoorenberg et al, 1999), but the BASFI is more discriminating with mild functional disability and more helpful in evaluating physical therapy clinical trials (Ruof & Stucki, 1999). The Bath Ankylosing Spondylitis Disease Activity Index (BASDAI) is a self-administered instrument that measures severity of fatigue, stiffness, and spinal and peripheral joint pain with visual analog scales (Garrett et al., 1994) (Figures 2 and 3). Functional evaluation in AS is an active area of research, and van der Heijde and associates (1999) recently conducted a survey of the most effective instruments.

A comparison of standard cervical spine measures with radiographic findings showed that all had good reliability and correlation except chin-to-chest distance. Cervical lateral flexion is the recommended measure for clinical trials (Viitanen, Kokko, Heikkila, & Kautiainen, 1998).

Table 3. Evaluation Techniques for Ankylosing Spondylitis

Schober test*
Ear tragus to wall distance (occiput)*
Lateral spinal flexion*
Intermalleolar spread*
Cervical rotation,* lateral flexion*
Smythe test
Height
Chest expansion
Finger to floor distance
Thomas test
Shoulder and knee ROM
Vital capacity

*Composite score for Bath Ankylosing Metrology Index.

Figure 1. Three common assessments for AS. The first is the distance of the occiput to wall or ear tragus to wall: note rigid forward head posture. (This can be self-monitored by cutting cardboard the goal distance and using it as a measure.) Another measure is the distance of finger tips to floor: note the flattened lower back, a classic sign of AS. (This can be self-monitored by standing along side a wall and marking fingertip level with a self-adhesive note or masking tape.) The third assessment is chest expansion. Patients can use all three of these measures to self-monitor their exercise program. *Source*: Courtesy of the Spondylitis Association of America, P.O. Box 5872, Sherman Oaks, CA 91413.

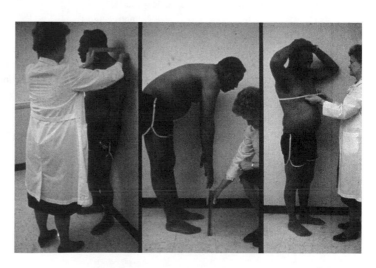

Psychosocial Interventions

Men with AS have been described by Gunther, Mur, Traweger, and Hawel (1994) as coping by downplaying stressful situations, comparing themselves with others such as patients with FMS, seeking alternative activities that offer gratification, and exhibiting less self-accusation and resignation than healthy control subjects. Participating in self-help groups lowers reliance on "powerful others" to control one's health. Members of these groups report greater satisfaction with available support and increased frequency of and compliance to exercise treatments (Barlow, Macey, & Struthers, 1992 and 1993).

Figure 2. Ankylosing Spondylitis Functional Index

Please place a mark on each line* below to indicate your level of ability with each of the following activities during the past week. (An aid is a piece of equipment that helps you perform an action or movement.)

1. Putting on your socks or stockings without help or aids (e.g., sock aid).
   easy _____ impossible

2. Bending forward from the waist to pick up a pen from the floor without an aid.
   easy _____ impossible

3. Reaching up to a high shelf without help or aids.
   easy _____ impossible

4. Getting up out of an armless dining room chair without using your hands or any other help.
   easy _____ impossible

5. Getting up off the floor from your back without help.
   easy _____ impossible

6. Standing unsupported for 10 minutes without discomfort.
   easy _____ impossible

7. Climbing 12 to 15 steps without using a hand rail or walking aid—one foot on each step.
   easy _____ impossible

8. Looking over your shoulders without turning your body.
   easy _____ impossible

9. Doing physically demanding activities (e.g., physical therapy exercises, gardening, or sports).
   easy _____ impossible

10. Doing a full day's activities whether at home or at work.
    easy _____ impossible

Note. From "A new approach to defining functional ability in ankylosing spondylitis: The development of the Bath Ankylosing Spondylitis Functional Index," by A. Calin, S. Garrett, H. Whitelock, L. G. Kennedy, J. O'Hea, P. Mallorie, and T. Jenkinson, 1994, *Journal of Rheumatology, 21,* 2281–2285. Copyright 1994 by the *Journal of Rheumatology.* Reprinted with permission.

*Actual patient questionnaires must have analog lines 10 cm long.

Figure 3. Ankylosing Spondylitis Disease Activity Index

Place a mark on each line* below to indicate your answer for each question relating to the past week.

1. Describe the overall level of fatigue or tiredness you have experienced.
   none _____ very severe

2. Describe the overall level of ankylosing spondylitis <u>neck, back, or hip</u> pain you have had.
   none _____ very severe

3. Describe the overall pain and swelling in joints <u>other than</u> the neck, back, or hips, you have had.
   none _____ very severe

4. Describe the overall level of discomfort you have had from any areas tender to touch or pressure.
   none _____ very severe

5. Describe the overall level of morning stiffness you have had from the time you wake up.
   none _____ very severe

6. How long does your morning stiffness last from the time you wake up?
   0 hours _____ 2 or more hours

Note. From "A new approach to defining disease status in ankylosing spondylitis: The Bath Ankylosing Spondylitis Disease Activity Index," by S. Garrett, T. Jenkinson, L. G. Kennedy, H. Whitelock, P. Gaisford, and A. Calin, 1994, *Journal of Rheumatology, 21,* 2286–2291. Copyright 1994 by the *Journal of Rheumatology.* Reprinted with permission.

*Actual patient questionnaires must have analog lines 10 cm long.

Behavioral therapy consisting of progressive muscle relaxation and cognitive restructuring has been shown to be effective in reducing pain intensity, anxiety, and psychophysiological symptoms and in encouraging emotional stabilization and increased feelings of well-being (Basler & Rehfisch, 1991).

Modalities

Although there is little data to support the use of any form of heat or cold for spondylarthropathies, most clinicians recommend superficial heat and cold. These are simple home treatments that patients find helpful in decreasing stiffness and pain. Heat in the form of a warm shower or hot bath is most commonly recommended. Fleece mattress covers and electric pads and blankets help decrease morning stiffness. Warm clothing around the neck and torso helps decrease stiffness.

Thermal and electric modalities serve as adjuncts to active treatment and can be used for other soft-tissue problems. Cold modalities are more effective in reducing joint and tendon inflammation, and heat is more effective for muscle stiffness. Both heat and cold can be effective for reducing muscle spasm. Transcutaneous electrical nerve stimulation (TENS) is the only modality that has some research to support its use (Gemignani, Olivieri, Rujo, & Pasero, 1991). Electrical (ionto) or sound (phono) interferential current is another form of TENS. There is no scientific justification for the use of ultrasound, iontophoresis, or electrical stimulation treatment for the spinal complaints of AS. Phoresis, however, may be helpful for treating peripheral enthesitis such as plantar fasciitis and bicipital tendonitis. Modality use in the clinic may be influenced by the patient's insurance plan. If only a few sessions are allowed, it is better to teach exercise and self-management skills than to use the time for a passive treatment. Massage is pleasant and may offer short-term relief of symptoms by increasing circulation and releasing tight fascia so that exercise can follow with fewer symptoms.

Mobilization Techniques

Mobilization techniques by therapists, osteopaths, or chiropractors should be chosen carefully. Fused joints and joints with pseudoarthrosis should never be mobilized. There is only anecdotal data to support the use of manual or mechanical traction, and spinal fracture is a potential complication. Patients frequently report the need "to be stretched," so safe independent or partner-assisted techniques should be taught to allow patients to do stretching at home (Figures 4 and 5). Patients report an increased sense of mobility with the use of home static traction units, lumbar rolls, thoracic wedges, and stretching maneuvers with the therapeutic Swiss Ball®.

External Supports

External supports such as assistive walking devices may be necessary for balance when the spine is extremely forward or when hip disease causes pain with weight bearing. Lumbosacral supports should only be used if physical activities

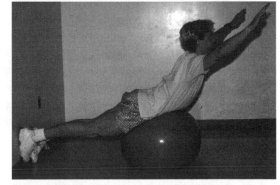

Figure 4. Use of a therapeutic ball to strengthen the spinal extensor muscles. *Source*: Courtesy of the Spondylitis Association of America, P. O. Box 5872, Sherman Oaks, CA 91413.

such as home chores or sports are painful. In the case of pseudoarthrosis or instability, rigid supports or collars may be needed.

Supportive footwear with shock-absorbing features is necessary to compensate for the loss of disc resiliency and to prevent or lessen lower-extremity enthesopathies, tendonitis, fasciitis, or other structural problems. Impact-absorbing insoles, heel cups, and shoes are recommended, and custom orthoses may be needed. Shoes designed for running have more shock absorption than those designed for walking. (See the Appendix for guidelines on selecting athletic shoes.)

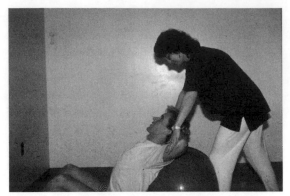

Figure 5. Using a therapeutic ball to assist in trunk mobilization. *Source*: Courtesy of the Spondylitis Association of America, P. O. Box 5872, Sherman Oaks, CA 91413.

Exercise

"Activity strengthens, no activity weakens, over-activity injures, and the right amount promotes well being" (Ostrow, 1985, p. 2). Research on the effect of exercise in AS has been conducted in Europe and Canada for individual and group programs. Notable improvement has been demonstrated in physical measures and in function, but no studies have investigated long-term outcome (Hidding, 1993; Kraag, Stokes, Groh, Helewa, & Goldsmith, 1990; O'Driscoll, Jayson, & Baddeley, 1978; Viitanen & Suni, 1995). Conclusions cannot be drawn regarding which type of exercise is best, although warm aquatic exercise is generally accepted as beneficial, and group exercise may be slightly better than individual exercise. To determine how much exercise is beneficial, Santos, Brophy, and Calin (1998) analyzed the responses of 4,282 patients with AS who completed a self-administered questionnaire on physical exercise. The authors compared patients who exercised 2 to 4 hr and 10 hr or more with patients who did not exercise. Patients who exercised 2 to 4 hr showed improved function and less disease activity than patients who did not exercise. Patients who exercised for 10 hr or more showed improved function but no difference in the level of disease activity. Santos and associates (1998) concluded that consistency in moderate exercise is more important than quantity of exercise and that patients who exercised were more likely to be followed by a rheumatologist, believe in the benefits of exercise, and have a higher level of education.

In Great Britain and in Europe in general, the therapeutic approach to AS is far more vigorous than in the United States. At the Royal National Hospital for Rheumatic Disease in Bath, England, patients participate in an intensive 3-week group physiotherapy program. In Austria, some spas offer a 6-week intensive exercise and sports program. In England and the Netherlands, evening community exercise programs for persons with AS are offered. These programs have demonstrated the value of active exercise (Hidding, 1993; O'Driscoll et al., 1978).

Home exercise with a method for self-monitoring is absolutely essential. Jane Barefoot, MCSP, a therapist in the United Kingdom who specializes in AS, advocates teaching patients the rationale for each exercise with detailed information on how to make it effective and information on normal joint range of motion (ROM) (Barefoot, 1993). She believes she obtains the best

Table 4. Realistic Exercise Prescription

Type of Exercise	Frequency
ROM (spinal and peripheral, including rib cage excursion)*	Briefly 2–3 times/day
Posture awareness	Constantly
Vigorous stretching	2–3 times/week
General strengthening	2–3 times/week
Cardiovascular conditioning (moderate physical activity or exercise)	30 min 3 times/week

*On the basis of weekly self-evaluation. *Note:* ROM=range of motion.

results by expecting the patient to put forth maximum effort and by praising the patient's effort, not the achievement.

Because self-management skills tend to improve outcomes in chronic disease, an independent program is best that allows the patient to modify the program according to symptoms without relying on a health professional's evaluation. It is helpful for the clinician to "contract" with the patient to fit exercise into his or her regular daily schedule. In Table 4, an exercise regimen is outlined on the basis of the literature for cardiovascular exercise and has a realistic time commitment (Gall, 1994).

To increase the likelihood of exercise compliance in AS, the program should be simple and enjoyable. This can be done by including brief exercise sessions for problem areas throughout the day (e.g., pectoral corner stretches or neck exercises on every trip to the toilet or during television commercial breaks). Progress and maintenance measurement techniques should be taught to the patient and performed monthly.

Increasing and maintaining an upright posture is essential. Postural dysfunction develops from assuming flexed positions that decrease pain and from daily activities most often done in flexion, such as desk work, driving, gardening, and watching television. Once the spine is slightly out of alignment, the extensor muscles must work harder to prevent further forward bending. The flexibility of the anterior muscles of the trunk, shoulder, and hips must be maintained, and the extensors must be strengthened.

The stretching program should involve an examination of all peripheral and spinal motions and soft-tissue flexibility. Pelvic motion and lateral trunk flexion are often limited early in the disease and should be given special attention. Stretching should be slow and sustained, and the hold–relax technique has been recommended in addition to exercising in warm water (Bulstrode, Barefoot, Harrison, & Clarke, 1987). Stretching exercises are shown and explained in a pull-out poster from the book *Straight Talk on Spondylitis* (Gitman & Rosenberg, 1992). (See appendix to this chapter for sample of a stretching program.)

A program of daily passive stretching of the hip joints during a 3-week inpatient course showed a major increase in the range of all movements of the hip joints except flexion, and these results were maintained by patients who performed them regularly after discharge (Bulstrode et al., 1987). Prone lying to tolerance can help maintain hip and spine extension.

The therapeutic exercise ball (Swiss Ball) is fun to use for stretching and strengthening. The ball provides a convex, nonrigid surface capable of weight bearing while sitting, side lying, prone lying, or supine (Figures 4 and 5). It is available in various sizes that are determined by the patient's height and can be purchased in some exercise stores and catalogs. Instruction from a therapist is advised, particularly for patients with rigid or semirigid spines.

A strengthening program is appropriate when a good flexibility and posture program is in place. Strengthening can be done with free weights, exercise tubing, the therapeutic ball, gym equipment, or a pool. Muscles most likely to need strengthening are the muscles that stabilize the scapula, extend the neck and spine, extend and abduct the hip, and extend the knee and the abdominal muscles.

Cardiovascular exercise is particularly important because of the potential loss of chest expansion and because of the fatigue and deconditioning that can accompany the disease (Calin et al., 1993). (For additional information on fatigue, see chapters 6 and 8 in this volume.) Physical fitness guidelines for general health have been modified by the Centers for Disease Control and Prevention ("Surgeon General's Report on Physical Activity and Health," 1996) to make compliance easier for deconditioned persons. The recommendations are for 30 min/day, three times a week, of moderate levels of exercise or activity. A moderate amount of physical activity (i.e., physical activity that uses approximately 1,500 kcal of energy per day or 1,000 cal a week) can be achieved in many ways. Patients can perform some activities at varying intensities; the suggested durations correspond to the expected intensity of effort. Patients may select activities that they enjoy and that fit into their daily lives. Because the amount of activity is a function of duration, intensity, and frequency, patients can obtain the same amount of activity in longer sessions of moderately intense activities (e.g., brisk walking) as in shorter sessions of more strenuous activities (e.g., swimming). Examples of moderate physical activity include gardening for 30 to 45 min, walking 1 3/4 miles in 35 min (20 min/mile) or 2 miles in 30 min (15 min/mile), washing and waxing a car for 45 to 60 min, basketball (shooting baskets) for 30 min, bicycling 5 miles in 30 min or 4 miles in 15 min, pushing a stroller 1 1/2 miles in 30 min, raking leaves for 30 min, participating in water aerobics for 30 min, swimming laps for 20 min, shoveling snow for 15 min, and walking up and down stairs for 15 min ("Surgeon General's Report on Physical Activity and Health," 1996). Patients with cardiac abnormalities should receive medical clearance before starting an aerobic program.

Pool exercises can be done during any stage of the disease. Buoyancy can promote relaxation in supine floating, assist stretching in many positions, offer resistance for strengthening, and is excellent for cardiovascular conditioning. Stretching can be assisted with simple flotation equipment.

Swimming is universally recommended because it exercises all the muscles in a non–weight-bearing environment, and it improves cardiovascular abilities and chest expansion. Swimming strokes may need to be adapted for patients with rigid spines and limited shoulder motion. For patients with severely limited neck and spine motion, a mask and snorkel will allow continuation of the breast stroke and freestyle stroke.

All patients should be encouraged to participate in ongoing community sports or exercise groups. Almost any sport or game is acceptable as long as it does not aggravate involved joints or tendons or cause impact trauma to the spine. The activities and sports chosen will depend on disease activity, availability of equipment, and the patient's sporting interest. Basketball and volleyball encourage extension and rotation but are high-impact sports because of the jumping and landing.

Tai chi is an ancient Chinese exercise form that uses flowing, rhythmic, deliberate movement to harmonize yang (active) and yin (passive) forces in the body and to free the flow of chi, the life force of the body. Tai chi exercises coordinate breath control with relaxation (passive) throughout the process of physical conditioning (active). The slow flowing exercises require an erect spine to facilitate the flow of chi. This makes them an ideal exercise form for persons with AS. The process teaches mindfulness and promotes relaxation. Koh (1982), a physician with AS, reported that practicing tai chi for 2½ years resulted in reduced pain, muscle spasm, stress, and malaise and improved strength, balance, chest movement, sleep, and capacity for relaxation.

All sports should be evaluated in terms of trauma to the spine and prolonged positioning in a flexed posture. In-line skating and roller skating are low-impact sports but involve a risk of falling. Contact sports like street hockey, rugby, football and sports in which a neck injury is possible such as diving and horseback riding are discouraged. Sports requiring prolonged trunk flexion such as bicycling and bowling should be minimized.

Stress Reduction and Self-Management

Stress reduction is a key tool for managing pain and can be achieved by learning effective communication, modifying environmental factors (e.g., job demands), or by doing relaxation exercises. Progressive relaxation, diaphragmatic breathing, meditation, visualization biofeedback, tai chi, and yoga are effective ways to learn how muscle tension and stress can amplify pain. Energy conservation training helps reduce fatigue and stress. Principles include planning, pacing, setting priorities, relaxing perfectionist standards, and organizing space to avoid unnecessary steps and work (Cordery & Rocchi, 1998).

Self-management is defined as "learning and practicing the skills necessary to carry on an active and emotionally satisfying life in the face of a chronic illness" (Lorig, 1993). Helping patients become self-managers requires moving beyond traditional didactic patient instruction with a sole focus on information transfer. Self-management requires the acquisition of a complex set of skills and attitudes. In addition to treatment-related behaviors, persons with AS must learn how to communicate with their health care team, make informed decisions, and use problem-solving skills to adapt to changes in their symptoms, roles, and emotions (Boutaugh & Brady, 1998). Teaching patients self-monitoring techniques such as height measurement, finger-to-floor distance, inches of chest expansion, and ear tragus to wall is critical to this process. Barlow and Barefoot (1996) evaluated the effectiveness of an intensive 3-week self-management course for persons with AS. They found improvement in depression, self-effectiveness, and severity at 3 weeks with trends toward continued improvement at the 6-month follow-up. Interestingly, gains in ROM and frequency of home exercise at 3 weeks were not maintained at 6 months. Therapists teaching self-management of AS must pay special attention to follow-through with exercise regimens. Access to patient education material and participation in support groups encourages independence in self-management.

ADL and Assistive Technology

Problems that interfere with ADL may be due to spinal rigidity, pain, spasm, or peripheral joint involvement. In women with milder cervical involvement, treatment is the same as for OA of the neck and FMS in which stiffness is a common complaint. (See chapters 5 and 6 in this volume.)

Assistive equipment or modified techniques can help relieve pain, provide support, encourage proper posture, and position small joints during activities. Devices may only be needed temporarily and can become an added expense, especially if they prove ineffective for their specific problem. For these reasons, patients should be encouraged to consult an occupational therapist to select items that are suitable before they buy them from a catalog. As with all ADL, patients should make every effort to use all the ROM and strength available. For example, patients who can reach with difficulty to don shoes may benefit more without a long-handled shoe horn that eliminates this functional stretch.

For persons with spinal involvement, proper positioning during activities, leisure, and sleep is crucial to prevent back deformities. Posture habits during activities such as watching television, reading, and desk work require careful evaluation. A reasonably functional life can be anticipated if proper posture is maintained (Wright & Moll, 1976).

Daily activities such as bathing, transferring, dressing, hygiene, toileting, driving, and vocational skills need special consideration because of stiffness that limits reaching the feet or overhead or because of the risk of losing balance. Resources to help patients problem solve to accomplish activities and increase safety include the "Guide to Independent Living for People With Arthritis" (Arthritis Foundation, 1988), which contains descriptions of each daily task and items and techniques to master them with the principles of joint protection and energy conservation; the Abledata database on the Internet (www.abledata.com), which lists more than 20,000 assistive devices or adaptive equipment with full resource information; and references on assistive devices and joint protection (Cordery & Rocchi, 1998; Mann, 1998; Melvin, in press; Slonaker, 1992) (Box 1).

Bathing and grooming. Several items can increase safety while bathing, including safety mats, grab bars, bathtub rails, liquid soap, soap on a rope, or soap holders. Patients who are unable to reach their feet find sitting in the shower and using a long bath sponge helpful. Bending to use the bathroom sink is often difficult or painful, and sitting on a stool to use the sink or resting on the forearms helps support the back. Some tools such as a mirror that hangs from the neck or extends from the wall can make use of a mirror easier without craning the neck forward.

Dressing. Use of modified Velcro® shoe closures, long shoe horns, and sock aids is indicated if a person is unable to reach the feet and to make fastening easier if there is peripheral involvement. Long-handled dressing sticks that have a hook can help manipulate garments on and off stiff lower extremities and shoulders.

Driving. Safety while driving is an important factor because cervical pain and ankylosis can reduce the visual driving field. Positioning the seat close to the pedals increases hip and knee flexion and brings the back more firmly against the seat for back support. Use of additional and wide-angled rear-view mirrors allows the patient to see blind spots without turning the neck. (Avoid mirrors that distort the distance of following cars.) Adapting the headrest so that it is in contact with the back of the head encourages proper posture when driving. Cruise control allows the legs to be stretched periodically. Persons with AS are eligible for disabled parking permits when fatigue or pain impair ambulation.

Desk and computer work. The workstation should be organized so that the lumbosacral and cervical spines are in a neutral position as much as possible and there is a minimal amount of strain on the shoulders. The following equipment may assist: slanted desks, drafting tables, book stands and copy holders, telephone headsets, and monitor stands that can tilt, rotate, swivel, raise, lower, retract, and extend. Ergonomic chairs with adjustable arm rests and back supports that slide up and down, swivel, and spring into flexion reduce strain on the shoulders, neck, and upper back. Patients should consider whether glasses may help avoid forward head posture to see the screen and should consider adjusting the monitor to be within focal distance at about 15° down from eye level and slanted for best visual convergence. (*Note.* New vision problems should be reported to the physician to determine if they are due to eye strain or symptoms of iritis.) Glare shields should be in place if there are reflections. Teaching patients how to identify their tissue tolerance, to build in stretch breaks, and to alternate tasks during high-intensity jobs so that they do not go past their tolerance can help control pain and fatigue. A principle of pain management is to be able to do a task *without an increase in pain* rather than no pain. Patients should organize their workstations so that this is possible.

Housework and outdoor chores. Long-handled tools for cleaning and scrubbing can augment limited reach and increase safety. Use of wheeled carts is beneficial for laundry, cleaning, gardening, working in the workshop, and keeping most frequently used products at a comfortable level to reduce lifting and bending. If a person cannot maintain an erect posture during a specific task, a soft neck collar or back support may be valuable solely as a postural reminder during the activity (Melvin, 1989), such as loading a dishwasher, scrubbing a bathtub or toilet, doing auto mechanics, reading, or using a computer.

For mowing the lawn, a good back support and a riding mower with vibration-absorbing cushions or gloves are recommended. Lightweight and long-handled tools or swivel-handled attachments for gardening and yard work as well as ergonomic handles can decrease back bending.

Child care. Place the car seat in a position that avoids extra twisting, and arrange a mirror to allow the patient to see the baby when there is limited cervical rotation. Use pillows to support the baby during nursing or feeding instead of rounding the back and chest. Teaching toddlers to climb up on a stepladder instead of reaching down to pick them up for dressing and hair care is extremely helpful.

Body Mechanics, Posture, and Positioning

With a growing emphasis on ergonomics equipment and education for the public, there is a wealth of information that can be applied to this patient population. Patients should be taught the principles of good posture and body mechanics and then encouraged to problem solve how to achieve these goals in specific activities.

Sitting. Patients must learn how to align the entire spine by keeping the head, neck, back, and feet in the best position by using various tilting and height-adjustable surfaces, footrests, and lumbar supports. Shallow chair seats allow the buttocks to sit fully back on the seat to allow optimal support. Pressure-sensitive contouring cushions can be used to relieve ischial pain or to accommodate contractures. There are two ergonomic chairs available to accommodate unilateral hip extension contractures with less than 90° flexion or fused hips. One has an adjustable split seat, and the other has a shallow seat pan. Both are made by Grahl Industries and are available through Office World (www.officeworld.com or 1-800-541-5059).

Patients with fused necks or backs find a high-backed comfortable chair at home with a swivel base helpful. This allows them to face others easily during conversations and to expand their visual field.

Standing. If prolonged standing is a problem, changing positions frequently by shifting weight, leaning, or putting one foot up on a step or ledge may reduce strain on the lower back. Impact-absorbing soles and antifatigue floor mats help reduce strain on the spine.

Lifting and carrying. General body mechanics principles should be stressed with the following additional considerations. Remain as upright as possible, and reduce stooping and bending forward as much as possible. Face objects to be lifted by rotating the body with the feet, not twisting the back or the knees. Because of the risk of falling off balance with a rigid spine, stand close to the object, establish a firm footing and a wide stance, and test the weight of the object before lifting. If it seems heavy, divide the object into smaller parts, get a secure grip on the load, then lift steadily by straightening the knees. Carry the object close to the body, or use a rolling cart to transport. Use larger joints if there is peripheral joint involvement.

Reaching. For patients with fused backs, special consideration is needed regarding safety precautions against falling. This is especially true during bending and reaching activities (e.g., dressing, gardening, or bathing) when a shift in the center of gravity can cause a loss of balance. These patients in particular are vulnerable to neck fractures (Wright & Moll, 1976). If there is limited spinal extension, there is a tendency to flex the knees and lean backwards to see higher, which places the person off balance and at risk for falling. Use a reacher, stable stepladder, or ladder to help prevent loss of balance when trying to reach an object on a shelf.

Sleeping. The patient should be aware of the best positions for sleeping; neutral alignment supine with cervical support rather than side-lying with legs bent is recommended. A firm mattress is preferred with the option of various air, water, and foam cushioning systems to distribute the body pressure. Eggcrate or "waffle" mattress pads tend to be difficult to move around on when changing positions, although bed mobility can be facilitated with grab bars, side rails, cloth ladders, or blanket cradles. Electric blankets or mattress covers help reduce stiffness. Hospital beds should be kept flat at night, should have only the back raised during the day, and should keep the knee section straight.

The pillow should properly support the cervical muscles to maintain a normal lordotic curve to the neck without causing cervical flexion. This supports the arch of the neck and allows the neck muscles to fully relax. The occipital skull should be touching or close to the mattress (Figure 6). Sleeping without a pillow flattens the lordotic curve and is not advised (Jackson, 1978). Buckwheat pillows provide conforming support to the lordotic curve. There are numerous cervical pillows available, but they should be

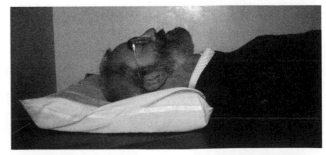

Figure 6. Patient demonstrating use of proper cervical support. The occiput should be touching or as close to the mattress as possible. The pillow should support the lordotic arch to allow the paraspinal muscles to relax. *Source:* Courtesy of the Spondylitis Association of America, P. O. Box 5872, Sherman Oaks, CA 91413.

evaluated by using these parameters before purchase. If the head and neck are fused in a forward position, additional pillows can be used for support. Reading while sitting up in bed is not recommended unless it can be done with the back and neck in good alignment. A book rest or stand or prism glasses can allow one to read while remaining flat in bed and keeping the cervical spine in alignment.

Pain often is most severe at night, so medications should be adjusted for maximum comfort. The stages of sleep may be disrupted by pain, stress, anxiety, or dietary factors. Nonrestorative sleep increases fatigue, depression, and anxiety. Patients who are waking not feeling rested should avoid stimulants like caffeine, alcohol, and nicotine; eat a light carbohydrate snack before bedtime; avoid highly acidic or spicy foods; and regulate the amount of fluids before bed to avoid too many nightly visits to the toilet (Melvin, 1989). (Other sleep hygiene principles described in chapter 6 in this volume likewise apply to persons with AS.)

AS is a member of the spondylarthropathies because it has a predilection for inflammatory arthritis of the axial joints, enthesopathy, iritis, and an association with HLA B-27. Environmental factors may influence the timing of onset, and genetic factors have a greater influence on prognosis. The course of AS is highly variable, with remissions and exacerbations, and may stop at any stage with residual pain-free deformity. Because the potential for permanent deformity is great and may occur quickly, patients should begin exercise, posture awareness, and education on self-management soon after diagnosis. Rehabilitation is critical in the treatment of this disorder and is rewarding because of its potential to prevent deformity and keep patients in the workforce. In addition, several functional outcome assessments developed for AS allow documentation of the effectiveness of therapy.

References

Amor, B., Santos, R. S., Nahal, R., Listrat, V., & Dougados, M. (1994). Predictive factors for the long-term outcome of spondyloarthropathies. *Journal of Rheumatology, 21*(10), 1883–1887.

Arnett, F. C. (1996). Ankylosing spondylitis. In W. J. Koopman (Ed.), *Arthritis and allied conditions* (13th ed., pp. 1197–1208). Baltimore: Williams & Wilkins.

Arthritis Foundation. (1988). *Guide to independent living for people with arthritis.* Atlanta, GA: Author.

Bakker, C., Rutten-van Molken, M., Hidding, A., van Doorslaer, E., Bennett, K., & van der Linden, S. (1994). Patient utilities in ankylosing spondylitis and the association with other outcome measures. *Journal of Rheumatology, 21*(7), 1298–304.

Barefoot, J. (1993). Stretch relax and a little bit more. In *Exercises for ankylosing spondylitis* (3rd ed.). Bath, England: Georgian Music Desktop Publishing.

Barlow, J. H., & Barefoot, J. (1996). Group education for people with arthritis. *Patient Education and Counseling, 27*(3), 257–267.

Barlow, J. H., Macey, S. J., & Struthers, G. (1992). Psychosocial factors and self-help in ankylosing spondylitis patients. *Clinical Rheumatology, 11*(2), 220–225.

Barlow, J. H., Macey, S. J., & Struthers, G. R. (1993). Health locus of control, self-help and treatment adherence in relation to ankylosing spondylitis patients. *Patient Education and Counseling, 20*(2–3), 153–166.

Basler, H. D., & Rehfisch, H. P. (1991). Cognitive-behavioral therapy in patients with ankylosing spondylitis in a German self-help organization. *Journal of Psychosomatic Research, 35*(2–3), 345–354.

Bluestone, R. (1992). Understanding the disease. In R. L. Swezey (Ed.), *Straight talk on spondylitis* (2nd ed., p. 1). Sherman Oaks, CA: Spondylitis Association of America.

Boutaugh, M., & Brady, T. (1998). Patient education for self-management. In J. L. Melvin & G. Jensen (Eds.), *Rheumatologic rehabilitation series: Volume 1: Assessment and management* (pp. 219–258). Bethesda, MD: American Occupational Therapy Association.

Brucker, J. (1992). Staying employed. In R. L. Swezey (Ed.), *Straight talk on spondylitis* (2nd ed., p. 47). Sherman Oaks, CA: Spondylitis Association of America.

Bulstrode, S., Barefoot, J., Harrison, R., & Clarke, A. K. (1987). The role of passive stretching in the treatment of ankylosing spondylitis. *British Journal of Rheumatology, 26,* 40–42.

Calin, A. (1985a). Ankylosing spondylitis. In G. S. Panayi (Ed.), *Clinics in rheumatic diseases* (Vol. 11, pp. 41–59). Philadelphia: Saunders.

Calin, A. (1985b). Ankylosing spondylitis. In W. M. Kelly, E. D. Harris, S. Ruddy, & C. B. Sledge (Eds.), *Textbook of rheumatology* (2nd ed., pp. 1017–1032). Philadelphia: Saunders.

Calin, A., Edmunds, L., & Kennedy, L. G. (1993). Fatigue in ankylosing spondylitis: Why is it ignored? *Journal of Rheumatology, 20,* 991–995.

Calin, A., & Elswood, J. (1988). The natural history of juvenile-onset ankylosing spondylitis: A 24 year retrospective case-control study. *British Journal of Rheumatology, 27*(2), 91–93.

Calin, A., & Elswood, J. (1989). Relative role of genetic and environmental factors in disease expression: Sib pair analysis in ankylosing spondylitis. *Arthritis and Rheumatism, 32*(1), 77–81.

Calin, A., & Fries, J.F. (1975). The striking prevalence of ankylosing spondylitis in 'healthy' W27 positive males and females: A controlled study. *New England Journal of Medicine, 293,* 835.

Calin, A., Garrett, S., Whitelock, H., Kennedy, L. G., O'Hea, J., Mallorie, P., & Jenkinson, T. (1994). A new approach to defining functional ability in ankylosing spondylitis: The development of the Bath Ankylosing Spondylitis Functional Index. *Journal of Rheumatology, 21,* 2281–2285.

Chamberlain, M. A. (1983). Socioeconomic effects of ankylosing spondylitis in females: A comparison of 25 females with 25 male subjects. *International Journal of Rehabilitation Medicine, 5*(3), 149–153.

Cohen, M. D., & Ginsburg, W. N. (1982). Late onset peripheral joint disease in ankylosing spondylitis. *Annals of Rheumatic Disease, 41,* 574.

Cordery, J., & Rocchi, M. (1998). Joint protection and fatigue management. In J. L. Melvin & G. Jensen (Eds.), *Rheumatologic rehabilitation series: Volume 1: Assessment and management* (pp. 279–322). Bethesda, MD: American Occupational Therapy Association.

Daltroy, L. H., Larson, M. G., Roberts, W. N., & Liang, M. H. (1990). A modification of the health assessment questionnaire for the spondyloarthropathies. *Journal of Rheumatology, 17,* 946–950.

Dougados, M., Gueguen, A., Nakache, J. -P., Nguyen, M., Mery, C., & Amor, B. (1988). Evaluation of a functional index and an articular index in ankylosing spondylitis. *Journal of Rheumatology, 15,* 302–307.

Dougados, M., Van Der Linden, S., Juklin, R., Huilfeldt, B., Amor, B., Calin, A., Cats, A., Dijkmans, B., Olivieri, I., Pasero, G., Veys, E., & Zeidler, H. (1991). The European spondyloarthropathy study group preliminary criteria for the classification of spondyloarthropathy. *Arthritis and Rheumatism, 34,* 1218–1227.

Gall, V. (1994). Exercise in the spondyloarthropathies. *Arthritis Care and Research, 7,* 215–220.

Garrett, S., Jenkinson, T., Kennedy, G. L., Whitelock, H., Gaisford, P., & Calin, A. (1994). A new approach to defining disease status in ankylosing spondylitis: The Bath Ankylosing Spondylitis Disease Activity Index. *Journal of Rheumatology, 21,* 2286–2291.

Gemignani, G., Oliveri, I., Rujo, G., & Pasero, G. (1991). Transcutaneous electrical nerve stimulation in ankylosing spondylitis: A double-blind study [Letter]. *Arthritis and Rheumatism, 4,* 788–789.

Gitman, S., & Rosenberg, M. (1992). Exercise is essential. In R. L. Swezey (Ed.), *Straight talk on spondylitis* (2nd ed., pp. 14–29). Sherman Oaks, CA: Spondylitis Association of America.

Gran, J. T., & Ostensen, M. (1998). Spondyloarthritides in females. *Balliere's Clinical Rheumatology, 12*(4), 695–715.

Guillemin, F., Briancon, S., Pourel, J., & Gaucher, A. (1990). Long-term disability and prolonged sick leaves as outcome measurements in ankylosing spondylitis: Possible predictive factors. *Arthritis and Rheumatism, 33*, 1001–1006.

Gunther, V., Mur, E., Traweger, C., & Hawel, R. (1994). Stress coping of patients with ankylosing spondylitis. *Journal of Psychosomatic Research, 38*(50), 419–427.

Hidding, A. (1993). Is group physiotherapy superior to individualized therapy in ankylosing spondylitis? A randomized controlled trial. *Arthritis Care and Research, 6*, 117–125.

Hunter, T., & Dubo, H. I. C. (1983). Spinal fractures complicating ankylosing spondylitis: A long-term followup study. *Arthritis and Rheumatism, 26*, 751–758.

Jackson, R. (1978). *The cervical syndrome* (4th ed.). Springfield, IL: Charles C. Thomas.

Jenkins, T. R., Mallorie, P. A., Whitelock, H. C., Kennedy, L. G., Garrett, S. L., & Calin, A. (1994). Defining spinal mobility in ankylosing spondylitis (AS): The Bath AS Metrology Index. *Journal of Rheumatology, 21*, 1694–1698.

Kennedy, L. G., Edmunds, L., & Cain, A. (1993). The natural history of ankylosing spondylitis: Does it burn out? *Journal of Rheumatology, 20*(4), 688–692.

Khan, M. A. (1994). Ankylosing spondylitis: Clinical features. In J. H. Klippel & P. A. Dieppe (Eds.), *Rheumatology* (1st ed., pp. 3.25.1–3.25.10). London: Mosby.

Koh, T. C. (1982). Tai chi and ankylosing spondylitis: A personal experience. *American Journal of Chinese Medicine, X*(1–4), 59–61.

Kraag, G., Stokes, B., Groh, J., Helewa, A., & Goldsmith, C. (1990). The effects of comprehensive home physiotherapy and supervision on patients with ankylosing spondylitis: A randomized controlled trial. *Journal of Rheumatology, 17*, 228–233.

Lorig, K. (1993). Self-management of chronic illness: A model for the future. *Generations*, 11–14.

Mann, W. (1998). Assistive technology for persons with arthritis. In J. L. Melvin & G. Jensen (Eds.), *Rheumatologic rehabilitation series: Volume 1: Assessment and management* (pp. 369–392). Bethesda, MD: American Occupational Therapy Association.

Martin, S. D., Zavadak, K., Noaker, J., Jacobs, M. A., & Poss, R. (1999). Hip surgery and rehabilitation. In J. Melvin & V. Gall (Eds.), *Rheumatologic rehabilitation series: Volume 5: Surgical rehabilitation* (pp. 81–120). Bethesda, MD: American Occupational Therapy Association.

Mau, W., Zeidler, H., Mau, R., Majewski, A., Freyschmidt, J., Stangel, W., & Deicher, H. (1988). Clinical features and prognosis of patients with possible ankylosing spondylitis: Results of a 10 year followup. *Journal of Rheumatology, 15*(7), 1109–1114.

Melvin, J. L. (1989). Ankylosing spondylitis. In J. L. Melvin (Ed.), *Rheumatic disease in the adult and child: Occupational therapy and rehabilitation* (3rd ed., p. 95). Philadelphia: F. A. Davis.

Melvin, J. L. (in press). Self-care strategies for persons with arthritis and connective-tissue diseases. In C. Christianson (Ed.), *Ways of living* (2nd ed.). Bethesda, MD: American Occupational Therapy Association.

O'Driscoll, S. L., Jayson, M. I., & Baddeley, H. (1978). Neck movements in ankylosing spondylitis and their response to physiotherapy. *Annals of Rheumatic Disease, 37*(1), 64–66.

Ostrow, S. (1985). Enjoying sports and activities. In R. L. Swezey (Ed.), *Straight talk on spondylitis* (p. 28). Sherman Oaks, CA: Spondylitis Association of America.

Resnick, D. (1989). Inflammatory disorders of the vertebral column: Seronegative spondyloarthropathies, adult-onset rheumatoid arthritis, and juvenile chronic arthritis. *Clinical Imaging, 13*, 253–268.

Roberts, W. N., Liang, M. H., Pallozi, L. M., & Daltroy, L. H. (1988). Effects of warming up on reliability of anthropometric techniques in ankylosing spondylitis. *Arthritis and Rheumatism, 31*, 549–552.

Ruof, J., & Stucki, G. (1999). Comparison of the Dougados Functional Index and the Bath Ankylosing Spondylitis Functional Index: A literature review. *Journal of Rheumatology, 26*(4), 955–960.

Santos, H., Brophy, S., & Calin, A. (1998). Exercise in ankylosing spondylitis: How much is optimum? *Journal of Rheumatology, 25*(11), 2156–2160.

Schweitzer, M. E., & Resnick, D. (1994). Spondyloarthopathies: Enthesopathies. In J. H. Klippel & P. Dieppe (Eds.), *Rheumatology* (pp. 27.1–27.6). London: Mosby.

Slonaker, D. (1992). Getting straight through the day and keeping straight through the night. In R. L. Swezey (Ed.), *Straight talk on spondylitis* (2nd ed., pp. 33–46). Sherman Oaks, CA: Spondylitis Association of America.

Some questions we knew you'd ask. (1992). In R. L. Swezey (Ed.), *Straight talk on spondylitis* (2nd ed., p. 53). Sherman Oaks, CA: Spondylitis Association of America.

Spoorenberg, A., van der Heijde, D., de Klerk, E., Dougados, M., de Vlam, K., Mielants, H., van der Tempel, H., & van der Linden, S. (1999). A comparative study of the usefulness of the Bath Ankylosing Spondylitis Functional Index and the Dougados Functional Index in the assessment of ankylosing spondylitis. *Journal of Rheumatology, 26*(4), 961–965.

Surgeon General's report on physical activity and health. (1996). *Morbidity and Mortality Weekly Report, 45*(27), 591–592.

van der Heijde, D., Calin, A., Dougados, M., Khan, M. A., van der Linden, S., & Bellamy, N. (1999). Selection of instruments in the core set for DC-ART, SMARD, physical therapy, and clinical record keeping in ankylosing spondylitis: Progress report of the ASAS Working Group: Assessments in ankylosing spondylitis. *Journal of Rheumatology, 26*(4), 951–954.

Van Der Linden, S., Valkenburg, H. A., & Cats, A. (1984). Evaluation of diagnostic criteria for ankylosing spondylitis: A proposal for the modification of the New York criteria. *Arthritis and Rheumatism, 27*, 361–368.

Viitanen, J. V., Kokko, M. L., Heikkila, S., & Kautiainen, H. (1998). Neck mobility assessment in ankylosing spondylitis: A clinical study of nine measurements including new tape methods for cervical rotation and lateral flexion. *British Journal of Rheumatology, 37*(4), 377–381.

Viitanen, J. V., Kokko, M. L., Lehtinen, K., Suni, J., & Kautiainen, H. (1995). Correlation between mobility restrictions and radiologic changes in ankylosing spondylitis. *Spine, 20*(4), 492–496.

Viitanen, J. V., & Suni, J. (1995). Management principles of physiotherapy in ankylosing spondylitis. *Physiotherapy, 81*, 322–329.

Walker, L. G., & Sledge, C. B. (1991). Total hip arthroplasty in ankylosing spondylitis. *Clinical Orthopedics, 262*, 198–204.

Wennenberg, B., Kopp, S., & Hollender, L. (1984). The temporomandibular joint in ankylosing spondylitis: Correlations between subjective, clinical and radiographic features in the stomatognathic system and effects of treatment. *Acta Odontologica Scandinavica, 42*(3), 165–173.

Wordsworth, B. P., & Mowat, A. G. (1986). A review of 100 patients with ankylosing spondylitis with particular reference to socio-economic effects. *British Journal of Rheumatology, 25*(2), 175–180.

Wright, V., & Moll, H. M. H. (1976). *Seronegative polyarthritis*. Amsterdam, Netherlands: Elsevier North-Holland.

APPENDIX A

Spondylitis Exercise Program

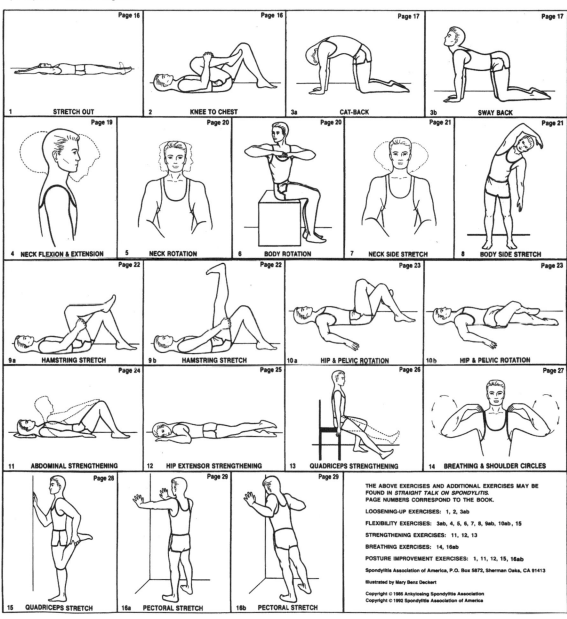

Page 16	Page 16	Page 17	Page 17
1 STRETCH OUT	2 KNEE TO CHEST	3a CAT-BACK	3b SWAY BACK
Page 19	Page 20	Page 20	Page 21 — Page 21
4 NECK FLEXION & EXTENSION	5 NECK ROTATION	6 BODY ROTATION	7 NECK SIDE STRETCH — 8 BODY SIDE STRETCH
Page 22	Page 22	Page 23	Page 23
9a HAMSTRING STRETCH	9b HAMSTRING STRETCH	10a HIP & PELVIC ROTATION	10b HIP & PELVIC ROTATION
Page 24	Page 25	Page 26	Page 27
11 ABDOMINAL STRENGTHENING	12 HIP EXTENSOR STRENGTHENING	13 QUADRICEPS STRENGTHENING	14 BREATHING & SHOULDER CIRCLES
Page 28	Page 29	Page 29	
15 QUADRICEPS STRETCH	16a PECTORAL STRETCH	16b PECTORAL STRETCH	

THE ABOVE EXERCISES AND ADDITIONAL EXERCISES MAY BE FOUND IN *STRAIGHT TALK ON SPONDYLITIS.* PAGE NUMBERS CORRESPOND TO THE BOOK.

LOOSENING-UP EXERCISES: 1, 2, 3ab

FLEXIBILITY EXERCISES: 3ab, 4, 5, 6, 7, 8, 9ab, 10ab, 15

STRENGTHENING EXERCISES: 11, 12, 13

BREATHING EXERCISES: 14, 16ab

POSTURE IMPROVEMENT EXERCISES: 1, 11, 12, 15, 16ab

Spondylitis Association of America, P.O. Box 5872, Sherman Oaks, CA 91413

Illustrated by Mary Benz Deckert

Copyright © 1985 Ankylosing Spondylitis Association
Copyright © 1992 Spondylitis Association of America

12

POLYMYOSITIS AND DERMATOMYOSITIS

Y. Lynn Yasuda, MSEd, OTR, FAOTA, Leslie Miller-Porter, PT, and Thomas D. Beardmore, MD

Polymyositis (PM) is an uncommon rheumatic disorder characterized by inflammation of skeletal muscle with resultant muscle degeneration, weakness, and atrophy. The disease is idiopathic in origin and is referred to as *dermatomyositis* (DM) when there is a typical skin rash. It is characterized by proximal muscle weakness of the shoulder girdle, pelvic girdle, trunk, and neck.

Population Affected

PM affects all races and age-equivalent groups with bimodal peaks between 5 and 14 years of age and 45 and 65 years of age (Medsger, Dawson, & Masi, 1970). The incidence of both PM and DM has been reported to be 1 case per million per year, with a combined incidence of 10 cases per million in the population (Oddis, Conte, Steen, & Medsger, 1990). Inflammatory muscle disease has a slightly higher incidence in women than in men and may have a more severe prognosis in women, African-Americans, patients who are more than 45 years of age at onset, and when there is cardiac or respiratory involvement (Plotz, Leff, & Miller, 1993).

Clinical Features and Prognosis

In PM and DM, weakness initially manifests as functional problems, such as rising from a seated position (particularly from low surfaces), climbing stairs (even stepping up on a curb), placing objects above the head, and doing upper-body grooming. Systemic features include arthralgias, fever, and muscle tenderness.

DM has a characteristic rash that occurs on the face, neck, and shoulders and over the extensor surfaces of the hands, elbows, and knees. The face, neck, and back rash may be exacerbated by sun exposure and in the periorbital regions may have a red or violet appearance referred to as a *heliotrope rash*. The rash that occurs on the extensor surfaces can present as red papules and later become scaly, erythematous, and atrophic. These are characteristic of DM and are called *Gottron's papules* or *Gottron's rash* after the physician that first described them.

Muscle pain may be present, but the primary complaint will be muscle weakness and the gradual or sudden loss of the ability to do physical activities. With severe disease, patients may be bedridden and have problems with swallowing and respiration that can be life threatening. Inflammatory muscle disease causes degeneration of the muscle and results in the elevation of muscle enzymes in the serum. These enzymes include creatine kinase (CK), aldolase, transaminases, and lactic dehydrogenase. Muscle biopsy will be abnormal and show muscle destruction and inflammatory changes; electromyography will be abnormal.

Anti Jo-1 antibodies are the most common of the myositis-specific autoantibodies. They are seen in 20% to 25% of all cases (Miller, 1997). These antibodies are antisynthetase antibodies directed against the protein component of transfer RNA synthetase; Jo-1 is directed against histidyl RNA synthetase. The antisynthetase antibodies are found exclusively in inflammatory myositis and act as serological markers of the disease. They are clinically associated with an increased incidence of interstitial lung disease (50–70%), Raynaud's phenomenon, nonerosive arthritis, fever, and dry cracked skin of the fingertips ("mechanic's hands"). This clinical complex has been labeled the *antisynthetase* or *Jo-1 syndrome* and is associated with a more severe prognosis. Mortality before the use of corticosteroids was 50%; recent information indicates a much higher survival rate of 80% after 5 years (Miller, 1997). Most deaths occur within the first year of treatment. Increased survival is attributed to corticosteroid treatment, but earlier diagnosis, better management of complications, and more sophisticated medical management additionally contribute to improved survival. Poorer prognosis is associated with increased age, associated malignancy, cardiac disease, PM, delayed diagnosis, severe weakness, lung disease, female gender, and antisynthetase antibodies.

Morbidity and functional outcome are difficult to determine. Reported studies have many inherent design faults that include being retrospective, uncontrolled, having a small sample size, and having a referral center bias rather than being community based. All of these factors would exclude milder cases and thus would indicate poorer outcomes. Recent studies show remission or complete recovery in 71% of children with DM and PM after 3 years and a 3% mortality rate (Van Rossum, Hiemstra, Prieur, Rijkers, & Kuis, 1994). When followed for a mean of 6.3 years, 85% of patients of all ages with PM and DM had insignificant or no disability (Maugars, Berthelot, Abbas, Mussini, Nguyen, & Prost, 1996). Patients with DM have a better functional prognosis than patients with PM. Generalized calcinosis tends to occur in childhood DM and is associated with a poor functional prognosis.

Diagnosis and Classification

Inflammatory myopathies are the most common forms of muscle disease that cause severe weakness in adults. However, they must be distinguished from drug-related myopathies and the hereditary dystrophies, which can cause weakness and may involve elevation of serum CK. By using clinical signs, symptoms, and laboratory investigations, the diagnosis of idiopathic PM or DM may be established with a sensitivity and specificity of greater than 95% (Tanimoto et al., 1995). Characteristic dermal rashes must be present for a diagnosis of DM. Serum enzymes such as CK (normal=20–220 IU/l) and aldolase (normal=0–8 IU/l) will usually be elevated and may be up to 100 times greater than normal. If the myositis has a sudden onset with extensive muscle necrosis, the muscle protein myoglobin may be in the serum or urine. Electromyography will show abnormali-

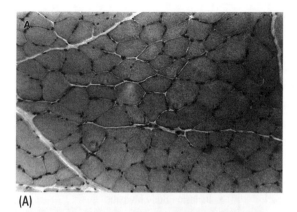

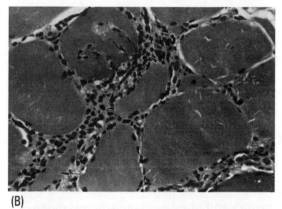

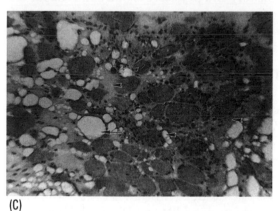

Figure 1. Histopathology of inflammatory myopathy. (A): Normal muscle with uniform fiber size and staining, absence of inflammatory cells, and connective and adipose tissue. (B): Recent-onset PM with fiber atrophy (*arrow*) and inflammatory cells (*arrowhead*). Reprinted from the Clinical Slide Collection on the Rheumatic Diseases, copyright 1991, 1995. Used by permission of the American College of Rheumatology. (C): Late-onset PM resistant to treatment with atrophic myofibrils, connective tissue (*arrowhead*), and adipose tissue (*arrow*) replacement of muscle.

ties consistent with inflammatory muscle disease, and biopsy of an affected muscle will show characteristic changes (Figure 1). The histopathology includes the presence of inflammatory cells within the muscle fascicles, atrophy of muscle fibers at the margins of the fascicles, and the presence of muscle fiber degeneration and regeneration. The pathology of advanced muscle disease, which is chronic or refractory to treatment, may indicate replacement of muscle fibers with fibrous connective tissue and fat. Careful selection of the site for muscle biopsy is important because there may be sampling errors if unaffected muscles are biopsied. Hence, it is important to biopsy a muscle that has evidence of weakness but continued function and to avoid muscles that have had injections or electromyogram needle insertion because these may create artifactual changes. Magnetic resonance imaging scans have some usefulness in the selection of involved muscles because there may be an increased signal in inflamed muscles (Fraser et al., 1991).

The clinical characteristics that are most useful in establishing diagnosis include proximal muscle weakness involving the shoulder girdle, pelvic girdle, and the flexor and extensor muscles of the neck and trunk (Table 1). However, in severe myositis, distal muscles may be involved in up to 20% of cases (Wortmann, 1992). Muscle atrophy; systemic symptoms of myalgia, arthritis, arthralgia; and a laboratory acute-phase response are useful for diagnosis but are not uniformly present. Antinuclear antibodies are commonly seen in patients with inflammatory muscle disease but do not have high sensitivity and specificity for diagnosis. Specific autoantibodies may be seen in inflammatory muscle disease and include the Jo-1 antibody (Wortmann, 1992).

Classification of inflammatory muscle disease (Table 2) includes the primary forms of

Table 1. Signs and Symptoms of Inflammatory Muscle Disease

- Skin rash on sun-exposed areas of face, neck, and shoulders; extensor areas of hands; elbows; and knees
- Proximal weakness of shoulders, hips, and neck extensors
- Elevation of muscle enzymes (CK, aldolase)
- Electromyogram abnormalities
- Muscle biopsy showing inflammatory myositis
- Autoantibodies (Jo-1)
- Systemic features (e.g., weakness, muscle atrophy, arthritis, acute-phase response, muscle pain)

Table 2. Types of Inflammatory Muscle Disease

- Polymyositis
- Dermatomyositis
- Polymyositis or Dermatomyositis with malignancy
- Polymyositis or Dermatomyositis of childhood
- Polymyositis or Dermatomyositis with another connective tissue disease
- Inclusion Body Myositis

PM and DM, myositis seen associated with malignancy, childhood PM or DM, overlap syndromes with other connective tissue disorders, and inclusion body myositis. The signs, symptoms, biopsy, and serological changes can be seen in both primary idiopathic PM and DM and in inflammatory myopathy associated with other diseases.

Myositis and Cancer

PM and DM is associated with malignancy primarily in patients more than 55 years of age and may occur before, after, or coincident with the diagnosis of cancer (Sigurgeirsson, Lindelof, Edhag, & Allander, 1992). Attention to the patient's history and physical examination is important in elderly patients to exclude malignancy. With treatment of the malignancy, the symptoms of PM and DM may abate.

Overlap With Other Connective Tissue Diseases

The myositis associated with connective tissue diseases such as rheumatoid arthritis and systemic lupus erythematosus, although clinically similar to PM, is frequently less severe, more easily treated, and results in less permanent disability. Myopathy in mixed connective tissue disease or scleroderma occasionally may be the predominant problem (Plotz et al., 1993). Childhood PM and DM may have distinct clinical and biopsy features, including the presence of inflammatory cells in a perivascular region and the development of cutaneous calcification (Ansell, 1991). (See volume 3, chapters 3 and 13, of this series for a discussion and case study of PM and DM in children.)

Inclusion Body Myositis

A treatment-resistant form of inflammatory myositis is inclusion body myositis (IBM) (Lotz, Engel, Nisnino, Stevens, & Litchy, 1989). This has recently been distinguished from the idiopathic variety because of its distinct histological feature of inclusion bodies within the myofibril cytoplasm seen on frozen section. Its presentation is different from that of idiopathic PM, and it occurs frequently in adult men who develop severe atrophy of the quadriceps muscles and forearms with more involvement of the distal musculature, less elevation of CK, a more insidious onset, and the presence of the inclusion body on biopsy. IBM is usually resistant to treatment and results in greater muscle atrophy and disability.

Drug-Induced Myopathy

When evaluating inflammatory muscle disease, it is always important to remember that drugs may cause weakness and myopathies. Drugs that are commonly responsible for myopathy include drugs that lower cholesterol, hydroxychloroquine, penicillamine, alcohol, corticosteroids, and zidovudine (AZT). The clinical and laboratory presentation will frequently be different for drug-induced myopathies. The biopsy will not usually show inflammatory changes, and the CK level is frequently not elevated. With corticosteroid myopathy, there is characteristic atrophy of type II fibers. The dystrophies (e.g., Duchenne's muscular dystrophy) will have a family history of weakness (particularly gender linked) and the typical presentation for hereditary myopathy. Although not usually confused with idiopathic PM, Duchenne's dystrophy may have high elevations of CK.

Medical Treatment

The initial medical treatment of inflammatory muscle disease is the use of corticosteroids. Although there are no controlled clinical trials to demonstrate their effectiveness, clinical experience demonstrates a prompt response of the disease markers and symptoms to steroid treatment. In mild and moderate disease, corticosteroids and outpatient treatment may be all that is needed. With more severe disease, inpatient treatment, higher doses, and parenteral corticosteroids are indicated. For this latter group, an initial dose of prednisone, 1 to 2 mg/kg/day (at least 60 mg/day for a 130-lb. woman) is commonly administered for 6 to 12 weeks (Adams & Plotz, 1995). Medical progress is measured by a lowering of CK and aldolase and an improvement in muscle strength. Subsequently, the corticosteroid dosage is gradually reduced to the lowest dose that maintains a clinical remission of the myopathy. Corticosteroid treatment will result in favorable results in 75% of patients. With severe disease, there may be involvement of respiratory, swallowing, and cardiac musculature. When this occurs, acute hospitalization in an intensive care unit may be needed to prevent cardiorespiratory failure.

Despite the usual steroid response, some patients will require additional treatment because of an incomplete response or corticosteroid toxicity (Adams & Plotz, 1995). In these patients, the use of azathioprine or methotrexate as a secondary treatment for myopathy is indicated, and a good response may occur. The addition of these drugs may permit use of a lower dose of steroids with less drug toxicity. Other treatments such as cyclophosphamide and plasmapheresis have been tried with a lack of a uniform response. More recently, the use of cyclosporin A and high-dose intravenous gammaglobulin has been popular (Villalba & Adams, 1996). Uncontrolled trials have shown that these drugs elicited a response in steroid-resistant cases, but high drug toxicity and high cost have limited their use.

Drug treatment of resistant PM and DM requires further study. IBM has a high incidence of treatment failure and occurs in a group of patients in which there is an additional need for new treatments. If the medical treatment of inflammatory muscle disease is successful, hospitalization and rehabilitation are not needed. However, for a small group of patients, rehabilitation becomes a major portion of their treatment program.

Corticosteroid side effects occur with high frequency and are the same as seen with other conditions. Side effects include hypertension, diabetes, weight gain, truncal obesity, moon facies, impaired wound healing, acne, hirsutism, cutaneous striae, thin friable skin, adrenal insufficiency, sodium retention, cataracts, osteoporosis, osteonecrosis, alteration in mood and behavior, euphoria, impaired sleep, and an increased risk of infection. Dose and duration of drug treatment are closely related to side effects. It is important that the minimally effective dose be used for the shortest possible time to avoid serious complications. If it is not possible to reduce the corticosteroid dose, then drug management for side effects is initiated.

Bone loss occurs in all patients who take more than 7.5 mg of prednisone daily for long periods. In elderly persons and those with risk factors, osteoporosis with fractures can occur. Treatment is indicated to prevent osteoporosis and includes adequate calcium and vitamin D intake, exercise, and hormone replacement therapy as indicated. Exercise may not be practical in this group of patients because they exhibit muscle weakness with increased fatigue and decreased endurance. Use of calcitonin and the bisphosphonates (e.g., alendronate) may be indicated in patients who have low bone mass and an increased risk of fractures.

Rehabilitation: Philosophy of Care

The rehabilitation program described herein was developed at Rancho Los Amigos National Rehabilitation Center, a rehabilitation center for the County of Los Angeles, CA. Patients are medically stabilized in an acute care hospital before referral to Rancho Los Amigos, where they are treated in the rheumatology unit until discharge to outpatient treatment.

Early symptoms of PM involve muscle weakness that may or may not progress. Because of the complex nature of disease-related problems faced by patients, frequent monitoring is necessary for both disease activity through clinical and laboratory findings and for patient activity by a team of professionals that may include a rheumatologist, an occupational therapist, a physical therapist, a social worker, and a psychologist. This team's continuous monitoring of the effects of the disease allows optimizing each patient's function throughout the disease course. The goals of the rehabilitation process are to optimize function, maximize mobility, protect weak muscles, and increase muscle strength with careful laboratory and clinical monitoring.

Occupational Therapy and Physical Therapy Evaluation

There are three parts to the comprehensive evaluation.

1. Occupational history
2. Musculoskeletal status
3. Functional status

Each of these areas will be described with an emphasis on the unique issues of the person with PM or DM.

Occupational History

Preonset. The patient's participation in home, work, or other community activities before onset of the disease will influence functional goal setting. A semistructured interview is used to find out what a typical day's activities involved for the patient. The information gathered will provide data on activities that are important to the patient and will be used to construct the treatment program.

Postonset. It is important to obtain information not only about the patient's typical daily activity level preadmission but also postonset if he or she has been admitted from home or another facility. During this interview, further evaluation of the patient's willingness to participate in a rehabilitation program is evaluated. The patient's description of how he or she functioned before admission may reveal that the patient or family members have under- or overestimated the patient's abilities. In this disease, where the course is unpredictable, lack of family member or patient understanding can lead to unrealistic expectations.

Musculoskeletal Status

Passive range of motion (ROM) evaluation is done to ensure that no loss of motion has occurred since the onset of disease. Joint pathology is not a typical manifestation of the disease. However, if notable weakness is present for a prolonged period, joint restrictions and tendon shortening may ensue.

Individual muscle testing is administered through the use of manual muscle or computerized testing (e.g., Cybex [Henley Health Care, Sugar Land, TX], Lido [Loredan Biomedical, West Sacramento, CA]) to find the level and distribution of weakness (Rancho Los Amigos Medical Center, 1978). The results of the testing provide baseline information that is necessary in monitoring the effects of the rehabilitation program.

Test grades and the presence of some tenderness in muscles or tendons are documented because both will guide the patient's rehabilitation program. In addition, grasp and pinch dynamometer strength testing is sensitive to subtle changes for muscles greater than grade 4 in the hand and allows comparison with norms in the general population (Mathiowetz, 1990). This strength information may be especially important for someone returning to competitive work or full-time homemaking.

Dysphagia and Respiratory Evaluation

Dysphagia reportedly occurs in 10% to 15% of persons with inflammatory muscle disease (Vencousky et al., 1988). If dysphagia is suspected, it is important to obtain a swallowing videofluoroscopy to determine the severity of the problem and its cause. In most cases, dysphagia occurs due to decreased strength of the pharyngeal musculature, tongue weakness, and disordered mobility of the esophagus (Kagen, Hochman, & Strong, 1985; Vencousky et al., 1988). Ventilatory insufficiency may occur due to diaphragmatic or intercostal muscle weakness. An evaluation of the person's pulmonary function will give the examiner important information about ventilatory ability.

Functional Status

Activities typically evaluated include sitting from supine, standing from sitting, ambulation, stair climbing, standing from the ground, and all personal care activities (e.g., feeding, dressing, toileting, and bathing). Observation of function confirms how weakness affects effort and ability to perform tasks. With the severely involved patient with PM, initial observation of function may be limited to activities in bed. This may include rolling side to side, feeding, hygiene, and grooming.

Initial and Ongoing Evaluation

The patient's musculoskeletal status, level of function, and occupational history will determine program goals. Additional behavioral factors are more elusive and equally important. The patient and family members' understanding of the condition will affect goal setting and active participation in the program. For example, if the patient believes that he or she will return to normal function soon, he or she may want to wait for full spontaneous recovery and may not be an active participant in establishing and working toward lesser functional goals that require the use of adaptive methods. Initial rehabilitation goals are determined from team members' reports on current medical, musculoskeletal, functional, and psychosocial status. These initial goals can be modified during the rehabilitation period as the patient's disease or the patient's adaptation to the disability changes. The length of the rehabilitation program depends on the patient's response to all therapies. During the acute phase of the disease, when response to medications could change the course of the disease, the following evaluations are done weekly: muscle testing of all key upper- and lower-extremity muscle groups, grasp and pinch measurements, evaluation of function, and the patient's subjective report of changes.

Program modifications to reduce stress on the muscles are indicated in the presence of any of the following: signs or subjective complaints of fatigue and weakness, muscle tenderness, loss of strength, and decreased function. An elevated but stable CK level without the presence of muscle tenderness, fatigue, and increased weakness is not typically an indicator to decrease a strengthening or functional training program.

Functional Approach to Therapy Management

Management of Weakness

Muscle test score implications. A symmetrical pattern of proximal weakness with greater strength distally in both upper and lower extremities is typical, but in some cases, distal strength can be diminished. Grades of 3+ or less on a 5-point scale are of special concern to the therapist. According to Beasley (1961), a muscle grade of 4 may indicate a 60% loss of normal muscle strength. Therefore, muscle strength grades of 4 or less on a 5-point scale are of special concern because this indicates a limitation on the consistent ability to perform daily self-care and repetitive or sustained activities such as those in the work and home environments.

Strengthening indications. Historically, active exercise in persons with inflammatory muscle disease was considered contraindicated because of the fear of aggravating the muscle inflammation. Data to support this supposition are scant. Recent studies have in fact shown that resistive exercise as part of a person's rehabilitation program resulted in increased muscle strength without a sustained rise in CK levels (Escalante, Miller, & Beardmore, 1993; Hicks, Miller, Plotz, Chen, & Gerber, 1993). These findings indicate that a carefully monitored resistive exercise program is an important aspect of the rehabilitation program.

Strengthening methods. The intensity of the program should reflect the person's strength (i.e., the weaker the muscle, the lower the intensity of the resistive exercise). For example, a grade 1 muscle group would receive active assisted ROM and isometric exercise, and a grade 2 muscle group would receive exercise in a gravity-eliminated position with increasing resistance. Muscle groups with strength grades of 3, 4, and 5 would benefit from exercise against gravity with resistance increased commensurate with the ability of the particular muscle group. The exercise program must be closely monitored and the intensity decreased if the person experiences muscle pain within 24 hr after the exercise or if loss of strength in a muscle group is detected.

Compensatory techniques. On admission to the occupational therapy and physical therapy program, patients are immediately placed in a functional program appropriate to their level of weakness. Assistive devices and specialized methods to perform tasks are instituted to enable patients to recognize that function is possible despite weakness. Patients are carefully monitored during this time to ensure that overuse problems do not occur.

Weak muscles may need to be protected while CK levels are increasing. Muscle grades below 2 can be protected with the use of orthoses to rest these muscles while allowing muscles of grade 3 or better to perform tasks. Other devices can be used to prevent grade 2 muscles from resistive activities while accomplishing functional tasks, such as devices for upper-extremity use (e.g., lightweight eating utensils, button hooks, loose-fitted clothing, mobile arm supports to protect weak scapular or shoulder muscles while eating, and performing light hygiene and desk activities) (Yasuda, Bowman, & Hsu, 1986) and devices for trunk, neck, and lower-extremity use (e.g., orthoses, reclining wheelchairs, cervical collars, trunk supports, ambulation aides, and elevated toilet and bath seats).

Management of Contractures

Contracture management is an important aspect of the rehabilitation program. Muscle weakness and limited mobility, if not counteracted with stretching and positioning, can easily result in loss of joint motion that can severely affect the person's ultimate functional outcome.

If the patient is treated early in the disease process, limitations in ROM may be averted because strength may be sufficient to allow active movement throughout the range. However, when strength is diminished to the extent that the patient cannot move through full normal ROM, limitations may ensue. Motions commonly at risk are shoulder flexion, abduction, and external rotation; elbow extension; finger flexion; hip and knee extension; and ankle dorsiflexion. Limitations are most often due to muscle weakness, muscle soreness (noted by pain when a muscle is stretched passively), and tendon shortening from positioning. Depending on the muscle grades, passive, active assisted, or active ROM is done daily. Pillows can be strategically placed in the following positions to prevent some common contracture problems when severe weakness exists: shoulders in external rotation and abduction to 90° in alternate periods and elbows alternately in flexion and full extension when in bed. Foot boards or ankle supports are used to place ankles in a neutral position, and patients can be encouraged to lie in a prone position to maintain or increase hip and knee extension range. With the more common upper-extremity problems seen with severely involved patients, the following orthoses are used: anterior elbow shells made of plaster or low-temperature thermoplastic material (for limited elbow extension); static wrist orthoses in functional extension (for limited wrist extension); and static wrist–hand platform orthoses in maximum wrist–hand extension (for finger flexor tendon shortening) (Hunter, Mackin, & Callahan, 1995). These orthoses are generally worn while in bed or whenever the patient is at rest.

Management of Dysphagia

If dysphagia is due to weakness, a soft diet is instituted, and patients are instructed to sit as erect as possible while eating, to eat slowly, and to alternate food with liquid. Instructions are given for the patient to remain in a sitting posture for at least 1 hr after a meal.

Cricopharyngeal achalasia (Kagen et al., 1985; Vencousky et al., 1988) is another less common cause of dysphagia. The cricopharyngeal muscle can become inflamed, swollen, and fibrotic due to the disease process (Darrow, Hoffman, Barnes, & Wiley, 1992; Dietz, Logeman, Sahgal, & Schmid, 1980; Vencousky et al., 1988). When this occurs, the opening to the esophagus is greatly decreased, and the food bolus is unable to pass below the level of the muscle. It is important to understand and identify this disorder because of the great potential for aspiration of contents into the airways that may cause asphyxiation, pulmonary infection, and damage to the bronchial tissue. Cricopharyngeal achalasia (diagnosed by videofluoroscopy) usually requires surgical intervention (Darrow et al., 1992; Dietz et al., 1980; Vencousky et al., 1988).

Management of Respiratory Problems

If ventilatory muscle weakness is identified, a diaphragm strengthening program consisting of inspiratory training or diaphragm weights is indicated (Sobush & Dunning, 1985). To optimize working conditions for the diaphragm, a binder can be applied around the person's abdominal region. In the presence of weak abdominal muscles, the patient may have difficulty producing a functional cough. Instruction on how to perform a manual assisted cough is important in helping the patient prevent aspiration of foods and liquids (Rancho Los Amigos Medical Center, 1980).

Endurance Training

Many of the patients who are diagnosed with inflammatory muscle disease have been inactive secondary to prolonged bedrest. Submaximal muscle training and activity programs should be instituted immediately to reverse the deconditioning that may have occurred during this period (Muller, 1970). Any respiratory insufficiency alerts the therapist to potential problems in endurance beyond those related to trunk and extremity weakness. This should be considered when patients report fatigue problems from the activity programs.

Management of Functional Problems

Functional training for mobility (e.g., rolling, sitting from supine, standing from sitting, transferring, wheelchair propulsion, and walking) progresses as the person's strength improves. With severe weakness and the inability to roll side to side and to sit independently, an electric bed is indicated that is adapted for the person to operate. The inability to stand or walk will necessitate a motorized wheelchair for independent mobility. Mobile arm supports can be attached to the chair to assist weak shoulder muscles and facilitate driving (Wilson, McKenzie, Barber, & Watson, 1984). Providing access to mobility as early as possible will help to give the person a sense of control and independence and thereby decrease fear and apprehension. As trunk and extremity strength improves, the person can be progressed to a manual wheelchair that can be propelled with lower extremities. (*Note.* If upper extremities have sufficient strength, they can assist.) When the patient is able to stand from a sitting position with minimal assistance, gait training can begin. Hip strength at this point may be between grades 2 and 3, and the person will exhibit a wide-based gait with a bilateral, lateral trunk lean (the trunk will deviate laterally over each stance limb) to compensate for hip abductor weakness and a posterior trunk lean to compensate for weak hip extensors. Patients at this level will require the use of a walker. As their muscle strength improves and their gait deviations lessen, they can progress to using crutches and eventually a cane. It is important that upper-extremity aids be used as long as gait deviations due to weak hip muscles are observed.

Assistive Equipment and Adaptive Methods

The following methods and equipment describe how daily routine tasks can be accomplished by patients with severe weakness and by those whose weakness and endurance improve.

When the patient is partially reclined in bed, the following can enable function.

- Feeding with suspension arm supports (attached to an over-bed frame) and built-up handled utensils, lightweight cups, and long straws (Figure 2)
- Managing a call buzzer by stabilizing the device within reach of weak proximal muscles
- Managing reading materials with a reading stand and a rubber-tipped stick to turn pages if necessary for weak hands
- Combing or brushing hair with a long-handled comb or brush and suspension arm supports
- Washing the face, hands, and upper body with a long-handled sponge (and a small sponge to prevent the need for wringing), a wash basin, an over-bed stand, and a small washcloth for drying
- Dressing sticks to allow for reaching distant items on an over-bed stand
- Participating in leisure activities with an over-bed stand (e.g., a card rack for playing cards, built-up handled writing or drawing implements, or spring-wire scissors to open small packages or letters or to open sugar and salt packets for hospital meals); large reading racks

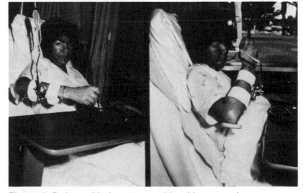

Figure 2. Patient with dermatomyositis with suspension arm supports attached to an over-bed frame to allow functional activities while still confined to bed most of the time. Reprinted from the ARHP Arthritis Teaching Slide Collection. Used with permission of the American College of Rheumatology.

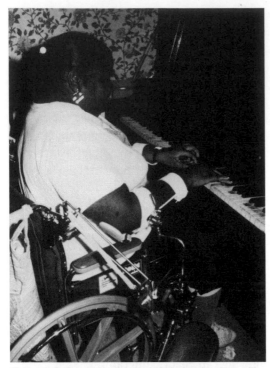

Figure 3. Patient with polymyositis playing the piano with bilateral mobile arm supports. *Note:* From "Occupational therapy management of a patient with severe polymyositis," by L. D. Deshaies, Y. L. Yasuda, and T. Beardmore, 1994, *Arthritis Care and Research, 7,* pp. 104–107. ©1994 American College of Rheumatology. Reprinted with permission.

make it possible to do picture puzzles or paint with suspension arm supports

When the patient is sitting reclined or upright in a wheelchair, the following can enable function.

- Mobile arm supports attached to the wheelchair to accomplish table-top activities similar to those in bed. The mobile arm support can be adjusted to operate the controls on a motorized wheelchair (Figure 3).

- A wheelchair lap board allows tabletop activities such as eating with mobile arm supports.

- A custom cut-out in the lap board is made for motorized wheelchair controls. Light home skills such as preparing meals can now be done. Additional equipment that may be needed for this includes a special cutting board with spikes to hold objects, serrated knives for easy cutting, and reachers to obtain objects from refrigerators, low cupboards, counter surfaces, and the floor.

- Dressing stick or reachers stored behind a wheelchair can assist with activities such as pulling open cupboard doors or opening drawers. The dressing stick can be used as a knob turner for some stove knobs.

- Lap boards are handy to transport meal items while in the wheelchair.

Progression of bed activities (with improved endurance, bed mobility, and hand strength) can be aided by the following.

Dressing. Dressing can be accomplished with the use of the following: a dressing stick to get clothing over shoulders or legs, button hooks to accomplish buttoning with weak hands, loose clothing with no back fasteners and with easy fasteners such as zippers or Velcro® closures, pants without fasteners (elasticized waists), front-closing bras, a sock aid to don socks or pantyhose, a reacher to obtain clothing in drawers, bed rails to roll side to side, an electric bed to sit with the assistance of motorized head raising, Velcro® closures on shoes, and a long-handled shoe horn to put on shoes.

Toileting (use of a bedpan in bed). Generally, if a patient is unable to sit upright, weakness of the trunk and extremities do not allow independent toileting in bed because this activity is generally too difficult, especially manipulating the bedpan. If a patient wants to perform perineal care, a long-handled toilet wiper (commercially available or a custom-made adaptation) is provided with hygienic cautions.

Complete bed bath. Generally, if the patient is unable to be upright, weakness of trunk and extremities does not allow thorough cleansing of the entire body. The patient may be able to clean the face, hands, anterior portion of upper body, and the perineum. If the patient wants to perform a complete bed bath without producing undue fatigue, muscle tenderness, and overuse problems, the following equipment may be provided: a reacher to dry the lower body, a wire toe washer with a terry cloth mitt (to wash between toes), and an extended washcloth to reach the bottoms of the feet and the back.

Bathing or showering in the bathroom (when sitting balance improves). The following equipment may be needed: bath bench and transfer board (e.g., "sliding board"), grab rails, and similar washing and drying equipment as used in bed. Simulation of the patient's home bathroom (including similar dimensions and furniture arrangement) is used to determine the techniques for bathing or showering.

Home and Community Activities

The following are examples of equipment that may be needed to perform activities in a wheelchair or when ambulatory.

Meal preparation. A lap board can be used in a wheelchair for easier cutting and stirring; a tray on the walker makes carrying items possible; for a person who can walk without ambulatory aides, a rolling cart prevents unnecessary trips, or an apron with pockets and a plastic waist band (to avoid the need for two hands to tie bows) can be used to transport small items; leather hoops on upper cupboard doors aid in reaching for both wheelchair and ambulatory patients; and reachers help to obtain items from upper cupboards or floor and can be used to open and close oven doors.

Laundry. A hamper on wheels for the ambulating person reduces the strain of carrying heavy loads.

Household cleaning for ambulatory patients. A long-handled sponge makes cleaning the bathtub easier, and a long-handled dustpan eliminates the need to squat or kneel. Special mops with a remote device to remove water from the mop head and a water bucket caddy on wheels limit sustained resistive upper-extremity work.

Increasing Daily Activities

When the patient gains muscle strength of grades 3+ to 4 throughout the trunk and extremities, the number of daily activities and the effort required to complete them can be increased using the following methods.

- Adapted equipment may be discarded at this time.
- Energy conservation and pacing techniques that have been taught throughout the rehabilitation process are reemphasized.
- Patients are instructed to monitor fatigue and note any increased weakness or muscle tenderness and to decrease activities accordingly.
- Examples of activities include shopping at the mall or grocery store or going to a restaurant.

Box 1
Resources

Organization Resources

Myositis Association of America
1420 Huron Court
Harrisonburg, VA 22801
540-433-1686 or 540-432-0206 (fax)
Internet address: www.myositis.org

This organization offers a newsletter, on-line consumer education, research updates, national conferences, and awareness programs.

The Arthritis Foundation
1330 West Peachtree Street
Atlanta, GA 30309
404-872-7100 or 1-800-283-7800
Internet address: www.arthritis.org

This organization provides an excellent booklet on PM and DM and on specific medications at no charge and aquatic and land-based exercise classes nationwide.

Muscular Dystrophy Association
National Headquarters
3300 East Sunrise Drive
Tucson, AZ 85718
1-800-572-1717
Internet address: www.mdausa.org

This organization offers extensive patient education and support services and is an excellent resource on adaptive technology.

National Support Group for Myositis
P.O. Box 890
Cooperstown, NY 14426
1-800-230-0441

National Support Group for Dermatomyositis
1119 Spring Garden Street
Bethlehem, PA 18017
215-974-9832

Myositis Support Group
Arthritis Foundation
1777 Reisterstown Road
 Suite 150
Baltimore, MD 21208
410-363-3345
e-mail: murphylm@aol.com

Dermatomyositis and Polymyositis Support Group
146 Newtown Road
Woolston, Southhampton SO2 9HR
England
Southhampton 449708

(continued)

Preparation for Discharge From Ongoing Therapy Programs

A home visit may be indicated to ensure that there are no environmental barriers affecting performance at home. This is especially important when there is major residual weakness necessitating the use of a motorized wheelchair. If the patient plans to return to work, a worksite visit may be indicated to ensure that the environment is appropriate to the available strength and endurance of the patient. Job modifications may need to be made or adapted equipment designed. Referrals to community resources, such as state agencies that provide vocational retraining or an occupational therapy driver education program for evaluation of driving from a wheelchair, may be made. Because this is a chronic disease with unpredictable exacerbations and remissions, patients must be routinely monitored by health care professionals knowledgeable in PM and DM.

Box 1 (continued)

The Arthritis Society
National Office
250 Bloor Street East, Suite 901
Toronto, ON M4W 3P2 Canada
416-967-1414 or 416-967-7171 (fax)
Internet address: www.arthritis.ca

This group offers specialized patient care programs, recreational exercise programs, resource libraries, aid in the establishment self-help groups, and consumer education material.

Internet Resources

- Myositis/Polymyositis (Sharon's Home Page): A personal web site that can link you with all other resources on these diseases and explores the causes, symptoms, treatments, research, and personal stories (www.myositis.com/index.html).
- A search for "polymyositis" on www.hotbot.com will link you to all web sites related to PM and DM.
- The Amazon Bookstore (www.amazon.com) lists all the books published on PM and DM.
- Abledata (www.abledata.com) is a national database for adaptive equipment and assistive devices

Case Study

There is little documentation in the literature regarding the rehabilitation of patients with severe PM. In an unpublished review of a 5-year period at Rancho Los Amigos National Rehabilitation Center, an average of 4 very severely involved patients with PM and DM were admitted per year, for a total of 20 patients over 5 years. None of these patients obtained complete muscle recovery during their hospital stay, which averaged approximately 11 weeks and ranged from 5 to 20 weeks. In fact, most had severe residual muscle weakness. However, the functional level of all of the patients increased. The level of independence that these patients achieved and their desire to maintain the functional gains after discharge testify to the need for rehabilitation programs for these patients.

The purpose of the following case is to illustrate the process through which a patient on an intensive rehabilitation program achieved functional improvement despite persistent muscle weakness (Deshaies, Yasuda, & Beardmore, 1994). The program was based on the rehabilitation team's close monitoring of the patient's medications, muscle enzyme level, muscle strength, and fatigue.

L.D. is an African-American woman 24 years of age who, before onset, was working part-time as a piano teacher at a local music studio, and teaching private piano students in her home, and attending school. Her career goals were to complete a baccalaureate degree in music and to earn the teaching credentials required to become a middle school music teacher.

L.D. was in good health up to the time that she experienced muscle pain that lasted for 4 days but resolved spontaneously. One month later, a second episode of progressive muscle pain and increasing weakness revealed a CK level of 35,000 mU/ml. Her condition continued to worsen, and, 2 months later, the diagnosis of PM was made. Treatment with prednisone and methotrexate was initiated. Despite a decrease in her CK level to 10,000 mU/ml, muscle weakness progressed.

L.D. was at home essentially confined to her bed at this time with a sitting tolerance of less than two hours. Two family members were needed to transfer her in and out of bed. She was able to feed herself once food was cut for her and to perform light hygiene once items were brought to her, but she was dependent in all bathing, dressing, and toileting tasks.

In this disabled state, L.D. was admitted to our rehabilitation center 5 months after the diagnosis was made. She had a CK level of 9,171 mU/ml. Her muscle strength at initial evaluation was in the 2–to 2 range (poor-minus to poor range) throughout the trunk, hips, and shoulder girdle. Distal musculature was in the 3 to 3+ range (fair to fair-plus range). Grip strength measured 15 lbs. bilaterally. Functional status was further compromised by her body weight of 250 lbs. Passive ROM was within normal limits, and no muscle tenderness or sensory or respiratory deficits were noted.

With L.D.'s severe muscle involvement, initial goals were limited to independence in motorized wheelchair mobility, feeding, hygiene, grooming, and the vocational skill of playing the piano.

In the first month of rehabilitation, L.D. was fitted with mobile arm supports that allowed use of her upper extremities despite her weak shoulders (Yasuda, Bowman, & Hsu, 1986). After the initial training, a daily program consisting of carefully selected and graded activities was initiated. The activities, beginning with tabletop tasks and progressing to those requiring upper-extremity elevation, were increased as L.D.'s endurance slowly improved. With equipment, she was able to manage her own hair care and makeup. She began playing a light-touch electronic keyboard placed at lap height.

With her limited active shoulder and hip motions, she was trained in the use of equipment with extended handles for lower-body bathing and dressing. After 1 week of practice, she was able to complete all dressing tasks, although not within a practical amount of time. After 3 months, L.D. decreased the time required for bathing and dressing from the original 90 min to 30 min.

By the fifth week, L.D.'s transfer status progressed from the use of a mechanical lift to independent sliding board transfers. Given this increased mobility and the long-handled equipment previously issued, she was able to shower independently by the end of the second month. She was issued a motorized wheelchair that allowed independence in mobility, and she was trained in home skills such as laundry and meal preparation.

She was now able to play a standard piano with the aid of her mobile arm supports (Figure 3). She found that the supports enabled her to reach areas of the keyboard that were otherwise inaccessible, and her playing endurance increased from 5 min to more than 1 hr.

In the third month, community reintegration activities from a wheelchair were initiated with an outing to a small, local supermarket. A preliminary visit to L.D.'s home was made by an occupational therapist and physical therapist to evaluate the architectural environment. Recommendations were made to allow accessibility in the home for L.D.

In the fourth month, community reintegration activities included a visit to the music studio where L.D. was hoping to return to work as a piano teacher. With minor modifications that her employer was willing to make for wheelchair accessibility, it was believed L.D. would be able to manage in her work setting with relative ease. A second home visit was made with L.D., her family members, and friends, who were given final training and education regarding L.D.'s abilities, limitations, and equipment.

When L.D. was discharged to her home, her CK level was still elevated but stable at 4,000 mU/ml; she continued on medications. Proximal musculature remained in grade 2-to 2 range, but the distal musculature had improved to 3+ to 4. Her grip strength had improved from 15 to 20 lbs., which was still greatly below the norm for her age (Mathiowetz, 1990).

Two weeks after discharge from the hospital, she returned to work 2 days a week at the music studio and resumed instructing private students in her home. L.D. has been followed regularly in our outpatient clinic to monitor her medications, muscle strength, and functional status. Several years after discharge, she continues to teach piano at least 30 hr a week from a motorized wheelchair.

Conclusion

Persons with PM and DM need a comprehensive rehabilitation program that addresses the distinct nature of muscle weakness that accompanies this condition. Clinicians have few documented guidelines for this population regarding when active use of weakened muscles should be decreased or halted and when to safely resume and progress activity (Deshaies et al., 1994; Feallock, 1965; Hicks, 1988; Melvin, 1989). Our experience with this population has shown us that a planned rehabilitation approach that enables function within the parameters of the disease process is the hallmark for enabling persons to participate in meaningful daily activities in the community throughout the course of the disease.

References

Adams, E. M., & Plotz, P. H. (1995). The treatment of myositis. *Rheumatic Disease Clinics of North America, 21,* 179–202.

Ansell, B. (1991). Juvenile dermatomyositis. *Journal of Rheumatology, 17,* 931–942.

Beasley, W. C. (1961). Quantitative muscle testing: Principles and applications to research and clinical services. *Archives of Physical Medicine and Rehabilitation, 2,* 398–417.

Darrow, D. H., Hoffman, H. T., Barnes, G. J., & Wiley, C. A. (1992). Management of dysphagia in inclusion body myositis. *Archives of Otolaryngology, Head and Neck Surgery, 118,* 313–317.

Deshaies, L. D., Yasuda, Y. L., & Beardmore, T. (1994). Occupational therapy management of a patient with severe polymyositis. *Arthritis Care and Research, 7,* 104–107.

Dietz, F., Logeman, J. A., Sahgal, V., & Schmid, F. R. (1980). Cricopharyngeal muscle dysfunction in polymyositis. *Arthritis and Rheumatism, 23,* 491–495.

Escalante, A., Miller, L., & Beardmore, T. D. (1993). Resistive exercise in the rehabilitation of polymyositis/dermatomyositis. *Journal of Rheumatology, 20,* 1340–1344.

Feallock, B. (1965). Dermatomyositis: case study. *American Journal of Occupational Therapy, 19,* 279–280.

Fraser, D. D., Frank, J. A., Dalakas, M., Miller, F. W., Hicks, J. E., & Plotz, P. (1991). Magnetic resonance imaging in the idiopathic inflammatory myopathies. *Journal of Rheumatology, 18,* 1693–1700.

Hicks, J. E. (1988). Comprehensive rehabilitative management of patients with polymyositis and dermatomyositis. In M. C. Dalakas (Ed.), *Polymyositis and dermatomyositis* (pp. 293–317). Stoneham, MA: Butterworth.

Hicks, J. E., Miller, F., Plotz, P., Chen, T., & Gerber, L. (1993). Isometric exercise increases strength and does not produce sustained creatine phosphokinase increases in a patient with polymyositis. *Journal of Rheumatology, 20,* 1399–1401.

Hunter, J. M., Mackin, D. J., & Callahan, A. D. (Eds.). (1995). *Rehabilitation of the hand* (4th ed., p. 1089). St. Louis: Mosby-Year Book.

Kagen, L. J., Hochman, R. B., & Strong, E. W. (1985). Cricopharyngeal obstruction in inflammatory myopathy (polymyositis/dermatomyositis): Report of three cases and review of the literature. *Arthritis and Rheumatism, 28,* 630–636.

Lotz, B. P., Engel, A. G., Nishino, H., Stevens, J. C., & Litchy, W. J. (1989). Inclusion body myositis. *Brain 112*(Part 3), 727–747.

Mathiowetz, V. (1990). Grip and pinch strength measurements. In L. R. Amundsen (Ed.), *Muscle strength testing* (pp. 163–177). New York: Churchill Livingstone.

Maugars, Y. M., Berthelot, J. M., Abbas, A. A., Mussini, J. M., Nguyen, J. M., & Prost, A. M. (1996). Long-term prognosis of 69 patients with dermatomyositis or polymyositis. *Clinical and Experimental Rheumatology, 14*(3), 263–274.

Medsger, T. A., Jr., Dawson, W. N., Jr., & Masi, A. T. (1970). The epidemiology of polymyositis. *American Journal of Medicine, 48,* 715–723.

Melvin, J. E. (1989). *Rheumatic disease in the adult and child: Occupational therapy and rehabilitation* (3rd ed.). Philadelphia: F. A. Davis.

Miller, F. W. (1997). Inflammatory myopathies: Polymyositis, dermatomyositis and related conditions. In W. J. Koopman (Ed.), *Arthritis and related conditions* (pp. 407–431). Baltimore: Williams & Wilkins.

Muller, E. A. (1970). Influence of training and of inactivity on muscle strength. *Archives of Physical Medicine and Rehabilitation, 51,* 449–462.

Oddis, C. V., Conte, C. G., Steen, V. D., & Medsger, T. A., Jr. (1990). Incidence of polymyositis-dermatomyositis: A 20-year study of hospital diagnosed cases in Allegheny County, PA 1963–1982. *Journal of Rheumatology, 17,* 1329–1334.

Plotz, P. H., Leff, R. L., & Miller, F. W. (1993). Inflammatory and metabolic myopathies. In H. R. Shumacher, Jr., J. H. Klippel, & W. J. Koopman (Eds.), *Primer on rheumatic diseases* (10th ed., pp. 127–131). Atlanta, GA: The Arthritis Foundation.

Rancho Los Amigos Hospital. (1978). *Guide for muscle testing of the upper extremity.* Downey, CA: Professional Staff Association of Rancho Los Amigos Hospital.

Rancho Los Amigos Medical Center. (1980). *Guideline for manual cough.* Downey, CA: Los Amigos Research and Education Institute.

Sigurgeirsson, B., Lindelof, B., Edhag, O., & Allander, E. (1992). Risk of cancer in patients with dermatomyositis or polymyositis: a population-based study. *New England Journal of Medicine, 326,* 363–367.

Sobush, D. C., & Dunning, M. (1985). Providing resistive breathing exercise to the inspiratory muscles using the pflex device. *Physical Therapy, 66*(4), 542–544.

Tanimoto, K., Nakano, K., Kano, S., Mori, S., Ueki, H., Nishitani, H., Sato, T., Kiuchi, T., & Ohashi, Y. (1995). Classification criteria for dermatomyositis and polymyositis. *Journal of Rheumatology, 22,* 668–674.

Van Rossum, M. A., Hiemstra, I., Prieur, A. M., Rijkers, G. T., & Kuis, W. (1994). Juvenile dermato/polymyositis: A retrospective analysis of 33 cases with special focus on initial CPK levels. *Clinical and Experimental Rheumatology, 12*(3), 339–342.

Vencousky, J., Rehak, F., Pafko, P., Jirasek, A., Valesova, M., Alusik, S., & Trnavsky, K. (1988). Acute cricopharyngeal obstruction in dermatomyositis. *Journal of Rheumatology, 15*(6), 1016–1018.

Villalba, L., & Adams, E. M. (1996). Update on therapy for refractory dermatomyositis and polymyositis. *Current Opinion in Rheumatology, 8*(6), 544–551.

Wilson, D. J., McKenzie, M. W., Barber, L. M., & Watson, K. L. (1984). Orthotic equipment. In *Spinal cord injury: A treatment guide for occupational therapists* (rev. ed., pp. 62–82). Thorofare, NJ: Slack.

Wortmann, R. L. (1992). Inflammatory diseases of muscle. In W. Kelley, E. Harris, S. Ruddy, & C. Sledge (Eds.), *Textbook of rheumatology* (4th ed., pp. 1159–1188). Philadelphia: Saunders.

Yasuda, Y. L., Bowman, K., & Hsu, J. D. (1986). Mobile arm supports: Criteria for successful use in muscle disease patients. *Archives of Physical Medicine and Rehabilitation, 67,* 253–256.

13

LESS COMMON RHEUMATIC DISEASES

Ranjana Sood, MD, James S. Louie, MD, Jeanne L. Melvin, MS, OTR, FAOTA, and Mary Lou Galantino, PhD, PT

This chapter reviews six categories of less common rheumatic diseases. The first two, infectious arthritis and crystalline-induced diseases, present with a monoarticular or single peripheral joint and are among the most treatable forms of arthritis (Freed, Nies, Boyer, & Louie 1980). The third group of diseases includes the spondylarthropathies and variants of ankylosing spondylitis that include reactive arthritis (Reiter's syndrome) and enteropathic arthritis. This group presents with inflammation in the bursa and entheses (the sites of ligament and tendon attachment to bone) as well as in the joint and is caused by both infectious and genetic elements. A fourth group, vasculitis, presents with a range of symptoms from fatigue and fever to major organ damage and is diagnosed by histological confirmation of acute and chronic inflammation in blood vessels. These diseases are mediated by immune factors, including antigen–antibody complexes and cytokines. The fifth group, infiltrative diseases, includes sarcoidosis, cancer, hypertrophic osteoathropathy, and amyloidosis. Finally, palindromic rheumatism, a disorder of brief recurring attacks of inflammation, is discussed in a category by itself.

Because these less common diseases present so variably over time, the final diagnosis is often delayed, and the referring diagnosis may be incorrect. Thus, the observations of experienced therapists are important in confirming or revising the diagnosis and in monitoring the progress of therapy.

Infectious Arthritis

Bacterial Arthritis

Infectious arthritis occurs when bacteria spread to the synovium from distant sites via the blood stream or by extension from an adjacent infection of bone, soft tissue, or a prosthetic device (i.e., a joint implant). The incidence in the general population (5/100,000) increases in patients with arthritis (35/100,000) and those with joint prostheses (60/100,000). Twenty-five percent of persons presenting with monoarticular arthritis in emergency departments of public hospitals have positive cultures for an infectious organism (Freed et al., 1980; Kaandorp, Van Schaardenburg, Krijnen, Habbema, & Van de Laar, 1995). Although most bacterial infections involve a single joint, 20% affect more than one joint (Baker & Schumacher, 1993). Patients present with fever and shaking chills, and the affected joint is painful, tender to touch and movement, swollen, and occasionally erythematous. Because delays in diagnosis and treatment lead to severe joint damage and functional disability, acute bacterial infection in a joint continues to be a serious cause of morbidity and mortality despite the availability of new and more potent antibiotics.

Most cases of septic arthritis are caused by gonococcus or Gram-positive organisms such as *Staphylococcus* and *Streptococcus*. Gram-negative organisms such as *Pseudomonas* and *Salmonella* constitute about 10% of bacterial arthritis and occur in the elderly persons and persons with host defenses compromised by disease or drugs. These include persons with diabetes, alcoholism, intravenous drug use, and rheumatoid arthritis (RA), particularly those with skin infections of the feet. Only 5% of cases are caused by mixed aerobic and anaerobic organisms. Infections caused by mycobacteria and fungi are responsible for less than 5% of joint infections. Polymicrobial infections caused by more than one organism occur after penetrating trauma or surgery (Mahowald, 1993).

Neisseria gonorrhoeae infections are the most common form of bacterial arthritis, particularly in young sexually active persons. Disseminated gonococcal infections (DGI) have a distinctive clinical presentation. These patients present with a 1-week history of fever, shaking chills, multiple skin lesions (e.g., macules, papules, vesicles, or pustules on an erythematous base; hemorrhagic bullae; erythema multiforme; or vasculitis), fleeting migratory polyarthralgias, and tenosynovitis. Affected persons may have genitourinary symptoms affecting the urethra, cervix, or anus. The current treatment regimen for DGI is ceftriaxone, a third-generation cephalosporin antibiotic, for 7 days and daily needle aspiration of accumulated synovial fluid. For other bacterial infection, despite appropriate antibiotic therapy, surgical drainage or debridement of infected tissue may be required.

In the early acute stages, complete rest or splinting to immobilize the infected joint may moderate the pain, but as the inflammation and fluid resolve with antibiotic therapy, the joint can be ranged gently, first passively then actively, to avoid contractures. If the range of motion (ROM) remains compromised, the therapist should alert the physician for surgery because loculations of pus will retard healing. Although complete functional recovery of the infected joint is expected, poor outcomes are predicted in older patients with longstanding joint disease or infected synthetic joints (Kaandorp, Krijnen, Moens, Habbema, & Van Schaardenburg, 1997).

Viral Arthritis

Viral infections present with less typical presentations and are more difficult to diagnose. Initially, multiple joints are involved in migratory patterns. Because techniques to culture viruses are expensive and laborious, clinical diagnoses are confirmed by identifying specific serum antibodies from the serum of the infected person. The acute infection is detected by measurement of immunoglobulin M (IgM) viral antibody titers, which are replaced within weeks by IgG titers that indicate chronic infection. Often the transient rise in IgM titers cannot be captured by serum studies. In the future, DNA hybridization tests to find bacterial DNA by using the polymerase chain reaction (PCR) will identify infections in a more timely manner.

Viral arthritis caused by Parvovirus B19, hepatitis B, rubella, or Epstein-Barr viruses, presents with a skin rash that lasts several days, followed by flu-like symptoms that include arthralgias and fever. Frank arthritis occurs in a small proportion of patients and typically involves the peripheral joints (Ytterberg, 1997). Parvovirus B19 presents with a "slapped cheek" rash in children and a rheumatoid-like symmetrical polyarthritis that involves the metacarpophalangeal (MCP), proximal interphalangeal, knee, wrist, and ankle joints that persists for weeks to months (Gran, Johnsen, Mykebust, & Nordbo, 1995). Hepatitis B virus presents with a symmetrical, small-joint polyarthritis that resolves before the development of jaundice (Inman, 1982). The joint involvement of rubella virus is polyarticular and asymmetrical and resolves within 2 weeks, but recurrences are possible. Infection from Epstein-Barr virus usually results in a transient arthritis of large joints (Gutierrez et al., 1992).

Lyme disease is one of a few human infections caused by spirochetes. The other spirochetal diseases include syphilis, leptospirosis, and relapsing fever. Lyme disease presents clinically in three stages: early local, early disseminated, and late persistent (Coyle & Schutzer, 1991). Oligoarticular arthritis, particularly in the knees, may be present along with severe flu-like symptoms. Successful drug therapy of the late persistent form requires appropriate antibiotic therapy for weeks before any clinical response.

In the acute early stages of viral arthritis, rest and proper positioning are essential. Cold modalities may reduce muscle spasm. In the subacute stage, gentle ROM is initiated. Once the acute inflammation resolves, restoration to functional pain-free joint mobility is expected. The prognosis for joints infected by viruses is complete functional recovery.

Human Immunodeficiency Virus

HIV is a retrovirus that is the etiological agent for AIDS. As HIV infects and destroys the helper subset of T lymphocytes (CD4), the normal immunity and host defenses are lost, and the patient becomes more susceptible to other serious infections and tumors.

An estimated 1 million persons were infected with HIV in the United States in 1996. (Chaisson & Moore, 1996). Since the epidemic began, more than 500,000 people in the United States have been reported to have AIDS. At least 300,000 of them have died (Centers for Disease Control and Prevention, 1997). Over the last few years, there has been a 7% increase in the incidence of AIDS among heterosexual women, whereas the incidence among white men has decreased by 16%.

Notably, there has a drastic disproportionate increase of African-American and Hispanic persons with AIDS. These two groups now constitute 54% of all men and 76% of all women with AIDS in the United States (CDC, 1997). This concentration among groups that are relatively socioeconomically disadvantaged will have future societal implications.

Therapists will likely treat increasing numbers of patients with AIDS in the future (Furth, Maloof, Flynn, & Shea, 1988). Several publications have addressed the role of rehabilitation for HIV infection and AIDS (Levinson & O'Connell, 1991; O'Dell, Hubert, Lubeck, & O'Driscoll, 1996; Methaler & Cross, 1988; O'Dell & Dillon, 1993; O'Dell, Levinson, & Riggs, 1996). The authors suggested that patients will fall into two broad categories. First, there are persons with unrelated disability and incidental HIV infection. The second category, and the primary focus of this section, consists of persons with disabilities stemming from HIV disease, including opportunistic infections or complications from treatment of HIV infection.

HIV and arthritis. Many musculoskeletal complaints are associated with HIV infection (Calabrese, 1989, 1997, and 1998; McReynolds, 1996) (Table 1). Although intermittent arthralgias of large

Table 1. Rheumatic Disease Manifestations Associated With HIV Infection

Joints	Wasting myopathy
Arthralgias of large joints	FMS
Oligoarthritis of lower-extremity joints with or without enthesopathy	**Nerves**
	Peripheral neuropathy
Oligoarthritis with psoriatic-like rash	**Glands**
Polyarthritis (nonerosive in large joints)	Parotid gland enlargement that simulates Sjögren's syndrome
Infectious arthritis and osteomyelitis	
AVN	Sicca syndrome
Reiter's syndrome	**Blood Vessels**
Overlap of Reiter's syndrome and psoriatic arthritis	Vasculitis with peripheral nerve involvement (e.g., polyarteritis nodosa)
Muscles	
Myositis with muscle weakness and CPK elevations	
Myelopathy secondary to anti-HIV drugs	
Myalgias with positive antinuclear antibodies simulating SLE (lupus-like syndrome)	

Note: AVN=avascular necrosis, CPK=creatine phosphokinase, SLE=systemic lupus erythematosus, FMS=fibromyalgia syndrome.

joints occur in one third of HIV-infected persons, another group presents with a highly inflamed oligoarthritis, enthesitis of the lower extremities, and a psoriasis-like rash. This "painful articular syndrome" is most likely to be referred to therapy because the arthritis progresses rapidly to contracture, responds poorly to nonsteroidal anti-inflammatory drugs (NSAIDs), and only occasionally responds to intra-articular steroids. The incidence of psoriatic arthritis is much higher in HIV-infected persons with psoriasis (32%) compared with noninfected persons with psoriasis (5–10%) (Reveille, Connant, & Duvic, 1990). Patients with HIV may develop an overlap syndrome of psoriatic arthritis and Reiter's syndrome with characteristic skin lesions from both syndromes (Calabrese, 1997).

The first report of HIV infection that presented with the complete triad of arthritis, urethritis, and conjunctivitis of Reiter's syndrome described the effect of immunosuppressive drugs on persons with HIV (Winchester, Bernstein, & Fischer, 1987). When NSAIDs did not control the articular symptoms, immunosuppressive agents including methotrexate and azathioprine accelerated the patient's immunodeficiency and progression to AIDS (Winchester et al., 1987). Currently, intra-articular corticosteroid injections are helpful to control the inflammation within selected joints (Altman, Centeno, Mahal, & Bieloryll, 1994; Gutierrez et al., 1992). More recently, with the capability to monitor HIV viremia by measuring HIV-RNA levels, the immunosuppressive nature of methotrexate and azathioprine may be more carefully monitored.

Another subgroup of HIV-infected presents with muscle weakness and elevations of serum creatine phosphokinase (CPK) as an inflammatory myositis. (Rehabilitation for these patients follows the guidelines for polymyositis in chapter 12 in this volume.)

A final group presents with marked parotid gland enlargement that simulates Sjögren's syndrome (Espinoza et al., 1989). The CD8 lymphocytes that infiltrate and enlarge the parotid glands regress dramatically with steroid therapy. In the interim, associated sicca syndrome with dry eyes and mouth requires artificial tears and scrupulous oral hygiene (Couderc et al., 1987).

Various forms of vasculitis have been seen in 1% of persons with HIV (Berman et al., 1988; Kaye, 1989). Isolated peripheral nerve involvement and polyarteritis nodosa with vasculitis of medium-size vessels have been described (Calabrese, 1989). Avascular necrosis (AVN) of bone is another complication of HIV. Treatment for AVN is the same as for patients with systemic lupus erythematosus (SLE). (See chapter 8 in this volume.)

HIV and myopathies. Numerous cases of myopathy that are clinically indistinguishable from polymyositis and dermatomyositis must be differentiated from a myopathic syndrome induced by the antiviral drug zidovudine (AZT). If the myopathy is related to AZT, the patient is usually switched to another antiviral agent (Espinoza et al., 1989; Munoz-Fernandez et al., 1991). Between 15% and 40% of patients taking AZT develop elevated serum CPK, whereas a much smaller percentage develop clinical myositis with myalgia or weakness (Calabrese, 1989).

Therapists should be alert for complaints of proximal muscle pain and difficulty stepping up on curbs or raising arms overhead. Rehabilitation intervention includes ROM exercises and gentle progressive strengthening similar to the treatment described for steroid-induced polymyopathy seen in SLE. (See chapter 8 in this volume.) Any increase in pain, weakness, or elevated muscle enzymes may indicate that the rehabilitation program is too aggressive and must be progressed more slowly. (See chapter 12 in this volume.)

HIV and fibromyalgia. About a third of those infected with HIV meet the criteria for fibromyalgia syndrome (FMS) (Buskila, Gladman, Langevitz, Urowitz, & Smythe, 1990). This is not surprising because FMS symptoms can be triggered by any chronic condition that induces fatigue or disturbs sleep. Accordingly, the treatment for HIV-related FMS includes the same interventions recommended for primary FMS: fitness training, sleep retraining, stress management, cognitive-behavioral pain management, good nutrition, fatigue management training, and deep breathing (Bennett, 1996; Galantino, & McCormack, 1992; Melvin, 1989; O'Dell et al., 1996). (See chapter 6 in this volume.) Antidepressant and antianxiety medications to improve sleep and secondarily to decrease pain are the primary medications used (Goldenberg, 1988). Hypnotics or sleeping pills are avoided because they succeed only for a couple of weeks, create dependence, and produce a rebound phenomenon when discontinued.

Patients with HIV-related arthritis can be managed with a combination of appropriate medication and rehabilitation with a focus on enhancing functional outcomes. The prognostic importance of HIV viremia is now unequivocal. Serum HIV-RNA levels are known to correlate with immune status after acute HIV infection (Cunningham, Dwyer, & Dowton, 1993) and the clinical response to antiretroviral therapy (Piatak et al., 1993). More recently, a direct relationship between serum HIV viremia and clinical outcome in HIV-infected patients has been demonstrated (Mellors et al., 1996; O'Brien et al., 1996). Furthermore, measurement of serum HIV-RNA levels has become a routine component of the developmental efforts for new antiretroviral therapies (MacDougal, 1996). It is likely that control of the viremia will prevent many of the rheumatic syndromes associated with HIV infection. Clearly, because these rheumatic presentations represent one of the many complications of HIV disease, it will be important to coordinate care with all the members of the health care team.

Rehabilitation strategies for HIV-related arthritic conditions. Rheumatic diseases have long been treated with a rehabilitation approach. Only recently have the roles of the occupational therapist and physical therapist been incorporated as instrumental in the management of HIV-related arthritic disorders (McReynolds, 1995 and 1996). The rehabilitation specialist may be the first to detect rheumatologic problems in an HIV-infected person. Therefore, rheumatologic problems as described above are important to include in a rehabilitation evaluation.

For treatment of acute arthritis, it is essential to provide the joint with localized rest, proper positioning, and orthotic immobilization to prevent dysfunctional contractures. For noninfectious arthritis with acute inflammation, cold modalities are preferred versus heat (Haralson, 1988). Phonophoresis with hydrocortisone at 1.5 W/cm^2 has been reported in case studies to decrease joint pain and increase ROM in HIV-infected patients (Ziskin, McDiarmis, & Michlovitz, 1990).

After control of acute inflammation, gentle ROM is initiated to maintain mobility, and isometric exercises can be added to maintain strength. *Therapists should observe appropriate body fluid precautions in the presence of HIV, especially when associated wound care is involved.*

For chronic arthritis, an orthosis may assist in providing support for a weak or unstable joint. Noninfectious joint inflammation usually responds to NSAIDs (Kaye, 1989). Treatments with azathioprine, methotrexate, and other immunosuppressive drugs require monitoring of HIV-RNA levels. Infectious arthritis is treated with antibiotics and proper positioning.

Musculoskeletal changes and pain associated with HIV arthritic conditions may result in major gait deviations. Proper implementation of orthoses and optimal footwear is most prudent to prevent further postural deficits. Modalities to modulate pain are incorporated into the rehabilitation approach. Early initiation of therapy and the appropriate splinting of inflamed tendons (enthesitis) may prevent complications associated with muscle atrophy, loss of ambulation, and joint laxity (Dimonte & Light, 1992).

Research on exercise for persons with active RA has demonstrated that joint disease can respond favorably to low- or non-impact aerobic exercise (Alpiner, Oh, Hinder, & Brander, 1995; Semble, 1995). The protocols used for RA are the most applicable to persons with concomitant HIV disease as long as specific neurological, cardiorespiratory, gastrointestinal, and musculoskeletal concerns are considered when prescribing an exercise program. The exercise protocol used by Alpiner and associates (1995) for persons with active RA advocates that patients begin with a 50% submaximal heart rate and progress to 60% to 65%. Shorter-interval training is recommended two to three times a day, three times a week, for 10 to 15 min. Obviously, this must be individually tailored to the patient with comorbid conditions. Side effects of medication must be considered in the design of the exercise program.

Crystalline-Induced Diseases

Various crystals can deposit in the synovium, cartilage, and other soft tissues. Metabolic and physical trauma can break down these crystalline deposits and induce acute inflammation within the tissues. The two most common crystals are monosodium urate monohydrate (MSUM) crystals that cause gout and calcium pyrophosphate dihydrate (CPPD) crystals that cause cartilage calcification or chondrocalcinosis (CC) and CPPD arthropathy. The CPPD is becoming a common referral to outpatient rehabilitation and hand therapy clinics.

Gout

Gout is a clinical syndrome resulting from the deposition of sodium urate crystals that incite acute inflammation and displace normal structures in joints, kidneys, and other body tissues. Uric acid precipitates as a crystal when serum uric acid levels increase beyond the solubility of 7 mg/dl. A primary form of gout presents in the postpubertal (9:1 men vs. women), most commonly in the fifth decade, and 10% report persistent limitations of activity (Becker & Levinson, 1997). Gout rarely occurs in women until after menopause. Secondary gout occurs when a coexistent disease increases the turnover of purines (overproduction) or retards the kidney excretion of the uric acid end products (underexcretion). Tophi or persistent deposits of urate in body tissues occur in primary forms.

The diagnosis of gout rests on the identification of MSUM crystals. The most expedient method is to examine clinical material aspirated from a tophus or from a joint with polarizing microscopy. When crystals are viewed in a microscope fitted with polarizing lenses and a red filter, urate crystals bend light into two rays (referred to as *birefringence*) and assume a yellow color when vertical and a blue color when horizontal. This method requires the red filter to be placed with the slow plane of light oriented vertically. An elevated serum uric acid level is not sufficient to confirm the diagnosis because only 10% of hospitalized persons with hyperuricemia have gout (Paulus, Coutts, Calabro, & Klinenberg, 1970).

Acute gouty arthritis. An acute attack of gout is exquisitely painful because the crystals induce a massive inflammatory response. Gout generally affects a single joint in the lower extremities, particularly the first metatarsophalangeal joint (podagra), ankle, or knee. The onset is rapid and is characterized by swelling, heat, and erythema in the affected joint.

Treatment involves maximal doses of anti-inflammatory drugs or colchicine to break the inflammatory cycle. Occasionally, intra-articular steroids are required, particularly if renal disease excludes the use of anti-inflammatory drugs and colchicine. Rest and occasionally splinting are advisable during the acute attack, especially if the site of the attack is the wrist or hand.

Chronic tophaceous gout. About 5 to 10 years after the onset of gout, tophi may develop, especially if treatment has been inconsistently followed (Figure 1). Tophi appear as subcutaneous lumps in the olecranon bursa and along the upper cartilage of the ear. When tophi occur around joints, cartilage and bone are eroded, and ROM is compromised. Frequently, tendon deposits restrict flexion of the fingers and movement of the wrists. Tophi may resorb with proper medication over a period of months to years. Tophi should be excised surgically when they compress nerves or other major structures or become infected

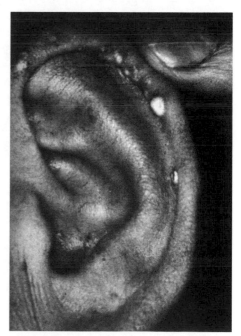

Figure 1. Chronic tophaceous gout. Note deposits of urate crystals (tophi) on the ear. Reprinted from the Clinical Slide Collection on the Rheumatic Diseases, copyright 1991, 1995, 1997. Used by permission of the American College of Rheumatology.

from repeated trauma. In the untreated patient, uric acid stones can induce acute obstruction or chronic renal disease. Medical management of chronic gout involves two classes of drugs to maintain a uric acid below 7 mg/dl. The uricosuric drugs (sulfinpyrazone or probenecid) lower serum uric acid levels by increasing the renal excretion of uric acid. High fluid intake is urged to minimize the risk of uric acid renal stone formation. Allopurinol is an enzyme-inhibiting drug that lowers serum uric acid levels by blocking xanthine oxidase, the enzyme that catalyzes purine breakdown by oxidizing hypoxanthine to xanthine and xanthine to uric acid. With the advent of these drugs to control the hyperuricemia, severe dietary restrictions are not necessary, although patients are advised to avoid foods that are particularly high in purine such as caviar (fish eggs) and sweetbreads (pancreas).

Therapists should encourage adherence to the medical regimen because gouty attacks can be prevented with compliance to therapies that decrease uric acid. Adaptive equipment and assistive devices for the hand may be necessary for patients with limited hand function secondary to the presence of tophi or to prevent pressure on tophi. Gait training to reduce weight-bearing stress on the lower extremities is indicated for patients with lower-extremity involvement.

Calcium Pyrophosphate Dihydrate (CPDD)

Chondro-calcinosis is the radiological affirmation of the deposition of CPPD crystals within fibrocartilage or hyaline cartilage. This process remains inactive until the crystals shed into synovial tissues and produce an inflammatory response that mimics gout (called pseudogout). Attacks of pseudogout are as frequent as attacks of gout. The resultant cartilage and bone abnormalities associated with intra-articular CPPD deposition are referred to as *pyrophosphate arthropathy*. Calcium pyrophosphate and other calcium crystals may be the inflammatory response characteristic of severe osteoarthritis (OA). CPPD is associated with hyperparathyroidism, hypothyroidism, and hemachromatosis.

CPPD tends to affect women more than men. The incidence of CPPD increases with age. Radiographic CC is rare in persons less than 50 years of age but increases from 10% to 15% in persons 65 to 75 years of age and from 30% to 60% in persons more than 85 years of age (Doherty, 1994).

The diagnosis of CPPD requires identification of the crystals by using polarizing microscopy with a red filter. The more rhomboid-like CPPD crystals are positively birefringent (i.e., they have the opposite orientation of urate crystals). Thus, CPPD crystals are blue when viewed in a vertical placement and yellow when horizontal. Characteristic radiographic findings of cartilaginous calcifications may indicate CPPD arthropathy but are not sufficient alone to make the diagnosis. Serum levels of calcium are helpful only when associated with hyperparathyroidism.

CPPD arthropathy is the most common cause of monoarticular synovitis in elderly persons. The knee is the most common site, followed by the wrist (particularly at the triangular fibrocartilage), shoulder, ankle, and elbow (Matteucci & Schumacher, 1996). Synovitis in two joints at one time is uncommon, and polyarticular presentation is rare. The synovitis is acute with swelling, redness, and heat similar to gout but often not quite as severe. Patients describe acute tenderness and inability to tolerate light touch or bed sheets on the joint. Acute attacks are self-limiting and resolve in 1 to 3 weeks. The more common mild attacks are often misdiagnosed as flare-ups of

OA. Attacks can be triggered by direct trauma, medical illness, surgery (especially parathyroidectomy), blood transfusion, parenteral fluid administration, thyroxine replacement therapy, and joint lavage (Doherty, 1997).

No specific intervention has proved effective in removing pyrophosphate deposits. Acute attacks often respond to aspiration of the crystals and intra-articular glucocorticoid injections. Some physicians use oral colchicine for acute attacks despite the inconsistent response. Splinting the acutely inflamed joints is often beneficial. Joint protection is indicated for chronic arthropathy. Use of thermal modalities and rest is the same as for OA. (See chapter 5 in this volume.)

Chronic pyrophosphate arthropathy characteristically affects the second and third MCP joints. Patients present with chronic pain, morning stiffness, stiffness after inactivity, limited motion, and impaired function. Typically, one or more joints is involved (Doherty, 1997). Because this disorder tends to affect older adults, concomitant OA is common. Chronic phosphate arthropathy is distinguished from OA by the pattern of joints involved (i.e., wrists, shoulders, ankles, and elbows are not common sites in OA), a monarticular or oligoarticular synovitis, synovial thickening in affected joints, periodic acute attacks, and knee involvement in multiple compartments including the patello-femoral joint.

Spondylarthropathies

The prototypical disease in this group is ankylosing spondylitis. (See chapter 11 in this volume.) Other diseases that exhibit inflammation of the entheses and joints of the axial and peripheral skeleton and are associated with the human lymphocyte antigen (HLA) B-27 include reactive arthritis (Reiter's syndrome), enteropathic arthritis, and psoriatic arthritis. (See chapter 10 on psoriatic arthritis.)

Reactive Arthritis (Reiter's Syndrome)

Reactive arthritis is a disease caused by a sterile joint inflammation after a sexually transmitted or gastrointestinal infection in a genetically susceptible person. The venereal bacteria include *Chlamydia* and *Ureaplasma*, and the enteropathic bacteria include *Salmonella, Shigella, Yersinia,* and *Campylobacter*. Anaerobic bacteria such as *Bacteroides* are important in transgenic animal models (Toivanen, 1994). As in ankylosing spondylitis, genetic susceptibility resides with the Class I gene HLA B-27, which occurs in 75% of cases (Khan & Khan, 1982). African-Americans are less frequently affected because apparently the African-American HLA B-27 gene protein binds bacterial antigen less effectively.

The original report of reactive arthritis described arthritis, urethritis, and conjunctivitis (Reiter, 1916). More commonly, men (6:1 versus women) present with an oligoarthritis or enthesitis of the lower extremities without urethritis or conjunctivitis. Asymmetrical sacroiliitis and spondylitis, oral ulcers, and skin rashes are detected in 10% to 20% of patients (McCord, 1977).

The typical skin lesion of reactive arthritis is keratoderma blenorrhagicum, also known as *pustulosis palmoplantaris* (Figure 2). These painless lesions occur in 12% to 14% of patients as vesicles

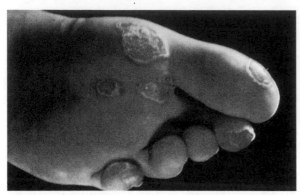

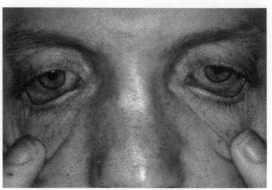

Figure 2. Reactive arthritis. Note characteristic skin lesions of keratoderma blenorrhagicum that are called *pustulosis palmoplantaris* when present on the soles. Reprinted from the Clinical Slide Collection on the Rheumatic Diseases, copyright 1991, 1995, 1997. Used by permission of the American College of Rheumatology.

Figure 3. Reactive arthritis. Ocular conjunctivitis is a common symptom. *Source*: Courtesy of James Louie, MD.

on erythematous bases and evolve into pustules and keratotic plaques but are nonscarring (Toivanen, 1994). They usually are found on the soles of the feet but may involve the hands, palms, penis, scrotum, trunk, and scalp. The rash is not contagious, and no special precautions are required in handling patients with these lesions.

Conjunctivitis (Figure 3) occurs in most patients after gastrointestinal infections and in 35% of patients with sexually transmitted infections (Keat, 1983). Small, shallow, painless ulcers of the glans penis and ureteral meatus follow sexually transmitted infections. In a few cases, extra-articular inflammation is detected in the eye, heart, gastrointestinal tract, and kidneys.

It is not clear whether the varying natural course of reactive arthritis depends on the fine structure of the gene or repeated infections. Avoiding gastrointestinal and sexually transmitted infections by not eating unrefrigerated dairy products and not engaging in unprotected intercourse is wise. NSAIDs are the mainstay of medical therapy to alleviate pain. If NSAIDs fail to control the arthritis, sulfasalazine or methotrexate are given. Local steroid injection of inflamed joints and entheses assists in controlling pain and tenderness. Anecdotes about the use of tumor necrosis factor (TNF)–soluble receptors are promising.

In addition to the systemic anti-inflammatory therapies, local rest is recommended to ameliorate pain. Splinting may be advisable. Acute enthesitis of the heel is treated with arch supports, heel cup inserts, and heel lifts to restrict stretching of the plantar fascia and Achilles tendons. In the chronic phase, mobilization, ROM, and isometric strengthening exercises are important to avoid heel cord shortening and fibrous ankylosis. Patients with spondylitis benefit from appropriate pain management, including posture instruction.

Enteropathic Arthritis

The clinical association of infectious and inflammatory bowel diseases with joint and tendon inflammation is another variant of a postinfectious arthritis. Interestingly, transgenic rats with HLA B-27 that are kept free of germs do not demonstrate gastrointestinal or joint inflammation until bacteria are introduced into their diets. These enteropathic diseases include inflammatory bowel diseases (IBD) (including ulcerative colitis and Crohn's disease), Whipple's disease, and intestinal bypass arthritis.

IBD. The prevalence of ulcerative colitis and Crohn's disease is 100/100,000 and 75/100,000, respectively (Mielants & Veys, 1997). Although each presents with different gastrointestinal manifestations and pathology, two patterns of arthritis occur: axial involvement and asymmetrical peripheral arthritis. The axial involvement includes sacroiliitis and spondylitis, precedes the intestinal symptoms by many years, and is frequently associated with HLA B-27. The peripheral arthritis usually coincides with the onset of the IBD. The peripheral arthritis presents in an asymmetrical, migratory pattern in the large and small joints of the lower extremities but is self-limited, nondestructive, and recurrent. A small subset (10%) develops enthesitis with pain and tenderness of the insertion of the Achilles tendon and plantar fascia and tenosynovitis of the digital flexors of the toe that results in inflammation throughout the digit (dactylitis or "sausage toe" deformity) (Weiner, Clarke, Taggart, & Utsinger, 1991).

Drug treatment is similar to that for ankylosing spondylitis and Reiter's syndrome. Sulfa-salazine is recommended because it addresses both the underlying bowel disease and the arthritis. Many physicians favor NSAIDs despite the theoretical exacerbation of gastrointestinal bleeding from the stomach. Oral corticosteroids reduce the peripheral inflammation but do not affect axial symptoms. In ulcerative colitis, colectomy cures the gastrointestinal disease and the peripheral arthritis, but axial symptoms persist. In Crohn's disease, treatment with a mono-clonal antibody to TNF (Remicade) aborts any flare-ups. Depending on the patient's symptoms, rehabilitation should follow the recommendations for Reiter's syndrome or ankylosing spondylitis. (See chapter 11 in this volume.)

Whipple's disease. Whipple's disease is a rare, chronic, systemic infectious disease that presents with intermittent arthralgias for years and the gradual onset of diarrhea, steatorrhea, weight loss, adenopathy, encephalopathy, uveitis, endocarditis, and nephritis. Men are affected 9:1 versus women (Fleming, Wiesner, & Shorter, 1988). The migratory polyarthritis occurs in 90% and does not associate with the intestinal symptoms, but it may associate with sacroiliitis (7%) and HLA B-27 (28%).

Synovial fluid analysis and intestinal biopsy specimens show periodic acid-Schiff material within macrophages, and electron microscopy demonstrates rod-shaped free bacilli that are identified by PCR to be an actinomycete called *Tropheryma whippelii* (Relman, Schmidt, Mac, Dermott, & Falkow, 1992). Antibiotic treatment results in dramatic improvement over a period of months. This elusive disease is unlikely to be referred for therapy, but middle-aged men with polyarthralgias, diarrhea, weight loss, and skin hyperpigmentation (50%) may prompt the experienced therapist to suspect this condition.

Intestinal bypass arthritis. Intestinal bypass surgery to control morbid obesity may be associated with a symmetrical, nonerosive peripheral polyarthritis that occurs several months after the surgery. Rarely, other extra-articular manifestations including inflammation of the skin, kidneys, and heart blood vessels can be seen. An immune response to bacterial overgrowth in the blind loop of the intestines is presumed to cause the disease. Antibiotics are helpful, and reanastomosis of the gut resolves the disease and its extra-articular manifestations. This condition occurs rarely and is not likely to be a source of referral to therapy.

Vasculitis

Polymyalgia Rheumatica

Polymyalgia rheumatica (PMR) is a syndrome of older persons who present with pain and stiffness of the shoulder and pelvic girdles. PMR occurs in 50/100,000 of white populations more than 50 years of age, and it is uncommon in African-American, Hispanic, and Asian-American populations. Women are affected twice as often as men (Hunder et al., 1990).

Some rheumatologists believe that PMR and temporal arteritis are manifestations of the same disease because the arteritis part of the continuum can occur as much as 20 years later (Healey, 1993). However, others detect only a 15% concordance of symptoms, signs, or histological evidence of temporal arteritis, so the relationship between these two syndromes remains unclear.

PMR presents abruptly with pain and stiffness in the neck, shoulder girdle, and occasionally in the thighs and hips as well. There is no objective weakness, but pain and stiffness make rising from a chair, getting out of bed, putting on clothes overhead, and styling or washing hair difficult. Pain likewise inhibits muscle strength. Other constitutional symptoms include malaise, weight loss, fever, myalgia, depression, morning stiffness, and pain at night with movement.

Diagnostic criteria include symmetrical proximal limb girdle myalgia associated with stiffness, onset during a period of 2 weeks or less, initial Westergren erythrocyte sedimentation rate (ESR) of 50 mm/hr or more, morning stiffness lasting 1 hr or longer, 50 years of age or older, depression or weight loss, bilateral upper-arm tenderness, and absence of other rheumatic diseases that cause the above symptoms (Healey, 1983).

PMR often is misdiagnosed as neck or back pain, OA, FMS, or bursitis. It is likely that an occupational therapist or physical therapist may be the first to encounter patients with PMR and should direct them to seek consultation with a rheumatologist or a knowledgeable physician.

The proximal muscle pains dramatically respond to low-dose prednisone (10 mg/day). If the ESR is greater than 100 mm/hr, some clinicians begin with 20 mg/day of prednisone. A prompt response to prednisone within days confirms the diagnosis. Half of the patients with PMR need long-term treatment with low-dose steroids to control their symptoms, and this predisposes postmenopausal elderly women to osteopenia and subsequent vertebral fractures. All women who are taking prednisone should likewise take calcium (1,500 mg/day) and vitamin D (800 IU/day) as well as exercise to counteract osteoporosis (Chuang, Hunder, Ilstrup, & Kurland, 1982). In addition, many patients with PMR will require counseling in energy conservation, conscious deep-muscle relaxation, methods to reduce postural strain, adaptive methods for activities of daily living (ADL), and assistive devices. Furthermore, all patients will need careful instruction in daily ROM programs and isometric shoulder exercises to prevent adhesive capsulitis and muscle atrophy capsulitis (Melvin, 1989).

Giant Cell (Temporal) Arteritis

Giant cell (temporal) arteritis is a granulomatous inflammation of the medium and large arteries to the head and neck, including the temporal arteries, that affects women (2:1 versus men) in an increasing percentage from 50 to 90 years of age (Weyand & Goronzy, 1997). The onset can be abrupt or insidious, with headaches, visual symptoms, and jaw claudication. The headaches present with severe lancinating pain that localizes to the scalp. Visual symptoms such as diplopia, ptosis, or transient blindness reflect ischemia of the optic nerve secondary to involvement of the ophthalmic or postciliary arteries. Psychological and neurological symptoms include confusion, depression, psychosis, hemiparesis, peripheral neuropathy, acute hearing loss, and brain stem strokes. Cardiac involvement includes angina pectoris, congestive heart failure, and myocardial infarction (Hunder et al., 1990).

Patients benefit from occupational therapy for the psychological and neurological symptoms and from training in adaptive methods to compensate for partial visual loss.

Patients with severe visual loss or blindness should receive specialized mobility and ADL training (Melvin, 1989). Fortunately, blindness and serious complications can usually be prevented with early detection of symptoms and maximal treatment with corticosteroids. Because corticosteroid therapy is required for years, trials with concomitant methotrexate and other steroid-sparing drugs are in progress.

Polyarteritis Nodosa

Polyarteritis nodosa (PAN) is a systemic vasculitis that affects the small and medium-sized vessels in the skin, joints, peripheral nerves, muscles, kidneys, and gastrointestinal tract. Marked constitutional symptoms are characteristic. PAN is an uncommon disease that occurs in adult men (2:1 versus women) from the mid-fourth to mid-sixth decades, with an annual incidence of 10/1,000,000. Although the cause is unknown, associations are reported with the intravenous use of methamphetamine ("speed") and with the hepatitis B virus. Skin involvement includes palpable purpura, livedo reticularis, or ulcerations. Joint manifestations range from arthralgias (50%) to frank arthritis (20%). Peripheral neuropathy (50–70%) occurs in patients with both sensory and motor involvement (mononeuritis multiplex). Rarely, seizures or hemiparesis signal central nervous system (CNS) involvement. Vasculitis of the upper or lower gastrointestinal tract induces abdominal pain and gastrointestinal bleeding. A segmental necrotizing vasculitis affects the kidneys (70%), and renovascular hypertension develops secondary to renal artery involvement. Vasculitis of the coronary arteries can result in myocardial infarction or congestive heart failure (Lightfoot et al., 1990).

There are no specific laboratory tests for PAN. P-ANCA (perinuclear-antineutrophilic cytoplasmic antibodies) with serum antibodies to myeloperoxidase, lactoferrin, elastase, and other cytoplasmic antigens occur in less than 20%. In the cases of microscopic PAN (which affects only small capillaries, venules, and arterioles), 50% to 80% will demonstrate P-ANCA. Other nonspecific tests include an elevated ESR, normocytic normochromic anemia, thrombocytosis, and diminished levels of serum albumin. Serum complement is decreased in 25% of patients who have diffuse cutaneous or renal disease. Serum rheumatoid factor is present in this group of patients. The subgroups of patients who demonstrate hepatitis B surface antigen are clinically indistinguishable. Biopsy specimens consist of necrotizing inflammatory lesions in small and medium-sized arteries.

The drug treatment of PAN focuses on the affected organ systems and the extent of involvement. Patients with limited disease are managed with prednisone. Usually, extensive disease involving visceral organs requires use of daily oral cyclophosphamide at a dose of 1 to 2 mg/kg/day for disease control in addition to the prednisone. Other steroid-sparing agents have been tried with variable results. Early diagnosis and treatment of PAN seems to correlate with improved survival rates.

Occupational therapy and physical therapy are indicated when arthropathy and peripheral neuropathy occur (Melvin, 1989). The pain of a sensory neuropathy may respond to transcutaneous electrical nerve stimulation (TENS), and care for a foot-drop deformity requires muscle reeducation, stretching, and possibly an ankle–foot orthoses. Occasionally, acute arthritis may require splints and instruction in ADL, ROM, and strengthening exercises. Patients with fatigue and weakness from systemic involvement may benefit from energy conservation training.

Relapsing Polychondritis

Relapsing polychondritis (RP) is a rare disorder of cartilage inflammation that affects men and women in the fourth or fifth decades of life. RP reduces life expectancy to a 5-year survival rate of 74% (Luthra & Michet, 1997). Death is caused by persistent inflammation and eventual collapse of the tracheobronchial tree and to infections attendant to steroid therapy.

The classic presentation is acute pain, swelling, and redness of the cartilage of the external ear, nose, and trachea. These episodes of chondritis continue from days to weeks and resolve without treatment but leave the cartilage misshapened and without resilience (Figure 4). After several episodes, untreated patients exhibit gnarled floppy ears, "saddle nose" (collapsed bridge) deformity (Figure 5), and tracheal stenosis leading to wheezing, hoarseness, and difficulty breathing. Vasculitis of the internal auditory artery or its cochlear or vestibular branch occurs in 30% of patients and leads to varying degrees of vertigo or neurosensory hearing loss (Luthra & Michet, 1997). A coexisting autoimmune disease such as RA, Sjögren's syndrome, biliary cirrhosis, or a vasculitis affecting the skin, eyes, heart, kidney, CNS, and peripheral nervous system occurs in one third of patients (McAdam, O'Hanlon, Bluestone, & Pearson, 1976).

Diagnosis requires three or more of the following clinical features: bilateral auricular chondritis, nonerosive inflammatory polyarthritis, nasal chondritis, ocular inflammation, respiratory tract chondritis, cochlear or vestibular dysfunction (e.g., neurosensory hearing loss, tinnitus, or vertigo), or cartilage biopsy confirming inflammation and cartilage destruction (McAdam et al., 1976).

Initially, the life-threatening manifestations of the disease require high doses of prednisone (1 mg/kg). As the inflammation resolves, the prednisone is maintained at 15 mg/day or the lowest possible dose for months.

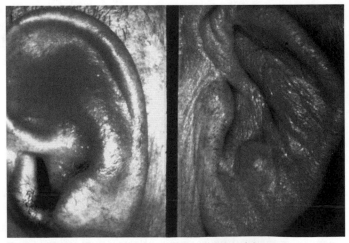

Figure 4. RP: note early inflammation of the cartilage of the ear (*left*) and collapse of the ear with chronic degeneration (*right*). Reprinted from the Clinical Slide Collection on the Rheumatic Diseases, copyright 1991, 1995, 1997. Used by permission of the American College of Rheumatology.

If a dose more than 15 mg/day is required, other immunosuppressive therapies such as azathioprine or cyclophosphamide are added. Occasionally, the chronic sequelae will require surgery to stent tracheal collapse, correct the saddle nose deformity, and replace the aortic valve.

Patients are rarely referred to occupational therapy or physical therapy because the rare joint manifestations are non-deforming. Patients with vestibular impairment may respond to vestibular rehabilitation exercises that are used with other diagnostic groups, such as exercises that gradually increase ROM and the frequency with which patients can tolerate head movement (Cohen, 1994).

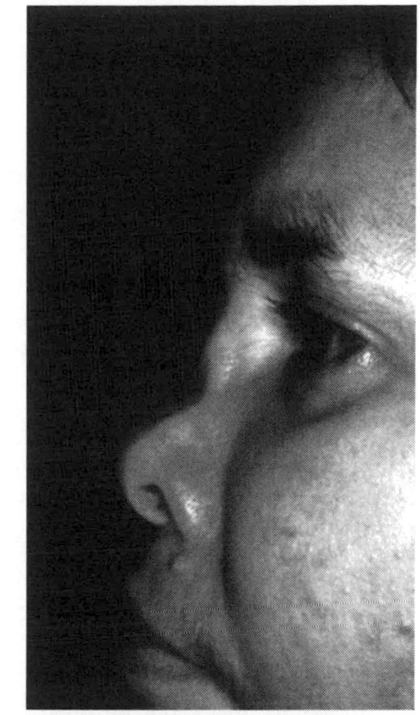

Wegener's Granulomatosis

Wegener's granulomatosis (WG) is a rare systemic granulomatous vasculitis that affects the upper and lower respiratory tract and the kidneys. WG occurs in all ages and races with a peak incidence in the fourth and fifth decades and a slight male predominance. The prevalence is not known. The pathology demonstrates a necrotizing granulomatous vasculitis.

Figure 5. RP: note the characteristic saddle nose deformity resulting from the collapse of the cartilage in the bridge of the nose. Reprinted from the Clinical Slide Collection on the Rheumatic Diseases, copyright 1991, 1995, 1997. Used by permission of the American College of Rheumatology.

Clinical presentations vary widely because the rhinitis, sinusitis, and nasal mucosal ulcerations of upper respiratory involvement and the cough and hemoptysis of lower respiratory involvement often are overshadowed by the marked constitutional involvement of arthralgias, weakness, fatigue, weight loss, and fever. Occasionally, otitis media with hearing loss and eye inflammation predominate. Musculoskeletal symptoms include arthralgias and myalgia, and frank arthritis is rare. Skin lesions include palpable purpura, subcutaneous nodules, and ulcerations. Nervous system involvement results in mononeuritis multiplex, stroke, and cranial nerve abnormalities.

Patients with WG have serum antibodies that react to proteinase 3, an enzyme that resides within the cytoplasmic component of neutrophils. These antineutrophilic cytoplasmic antibodies (C-ANCA) occur in 80% to 90% of patients with active generalized disease. Other laboratory abnormalities include an elevated ESR, cells, urinary cellular casts and protein, and infiltrates in the chest and sinus films (Leavitt et al., 1990). Biopsy of affected tissue reveals a necrotizing granulomatous inflammatory process affecting small arteries and veins.

Current treatment of WG has increased the life span from 6 months to more than 15 years. Prednisone (60 mg/day) and oral cyclophosphamide (1–2 mg/kg/day) are given until the clinical parameters improve and then are tapered to minimal doses. Most patients will require medication for several years. Neurological involvement resulting in foot drop is usually the primary reason for occupational therapy or physical therapy. Gastroc-soleus stretching, muscle reeducation, and an ankle–foot orthosis are indicated.

Infiltrative Diseases

Sarcoidosis

Sarcoidosis is a systemic, granulomatous disease affecting persons between 20 and 40 years of age with an increased incidence in women, African-Americans, and Northern Europeans (Schumacher, 1997).

In sarcoidosis, the lungs are affected in 90% of patients. Arthritis presents in both acute and chronic forms. The acute form is referred to as Löfgren's syndrome and features an inflammatory polyarthritis with marked fever, weight loss, fatigue, and tender pretibial skin nodules called *erythema nodosum*. Chest X-rays depict bilateral hilar adenopathy. The chronic form of arthritis is oligoarticular, less inflammatory, and is associated with granulomatous infiltration of multiple tissues, including a dactylitis (Figure 6), laryngeal or nasal cartilage involvement, uveitis, parotid gland enlargement, myositis, mononeuritis multiplex, and facial palsies. Cardiac involvement leads to arrhythmias, cardiomyopathy, and sudden death. Neurosarcoidosis results in seizures and neuroendocrine disorders (Schumacher, 1997).

Musculoskeletal manifestations respond to NSAIDs. Major organ involvement requires the use of corticosteroids. The acute arthritis is self-limited, but ROM and splinting may help for the first weeks. Chronic arthritis will require a comprehensive program of exercise, joint protection training, and fatigue management training because current medical management poorly controls granulomatous infiltration. Major organ involvement requires the use of corticosteroids. Patients with major lung involvement need fatigue management training with an emphasis on energy conservation.

Cancer

Hypertrophic osteoarthropathy. Hypertrophic osteoarthropathy (HOA) is a syndrome characterized by a proliferation of skin and periosteum in the distal parts of the extremities. The digits are "clubbed" with bulbous swelling about the nails. In advanced stages, the periosteal growth extends to the tubular bones, is tender to pressure in a periarticular distribution, and occasionally is associated with synovial effusions (Altman, 1997).

HOA is classified into primary and secondary forms. In the heritable primary form, the skin hypertrophy creates a coarse appearance on the forehead and face, which gives a similar facial appearance to all of the family members with the disorder. In the secondary form, the osteoarthropathy is associated with cancers of the pleura and lung, although other diseases such as pulmonary fibrosis, cirrhosis, infectious endocarditis, and Graves disease are additionally associated. It has been postulated that fibroblast growth factors may mediate the proliferative changes (Fontenay-Roupie et al., 1995).

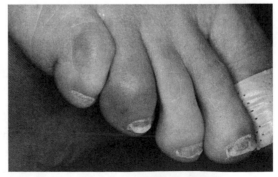

Figure 6. Sarcoidosis. Digital arthritis can present as a dactylitis or sausage toe deformity. *Source*: Courtesy of James Louie, MD.

Patients who complain of severe bone pain, exhibit clubbing of the fingers and toes, and are tender when the distal long bones of the extremities are squeezed may have cancer. The clubbing deformity of the digits begins with soft tissue at the nailbeds that has a rocking sensation when palpated. Periosteal tenderness is elicited proximal to the wrists or ankles or in other areas devoid of muscle. The periosteal proliferation can be confirmed by X-ray. Synovial effusions are noninflammatory. Occasionally, painful osteoarthropathy responds to NSAIDs, but surgical removal of the associated cancer is the definitive treatment for this disorder.

Patients with persistent periarticular pain in a setting where the underlying disease cannot be surgically treated may be referred to occupational therapy or physical therapy for appropriate ADL adaptation and exercise. Splinting to immobilize affected joints affords minimal pain relief.

Amyloidosis. Amyloidosis is a syndrome characterized by the extracellular deposition of a highly insoluble protein complex within multiple tissues. Aside from heritable forms, there are several subsets of this disease: AL (or primary) amyloid occurs in a monoclonal gammopathy and indicates proliferation of a single B lymphocyte line, and AA (or secondary) amyloid is associated with chronic inflammatory diseases. AA amyloid is more prevalent in western Europe, whereas AL amyloid is more common in the United States. A third form of amyloid deposition is associated with chronic renal disease in which β-2 microglobulin protein deposits around the joints (Benson, 1997).

AL amyloid has a more diverse presentation with deposits of immunoglobulin light chain in the kidneys, heart, gastrointestinal tract, nerves, lungs, blood vessels, and joints. Deposition of amyloid in the kidneys produces a nephrotic syndrome with massive protein loss in the urine. Cardiac amyloid is more a subtle restrictive cardiomyopathy that leads to arrhythmias and heart failure. In AL amyloid, which is always associated with multiple myeloma or other monoclonal gammopathies, amyloid infiltrates the skeletal muscles and produces an enlarged tongue carpal tunnel syndrome, and the "shoulder pad sign." Periarticular joint infiltration causes severe limitation of motion and is uncomfortable (Katz, Peter, Pearson, & Adams, 1973). Neuropathic involvement is usually sensorimotor and can present as carpal tunnel syndrome or other peripheral neuropathies.

Treatment of amyloidosis focuses on reducing the plasma cell clone and treating the chronic inflammatory disease. In AL amyloidosis, prednisone and melphalan often dramatically reverse the nephrotic syndrome, but no controlled studies are available. In AA amyloidosis, prednisone or cytotoxic drugs are used to control the chronic inflammatory disease, and antibiotics and surgical excision decrease the inflammation of osteomyelitis and other chronic infections. Rarely, amyloid deposits resolve as the inflammation of the chronic disease is controlled.

Therapists are more likely to see patients with an AA amyloidosis when it occurs in association with chronic inflammatory diseases such as RA, juvenile chronic polyarthritis, or osteomyelitis. Rehabilitation focuses on self-management of ROM, strength, and pain. Wrist splints may help alleviate carpal tunnel syndrome.

Palindromic Rheumatism

Palindromic rheumatism (PR) is characterized by recurring, afebrile attacks of acute arthritis or periarthritis in a single joint that last a few hours to several days and are followed by symptom-free intervals ranging from days to months (Hench & Rosenberg, 1944). The usual onset is between the third and sixth decades, and men and women are affected equally. The etiology and pathogenesis of this disease remains unclear.

Joint pain begins suddenly in one or two joints and resembles an acute attack of gout. Attacks start late in the afternoon, and the intensity of pain peaks within hours to days. Objective signs of inflammation, including swelling, warmth, and redness overlying the affected joint, are necessary for the clinical diagnosis. The commonly affected joints are knees, wrists, and shoulders, but attacks are additionally reported in the vertebral column and temporomandibular joints.

The clinical course is quite variable. Most patients continue to experience intermittent attacks without any chronic synovitis. Generally, patients are seronegative for rheumatoid factor, but one third of patients will progress to classic RA with rheumatoid nodules and serum rheumatoid factor, and another 4% will develop other rheumatic diseases such as WG or Whipple's disease (Guerne & Weisman, 1992).

NSAIDs appear to be effective for partial relief of joint pain and rarely can induce a long-lasting remission. Injectable gold and other disease-modifying antirheumatic drugs including methotrexate, D-penicillamine, antimalarials, and sulfasalazine may be helpful, particularly in patients developing RA.

Occupational therapy and physical therapy will not be necessary in the intermittent form of the disease because the acute arthritis usually resolves within 1 week. Patients that progress to classic RA should be treated accordingly. (See chapter 7 in this volume.)

Conclusion

This chapter reviews the less common rheumatic diseases and identifies the current role of rehabilitation in the management of these patients. For most of these diseases, there is a dearth of published rehabilitation literature, so therapists treating these patients can help further define the role of rehabilitation by publishing case studies of successful clinical interventions. Therapists are some of the members of the health care team who monitor these patients for disease progression, signs of infection, and medication side effects. The combination of rehabilitation with drug therapy enhances the effectiveness of managing these potentially devastating rheumatic diseases.

References

Alpiner, N., Oh, T., Hinder, S., & Brander, V. A. (1995). Rehabilitation in joint and connective tissue diseases and systemic diseases. *Archives of Physical Medicine and Rehabilitation, 76*(Suppl. 5), S32–S40.

Altman, E. M., Centeno, L. V., Mahal, M., & Bieloryl, L. (1994). AIDS-associated Reiter's syndrome. *Annals of Allergy, 72,* 307–316.

Altman, R. D. (1997). Hypertrophic osteoarthropathy. In W. J. Koopman (Ed.), *Arthritis and allied conditions* (pp. 1751–1758). Baltimore: Williams & Wilkins.

Baker, D. G., & Schumacher, H. R. (1993). Acute monoarthritis. *New England Journal of Medicine, 329,* 1013–1020.

Becker, M. A., & Levinson, D. J. (1997). Clinical gout and the pathogenesis of hyperuricemia. In W. J. Koopman (Ed.), *Arthritis and allied conditions* (pp. 2041–2071). Baltimore: Williams & Wilkins.

Bennett, R. M. (1996). Multidisciplinary group programs to treat fibromyalgia patients. *Rheumatic Disease Clinics of North America, 22,* 351–368.

Benson, M. D. (1997). Amyloidosis. In W. J. Koopman (Ed.), *Arthritis and allied conditions* (pp. 1661–1687). Baltimore: Williams & Wilkins.

Berman, A., Espinoza, L. R., Diaz, J. D., Aguilar, J. L., Rolando, T., Vasey, F. B., Germain, B. F., & Lockey, R. F. (1988). Rheumatic manifestations of human immunodeficiency virus infection. *American Journal of Medicine, 85,* 59–64.

Buskila, D., Gladman, D. D., Langevitz, P., Urowitz, S., & Smythe, H. A. (1990). Fibromyalgia in human immunodeficiency virus infection. *Journal of Rheumatology, 17,* 1202–1206.

Calabrese, L. H. (1989). Rheumatic manifestations of infection with the human immunodeficiency virus. *Seminars in Arthritis and Rheumatism, 18,* 225–239.

Calabrese, L. H. (1997). Human immunodeficiency virus infection and rheumatic disease. *Bulletin on the Rheumatic Diseases, 46*(8), 2–5.

Calabrese, L. H. (1998). Rheumatic aspects of acquired immunodeficiency syndrome. In J. H. Klippel & P. A. Dieppe (Eds.), *Rheumatology* (pp. 6:7.1–6:7.12). St. Louis: Mosby-Year Book.

Centers for Disease Control and Prevention. (1997). *Fact sheet: HIV and AIDS trends* [On-line]. Available: www.cdcnac.org/abstracts/trends.html

Chaisson, R. E., & Moore, R. D. (1996). Natural history of opportunistic disease in a HIV infected urban clinical cohort. *Annals of Internal Medicine, 124*(7), 633–642.

Chuang, T. Y., Hunder, G. G., Ilstrup, D. M., & Kurland, L. T. (1982). Polymyalgia rheumatica: A 10 year epidemiologic and clinical study. *Annals of Internal Medicine, 97,* 672–680.

Cohen, H. (1994). Vestibular rehabilitation improves daily life function. *American Journal of Occupational Therapy, 48,* 919–925.

Couderc, L. J., D'Aqay, M. F., Danon, F., Harzie, M., Brocheriou, C., & Clauvel, J. P. (1987). Sicca complex and infection with human immunodeficiency virus. *Archives of Internal Medicine, 147,* 898–901.

Coyle, P. K., & Schutzer, S. E. (1991). Neurologic presentations in Lyme disease. *Hospital Practice, 26*(11), 55–70.

Cunningham, A. L., Dwyer, D. E., & Dowton, D. N. (1993). Viral markers in HIV infection and AIDS. *Journal on Acquired Immune Deficiency Syndrome, 6*(Suppl.), S32–S35.

Dimonte, P., & Light, H. (1992). Pathomechanics, gait deviations, and treatment of the rheumatic foot. *Physical Therapy, 62,* 1148.

Doherty, M. (1997). Crystal arthropathies: Calcium pyrophosphate dihydrate. In J. H. Klippel & P. A. Dieppe (Eds.), *Rheumatology* (pp. 8:16.1–8:16.12). St. Louis: Mosby.

Espinoza, L. R., Aguilar, J. L., Berman, A., Gutierrez, F., Vasey, F. B., & Germain, B. F. (1989). Rheumatic manifestations associated with human immunodeficiency virus infection. *Arthritis and Rheumatism, 32,* 1615–1622.

Fleming, J. L., Wiesner, R. H., & Shorter, R. G. (1988). Whipple's disease: Clinical biochemical, and histopathologic features and assessment of treatment in 29 patients. *Mayo Clinic Proceedings, 63,* 539–551.

Fontenay-Roupie, M., Dupuy, E., Berrou, E., Tobelem, G., & Bryckaert, M. (1995). Increased proliferation of bone-marrow derived fibroblasts in primitive hypertrophic osteoarthropathy with severe myelofibrosis. *Blood, 85,* 3229–3238.

Freed, J. F., Nies, K. M., Boyer, R. S., & Louie, J. S. (1980). Acute monoarticular arthritis: A diagnostic approach. *JAMA, 243,* 2314–2316.

Furth, P. A., Maloof, M., Flynn, J. P., & Shea, F. (1988). Rehabilitation and AIDS: Primary care and system support. *Maryland Journal of Medicine, 37,* 469–471.

Galantino, M. L., & McCormack, G. (1992). Pain management. In M. L. Galantino (Ed.), *Clinical assessment and treatment in HIV disease: Rehabilitation of a chronic Illness* (pp. 104–114). Thorofare, NJ: Slack.

Goldenberg, D. L. (1988). Fibromyalgia and other chronic fatigue syndromes: Is there evidence for chronic viral disease? *Seminars in Arthritis and Rheumatism, 18,* 111–120.

Gran, J. T., Johnsen, V., Mykebust, G., & Nordbo, S. A. (1995). The variable clinical picture of arthritis induced by human parvo virus B19. *Scandinavian Journal of Rheumatology, 24,* 174–179.

Guerne, P. A., & Weisman, M. H. (1992). Palindromic rheumatism: Part of or apart from the spectrum of rheumatoid arthritis. *American Journal of Medicine, 93,* 451–460.

Gutierrez, V. F. J., Martinez-Osuna, P., Seleznick, M. J., et al. (1992). Rheumatologic rehabilitation for patients with HIV. In J. Mukand (Ed.), *Rehabilitation in patients with HIV disease* (pp. 77–93). New York: McGraw Hill.

Haralson, K. (1988). Physical modalities. In B. F. Banell & V. Gall (Eds.), *Physical therapy management of arthritis* (pp. 77–106). New York: Churchill Livingstone.

Healey, L. A. (1993). Polymyalgia rheumatica. In H. R. Schumacher, J. H. Klippel, & W. J. Koopman (Eds.), *Primer of the rheumatic diseases* (10th ed., pp. 148–149). Atlanta, GA: Arthritis Foundation.

Hench, P. S., & Rosenberg, E. F. (1944). Palindromic rheumatism: A "new" often recurring disease of joints (arthritis, periarthritis, para-arthritis) apparently producing no articular residues. *Archives of Internal Medicine, 73,* 293–321.

Hunder, G. G., Bloch, D. A., Michel, B. A., Stevens, M. B., Arend, W. P., Calabrese, L. H., Edworthy, S. M., Fauci, A. S., Leavitt, R. Y., Lie, J. T., et al. (1990). The American College of Rheumatology 1990 Criteria for the Classification of Giant Cell Arteritis. *Arthritis and Rheumatism, 33,* 1122–1128.

Inman, R. (1982). Rheumatic manifestations of hepatitis B infection. *Seminars in Arthritis and Rheumatism, 11,* 406–420.

Kaandorp, C. J. E., Krijnen, P., Moens, H. J. B., Habbema, J. D. F., & Van Schaardenburg, D. Y. (1997). The outcome of bacterial arthritis. *Arthritis and Rheumatism, 40,* 884–892.

Kaandorp, C. J. E., Van Schaardenburg, D. Y., Krijnen, P., Habbema, J. D. F., & Van de Laar, M. A. F. J. (1995). Risk factors for septic arthritis in patients with joint disease. *Arthritis and Rheumatism, 38,* 1819–1825.

Katz, G. A., Peter, J. B., Pearson, C. M., & Adams, W. S. (1973). The shoulder pad sign: A diagnostic feature of amyloid arthropathy. *New England Journal Medicine, 288,* 354–355.

Kaye, B. R. (1989). Rheumatologic manifestations of infection with human immunodeficiency virus (HIV). *Annals of Internal Medicine, 111,* 158–167.

Keat, A. (1983). Reiter's syndrome and reactive arthritis in perspective. *New England Journal Medicine, 309,* 1606–1615.

Khan, M. A., & Khan, M. K. (1982). Diagnostic value of HLA B27 testing in ankylosing spondylitis and Reiter's syndrome. *Annals of Internal Medicine, 96,* 70–76.

Leavitt, R. Y., Fauci, A. S., Bloch, D. A., Michel, B. A., Hunder, G. G., Arend, W. P., Calabrese, L. H., Fries, J. F., Lie, J. T., Lightfoot, R. W., Masi, A. F., McShane, D. J., Mills, J. A., Stevens, M. B., Wallace, S. L., & Zvaifler, N. J. (1990). American College of Rheumatology 1990 Criteria for the Classification of Wegener's Granulomatosis. *Arthritis and Rheumatism, 33,* 1088–1093.

Levinson, S. F., & O'Connell, P. G. (1991). Rehabilitation dimensions of AIDS: A review. *Archives of Physical Medicine and Rehabilitation, 72*, 690–696.

Lightfoot, R. W., Michel, B. A., Bloch, D. A., Hunder, G. G., Zvaifler, N. J., McShane, D. S., Arend, W. P., Calabrese, L. H., Leavitt, R. F., Lie, J. T., Masi, A. F., Mills, J. A., Stevens, M. B., & Wallace, S. L. (1990). The American College of Rheumatology 1990 Criteria for the Classification of Polyarthritis Nodosa. *Arthritis and Rheumatism, 33*, 1088–1093.

Luthra, H. S., & Michet, C. S. (1997). Relapsing polychondritis. In J. H. Klippel & P. A. Dieppe (Eds.), *Rheumatology* (pp. 5:27.1–5:27.4). St. Louis: Mosby-Year Book.

MacDougal, D. S. (1996). Indinavir: Lightening the load. *Journal of the International Association of Physicians in AIDS Care*, 6–11.

Mahowald, M. (1993). Infectious arthritis A: Bacterial agents. In H. R. Schumacher, J. H. Klippel, & W. J. Koopman (Eds.), *Primer on the rheumatic diseases* (10th ed., pp. 192–197). Atlanta, GA: Arthritis Foundation.

Matteucci, B. M., & Schumacher, H. R. (1996). Systemic arthritic conditions of the upper extremities: Inflammatory. In C. A. Peimer (Ed.), *Surgery of the hand and upper extremity* (pp. 1617–1632). New York: McGraw-Hill.

McAdam, L. P., O'Hanlon, M. A., Bluestone, R., & Pearson, C. M. (1976). Relapsing polychondritis: Prospective study of 23 patients and a review of the literature. *Medicine, 55*, 193–215.

McCord, W. C. (1977). Acute venereal arthritis: Comparative study of acute Reiter syndrome and acute gonococcal arthritis. *Archives of Internal Medicine, 137*, 858–862.

McReynolds, M. A. (1995). Rehabilitation management of the lower extremity in HIV disease. *Journal of the American Podiatric Medicine Association, 85*, 394–402.

McReynolds, M. A. (1996). The rheumatological manifestations of HIV disease. In M. L. Galantino (Ed.), *Issues in HIV rehabilitation*.

Mellors, J. W., Rinaldo, C. R., Gupta, P., White, R. M., Todd, J. A., & Kingsley, L. A. (1996). Prognosis in HIV-1 infection predicted the quantity of virus in plasma. *Science, 272*, 1167–1170.

Melvin, J. L. (1989). *Rheumatic disease in the adult and child: Occupational therapy and rehabilitation* (3rd ed.). Philadelphia: F. A. Davis.

Methaler, J. M., & Cross, L. L. (1988). Traumatic spinal cord injury complicated by AIDS-related complex. *Archives Physical Medicine Rehabilitation, 69*, 219–222.

Mielants, H., & Veys, E. M. (1997). Enteropathic arthritis. In W. J. Koopman (Ed.), *Arthritis and allied conditions* (pp. 1245–1263). Baltimore: Williams & Wilkins.

Munoz-Fernandez, S., Cardenal, A., Balsa, A., Quiralte, J., del Arzo, A., Pena, J. M., Barbado, F. J., Vàsquez, J. J., & Gijón, J. (1991). Rheumatic manifestations in 556 patient with human immunodeficiency virus infection. *Seminars in Arthritis and Rheumatism, 21*, 30–39.

O'Brien, W. A., Hartigan, P. M., Martin, D., Esinhart, J., Hull, A., Benoit, S., Rubin, M., Simberkoff, M. S., & Hamilton, J. D. (1996). Changes in plasma HIV-1 RNA and CD4 lymphocyte counts and the risk of progression to AIDS. *New England Journal Medicine, 334*, 426–431.

O'Dell, M. W., Dillon, M. E. (1993). Rehabilitation in adults with human immunodeficiency virus related diseases. *American Journal of Physical Medicine and Rehabilitation, 71*, 183–190.

O'Dell, M. W., Hubert, H. B., Lubeck, D. P., & O'Driscoll, P. (1996). Physical disability in cohort of persons with AIDS. *AIDS, 10*, 667–673.

O'Dell, M. W., Levinson, S. F., & Riggs, R. V. (1996). Focused review: physiatrics management of HIV-related disability. *Archives of Physical Medicine and Rehabilitation, 77*(Suppl.), S66–S73.

Paulus, H. E., Coutts, A., Calabro, J. J., & Klinenberg, J. R. (1970). Clinical significance of hyperuricemia in routinely screened hospitalized men. *JAMA, 211*, 277–281.

Piatak, M., Saag, M. S., Yang, L. C., Clark, S. J., Kappes, J. C., Luk, K. C., Hahn, B. H., Shaw, G. M., & Lifson, J. D. (1993). High levels of HIV-1 in plasma during all stages of infection determined by competitive PCR. *Science, 259*, 1749–1754.

Reiter, H. (1916). Uber eine bisher unerkannte Spirochateninfektion (Spirochaetosis arthritica). *Deutsche Medicine Wochenschr, 42*, 1535–1536.

Relman, D. A., Schmidt, T. M., MacDermott, R. P., & Falkow, S. (1992). Identification of the uncultured bacillus of Whipple's disease. *New England Journal Medicine, 327*, 293–301.

Reveille, J. D., Connant, M. A., & Duvic, M. (1990). Human immunodeficiency virus-associated psoriasis, psoriatic arthritis and Reiter's syndrome: A disease continuation. *Arthritis and Rheumatism, 33*, 1574–1578.

Schumacher, H. R., Jr. (1997). Sarcoidosis. In W. J. Koopman (Ed.), *Arthritis and allied conditions* (pp. 1689–1695). Baltimore: Williams & Wilkins.

Semble, E. (1995). Rheumatoid arthritis: New approaches for evaluation and management. *Archives of Physical Medicine and Rehabilitation, 76*, 190–201.

Toivanen, A. (1994). Reactive arthritis. In J. H. Klippel & P. A. Dieppe (Eds.), *Rheumatology* (pp. 4.9.1–4.9.7). St. Louis: Mosby.

Weiner, S. R., Clarke, J., Taggart, N. A., & Utsinger, P. D. (1991). Rheumatic manifestations of inflammatory bowel disease. *Seminars in Arthritis and Rheumatism, 20*, 353–366.

Weyand, C. M., & Goronzy, J. J. (1997). Polymyalgia rheumatica and giant cell arteritis. In W. J. Koopman (Ed.), *Arthritis and allied conditions* (pp. 1605–1616). Baltimore: Williams & Wilkins.

Winchester, R., Bernstein, D. H., & Fischer, H. D. (1987). The co-occurrence of Reiter's syndrome and acquired immunodeficiency syndrome. *Annals of Internal Medicine, 106*, 19–26.

Ytterberg, S. R. (1997). Viral arthritis. In W. J. Koopman (Ed.), *Arthritis and allied conditions* (13th ed., pp. 2341–2360). Baltimore: Williams & Wilkins.

Ziskin, M., McDiarmis, T., & Michlovitz, S. (1990). Therapeutic ultrasound. In S. L. Michlovitz (Ed.), *Thermal agents in rehabilitation* (pp. 353–366). Philadelphia: F. A. Davis.

Appendix A

Recommending Shoes and Foot Orthoses for Persons With Rheumatic Disease

Jeanne Melvin, MS, OTR, FAOTA, and Dennis Janisse, CPed

There is an old saying: "When the feet hurt, everything hurts." Proper footwear is an important part of pain management for persons with arthritis.

The Right Footwear for Persons With Arthritis

Ideally, everyone who wants to prevent foot problems and reduce stress to weight-bearing joints should wear comfortable shoes, ones with a good arch support, a cushion sole instead of a leather sole, and adequate length, width, and toe depth (sufficient to allow curling of the toes). Many walking and casual laced shoes offer these features. If a nonathletic, sturdy shoe allows a person to walk pain free for a couple of hours, it is probably sufficient for his or her needs. But if a person using even a walking shoe finds that the feet hurt after a couple of hours walking, he or she should consider using an athletic running shoe or foot orthoses.

Most persons with osteoarthritis do well with a comfortable shoe or running shoe as described above. When they have a stiff or painful first metatarsophalangeal (MTP) joint, an extended steel shank and rocker sole may be helpful in reducing the amount of motion needed in the toes for push-off when walking. Hallux valgus requires a shoe with a wide toe box that does not cause pressure on the first MTP joint or push the toes laterally. Of course, all of the foot problems that affect the general population (e.g. flat feet, pes cavus, Morton's neuroma) can likewise affect persons with arthritis.

Persons with rheumatoid arthritis, juvenile rheumatoid arthritis, systemic lupus erythematosus, systemic sclerosis, and psoriatic arthritis who are prone to developing dynamic foot deformities generally benefit from the extra support of a running shoe. In the early stages of active MTP joint synovitis, patients generally need custom foot orthoses to support the arch and reduce weight-bearing pressure on the MTP joints. Patients with subtalar synovitis may need the support of a heel-cup orthosis to reduce inversion and eversion. Patients with severe deformities may need in-depth shoes or custom-molded shoes.

Which shoe is best for a specific person? How do you find the best shoe from the myriad selections now available? When are athletic shoes not sufficient or the best choice? And when are foot orthoses needed?

Athletic Shoes

Athletic shoes have become the most popular type of shoe in North America. This is fortunate for persons with arthritis and foot pain because these are generally the best shoes for support and reducing impact on joints, and they are stylish as well. Even Velcro® closures and elastic shoe laces, which are easier for arthritic fingers to use, are common today.

Of all the shoes commercially available, athletic shoes designed for running are considered to have the best heel support and sole cushion for reducing impact to the joints during walking. Many have a mild rocker sole that facilitates push-off. Because of these features, athletic shoes are recommended over walking shoes. For persons who need foot orthoses, most athletic shoes offer the advantage of a removable insole to make space for the orthosis (see Box 1 for guidelines for self-fitting shoes).

Laces

The location of the laces (high or low) can make a great difference in the stability of the foot in the shoe and in the ease or difficulty of donning the shoe. Some shoes are made with Velcro® closures, and shoes that are not can have them added at a shoe repair shop. There are also elastic shoe laces that are curled like a corkscrew that eliminate the need for tying. Information on adaptive lace is available from Abledata [www.abledata.com].

Foot Orthoses and Shoe Adaptations To Reduce Pain and Stress and Improve Gait

Internal Shoe Modifications and Indications

Custom-made foot orthosis (CFO). These insertable orthoses are made from a mold of the patient's foot. For persons with inflammatory arthritis, the most well-tolerated CFO is made of a combination of soft materials (Plastazote®) and semiflexible materials (leather and cork). CFOs can be designed to accommodate deformity by distributing pressure over the entire plantar surface and to be functional by altering the biomechanics of the foot to reduce deforming forces and improve stability and gait. The surface is referred to as the *shell*, and the material between the shell and the shoe is referred to as the *posting*.

Some design features that are commonly used for persons with arthritis are

- a metatarsal pad that reduces weight-bearing stress to the MTP joint by shifting the pressure of weight bearing proximally to the painful metatarsal heads,
- a medial wedge in the posting to help correct valgus deformity or a lateral wedge to reduce varus deformity, and
- heel modifications to reduce pressure on heel spurs.

Box 1
Guidelines for Self-Fitting Athletic Shoes in a Store

Shoes should be comfortable at the time of purchase, and patients should be encouraged not to purchase shoes that need to be "broken in." After buying new shoes, patients should be encouraged to wear them for gradually increasing periods of time and to check their feet after wearing them to make sure there are no areas of redness, tenderness, or skin breakdown. The following are some guidelines for buying shoes in a shoe store.

- The type of socks you wear may affect the fit of the shoe. When buying new shoes, take your socks with you.

- If you use orthoses, take them with you.

- Women sometimes find that men's shoes are wider and accommodate certain orthoses or swelling better than women's shoes.

- Request a pair of each brand in your size. (Typically there are 3–6 brands or styles from which to choose.).

- Systematically cross-compare each shoe with the other. Try on the left shoe of brand A and the right shoe of brand B.

Select the best-fitting shoe of the two. Then compare that shoe to brand C by walking in one of each. Select the best fitting of the two. Continue this process with each brand in your size. Ultimately, the last best one wins the cross-comparison. Because different people have feet of different sizes and shapes, try on both the left and right shoes of the winning brand or style. Walk in the "best" pair, and make sure they are comfortable on *both* feet. Be sure the shoe is long enough and that the arch and midfoot sections are comfortable and that the toes can curl and straighten.

- The first MTP joint (the base of the large toe) should be at the widest part of the shoe.

- The shoe should be longer than your longest toe to allow the foot to slide forward during push-off.

- The heel should be snug.

- The top part of the shoe (the vamp) should be comfortable when laced securely.

When subtalar pain and instability are a problem, a rigid polyethylene CFO with an extension that cups the heel is used in combination with a lateral posting wedge to reduce subtalar motion (inversion and eversion).

Heel lifts. When a person has a leg-length discrepancy, a heel insert may help determine how large the heel extension should be to restore balance to the pelvis and spine. Extensions must be added to the external heel of the shoe.

Heel cushions. Sponge inserts with a hole to relieve pressure over heel spurs are helpful for many patients, but they may require a shoe with extra depth (Clark, 1996).

Heel cups. Prefabricated rubber or plastic heel cups can help reduce pain associated with Achilles enthesitis, plantar fasciitis, or subcalcaneal spurs. They mold the soft tissues to provide greater protection between the tender point and the shoe during weight-bearing (Clark, 1996).

External Shoe Modifications and Indications

Rocker sole. The function of a rocker sole is to literally "rock" the foot from heel-strike to toe-off without bending the shoe. It reduces the amount of motion required in the ankle and MTP joints to accomplish push-off and therefore is a helpful adaptation for persons with ankle synovitis or surgical fusions and limited or painful MTP joints. There are six different styles of rocker soles depending on the foot problem (Janisse, 1995). Many walking and running athletic shoes are made with a mild or generic rocker sole (Nawoczenski, Birke, & Coleman, 1988).

Extended steel shank. This is a strip of spring steel inserted between the layers of the sole that extends from the heel to the toe of the shoe. It is commonly used in combination with a rocker sole to prevent the shoe from bending. This is helpful for persons with limited MTP motion (e.g., hallux rigidus).

Metatarsal bar. This bar is an addition to the sole that shifts weight-bearing pressure proximal to the MTP joints instead of directly onto the metatarsal heads.

Stabilization flare. This is an addition to the heel, or to both the heel and sole, to stabilize the hindfoot or midfoot. It can be either medial or lateral, but the most common use in arthritis is a medial flare to support a valgus heel deformity.

Solid ankle cushion heel (SACH). A SACH is a wedge of shock-absorbing material that is added to the heel of the shoe. Its purpose is to provide a maximum amount of shock absorption under the heel. It is commonly used in conjunction with a rocker sole to improve gait for persons with limited or fused ankles.

Wedge. Sole material in a wedge shape is sometimes added to the heel or heel and sole to redirect the weight-bearing position of the foot. It can be useful in accommodating a fixed deformity by essentially bringing the ground to the foot. A medial wedge is indicated in cases of extreme pronation, whereas a lateral wedge can be used for ankle instability or a varus heel deformity.

Extensions. This is sole material added to increase the thickness of the sole and heel to accommodate a leg-length discrepancy or added to adjust the heel to accommodate a plantar flexion contracture.

Prescription Shoes

When a person has severe or fixed-toe deformities that cannot be accommodated comfortably in even adapted commercial shoes, there are three other options. First, patients may use in-depth shoes that have extra depth in the shoe to accommodate custom shoe orthoses. Second, in-depth shoes with uppers that can be heat molded to reduce pressure on specific toes or bony prominences were found to reduce pain in 25 patients fitted with these shoes, and 80% of these subjects reported that they "walk better" (Moncur & Ward, 1990). Third, in cases of extreme deformity, custom-made shoes or sandals can be constructed from a mold of the person's foot (Deland & Wood, 1993).

References

Clark, B. M. (1996). Foot management and ambulatory aids. In *Clinical care in the rheumatic diseases*. Atlanta, GA: Arthritis Foundation.

Deland, J. T., & Wood, B. (1993). Foot pain. In W. N. Kelly, E. D. Harris, S. Ruddy, & C. B. Sledge (Eds.), *Textbook of rheumatology* (4th ed., pp. 459–470). Philadelphia: Saunders.

Janisse, D. J. (1995). Prescription insoles and footwear. *Clinics in Podiatric Medicine and Surgery, 12*(1), 41–61.

Moncur, C., & Ward, J. R. (1990). Heat-moldable shoes for management of forefoot problems in rheumatoid arthritis. *Arthritis Care and Research, 3*(4), 222–226.

Nawoczenski, D. A., Birke, J. A., & Coleman, W. C. (1988). Effect of rocker sole design on plantar forefoot pressures. *Journal of the American Podiatric Medical Association, 78*, 455.

Index